Rural Health in the United States

Rural Health in the United States

Edited by

Thomas C. Ricketts, III

North Carolina Rural Health Research and Policy Analysis Program
Cecil G. Sheps Center for Health Services Research
The University of North Carolina, Chapel Hill

New York Oxford
OXFORD UNIVERSITY PRESS
1999

Oxford University Press

Oxford New York
Athens Auckland Bangkok Bogota Buenos Aires Calcutta
Cape Town Chennai Dar es Salaam Delhi Florence Hong Kong Istanbul
Karachi Kuala Lumpur Madrid Melbourne Mexico City Mumbai
Nairobi Paris São Paulo Singapore Taipei Tokyo Toronto Warsaw

and associated companies in
Berlin Ibadan

Published by Oxford University Press, Inc.
198 Madison Avenue, New York, New York 10016

Library of Congress Cataloging-in-Publication Data
Rural health in the United States / [edited by] Thomas C. Ricketts III
p cm. Includes bibliographical references and index.
ISBN 0-19-513127-4 —ISBN 0-19-513128-2 (pbk).
1. Rural health—United States. 2. Rural health services—United States.
3. Medicine, Rural—United States.
I. Ricketts, Thomas C.
[DNLM: 1. Rural Health Services—United States. 2. Rural Health—United States.
WA 390 R95145 1999] RA771.5.R859 1999
362.1'04257'0973—dc21 DNLM/DLC for Library of Congress 98-52112

2 4 6 8 9 7 5 3 1

Printed in the United States of America
on acid-free paper

Foreword

This volume is a long-awaited update to *Health Care in Rural America*, published in 1990 by the U.S. Office of Technology Assessment. *Health Care in Rural America* proved to be an important tool in the debates over significant rural health legislation, such as changes in Medicare Prospective Payment rules and the creation of Rural Health Outreach and Rural Health Networks programs. This Office is very grateful that this updated volume has been developed.

We at the federal Office of Rural Health Policy, in HRSA, want to thank the book's editor, Tom Ricketts, for his two-year long effort to make the current book, *Rural Health in the United States*, a reality. Although this is a book that includes the work of many outstanding researchers in rural health policy, without Tom's coordination and willingness to see this through, the parts might not have been assembled as effectively as they are. He and his team not only made important contributions to the book, but oversaw the daunting task of coordinating its creation with numerous research centers, federal agencies, and national organizations. In doing so, they have compiled a useful, comprehensive reference guide to rural health care delivery.

I am sure that this new book will also be a valuable tool for future policy making, and I and the rural health community are grateful to Tom and to everyone who contributed to *Rural Health in the United States*.

Wayne Myers, M.D.
Director, Office of Rural Health Policy, HRSA, DHH

Preface

When confronted with the realities of the size and scope of the rural population in the United States, it is hard to think of these 61 million people as a disadvantaged group. Their numbers exceed the total population of many nations, including Great Britain, France, Spain, and Italy. Yet, in many ways, but specifically in health care access, rural Americans are distinctly disadvantaged. Rural Americans make up 20% of the nation's population, but only 9% of the nation's physicians practice in rural counties. Medicare beneficiaries in nonmetropolitan counties receive 15% less in the way of all physician services and a striking 40% less in cardiology. Rural patients see doctors less often and usually later in the course of an illness. When a person living in a rural area goes into the hospital, it is usually for a longer stay even though the hospital will be paid less for that patient if the hospital is located in a rural area. This pattern evolved early in this century and despite major efforts to change the distribution of resources, rural communities lag well behind their city cousins in health care. The U.S. Congress, state legislatures, and regional governments recognize this disparity but the solution to the imbalances continues to elude them.

The facts of this disparity between rural and urban remain and this book is intended to bring those facts once again to the attention of the people who can make a differences in policies. *Rural Health in the United States* is also meant to inform rural communities themselves, to provide them with the information they need to effectively argue for change. Facts, data and statistics cannot create solutions: they must be turned into information on which arguments can be based and comparisons drawn to support options that are favorable for change. This book is designed to take data and turn them into information that can be used to create the policies that help Americans—especially rural Americans—build a better and more effective health care delivery system.

Most who are involved in the field of rural health policy analysis or rural health research are familiar with the report published in 1990 by the U.S. Office of Technology Assessment, *Health Care in Rural America*. The report was the result of 2 years of concentrated work by a talented and dedicated OTA staff and has served as the primary reference tool for rural health policy makers, journalists, analysts, and researchers ever since. Almost 10 years have passed since the report's release and much of the data and information it contained have changed. That same decade witnessed the development of several policy initiatives including legislation to assist rural hospitals, strengthen efforts to place professionals in rural areas, and modify payment systems to be more equitable to rural citizens that were supported by that report. Despite these efforts, many of the same problems that confronted rural America in the 1980s remain in the 1990s, despite the best efforts of interested policy makers and their supporters.

The Office of Rural Health Policy sought to provide current policy-relevant information by supporting the creation of an information service in the National Agriculture Library—the Rural Information Center, Health Services (RICHS). The RICHS staff collected published articles, reports, working papers, findings, and policy briefs issued by rural health services researchers, rural policy analysts and other authoritative sources, and developed a number of focused, annotated bibliographies. In addition, RICHS has served as a clearinghouse for those interested in rural health issues. This "virtual" reference source was effective as a clear demand emerged for a comprehensive reference book that would more efficiently answer the many specific questions often directed to RICHS, ORHP, and its network of research centers. Likewise, many of the summary tables, charts, maps, and graphs presented in the OTA report had not been updated by researchers and were not available to either RICHS or ORHP. By 1996, ORHP made the decision to assign the task of updating the OTA report to its research centers. In 1997 the Office of Rural Health Policy (ORHP) in the Health Resources and Services Administration (HRSA) and its research and policy analysis centers at the Universities of Minnesota, North Carolina, Southern Maine, and Washington, and Project Hope, recognized the great value of the OTA compendium and set out to update its contents. The Rural Health Research Program at the Cecil G. Sheps Center for Health Services Research at The University of North Carolina at Chapel Hill assumed the task of coordinating the work of the research centers to create a comprehensive and contemporary document.

The goal of the project was to create a comprehensive reference book as practically useful as *Health Care in Rural America,* but more "user-friendly," with less text detail and more graphical detail, making use of figures, tables, and maps. The OTA book was encyclopedic in its treatment of publicly funded programs and included background material and historical trend data on the growth of publicly supported rural programs and the distribution of resources in rural America. The current volume is intended to summarize policy initiatives in a more concise way while covering all aspects of rural health care. Where *Health Care in Rural America* placed a heavy emphasis on federal programs, *Rural Health in the United States* includes all of the major federal programs and projects, but attempts to include more attention to the broader set of resources and the private market changes affecting rural health care delivery. The OTA book proved to be very popular. The Office distributed its first printing of 2,000 copies free of charge to key policy makers and sold out two additional printings through 1993. To tap this level of interest inside and outside of government, it was decided that the book would be published by a commercial firm, and Oxford University Press was chosen because of its proven track record in publishing important books in the health policy field and its willingness to work with our graphics-intensive format.

The task of dividing the rural health policy field into a limited number of chapter headings was not straightforward. Some areas had the focused attention of policy makers and were clearly delineated as "domains" such as hospitals, health professions, and maternal and child health issues. In other areas, such as emergency medical services (EMS), little progress had been made in the decade since the OTA report or it was not a "hot" political issue but one that was likely to rise in importance in the future. The final set of chapters represents a consensus view of issues in rural health policy that the contributing authors felt will be important in the near future.

Key investigators at the five centers were assigned the task of authoring chapters, which were shared across all centers as they evolved. Nationally recognized experts were recruited to review and comment on chapter drafts. Twenty-three outside experts worked exceptionally hard to improve and correct the chapters and to focus the work. A managing editor in the North Carolina center responsible for integrating the chapters in a way that would make the book more of a unified effort than a collection of separate issue-focused chapters. The process of negotiating with a publisher was also an important step along the way. The book was to be primarily a public document with no copyright restrictions, thus the choice of a publisher hinged on a willingness to produce the book under that condition. In keeping with the goal of producing a user-friendly product, the ability to publish the book with full-color maps was also an important criterion for selection of a publisher. The experience of Oxford University Press in these two critical areas was instrumental in their selection by the rural research centers and ORHP.

The goal of ORHP and the collaborating centers was to assemble the basic facts and trends that affect the health and health care resources of rural people. The strategy of creating a single reference volume that depended upon data and the visual representation of data using charts, graphs, and maps might have seemed obvious after the commitment was made to do this. However, the effort to make that commitment required the focused leadership of the Director of Research Programs in ORHP and the dedicated resources of the Office through its funding and coordination to make this book happen.

Chapel Hill, N.C. T.C.R.

Acknowledgments

This book would not have been developed without the leadership and vision of Pat Taylor, Ph.D., Director of Research Programs in the federal Office of Rural Health Policy in the Health Resources and Services Administration. While many people in the field of rural health policy may have suggested the need to update *Health Care in Rural America*, Pat Taylor was the only person to step forward with the focused vision to move this project toward reality. Putting the book together required a careful process of persuasion to make the otherwise very independent academic researchers collaborate to create a unified piece of work. Pat was able to do this with a style that moved the group's members along without their feeling pushed or overly prodded.

The Office of Rural Health Policy added the important stimulation of funding for the centers to support this work: all of the centers were able to include work on the book in their formal research agendas. This structure reflects Pat's commitment to this project as well as the support of the former Director of ORHP, Jeff Human, and acting director, Dena Puskin.

The flow of materials from multiple authors representing individual centers and, in some instances, cooperative projects between centers, had the potential of becoming very complex and unwieldy. However, the project's managing editor, Heather McCary Edin, kept the project and the authors organized and motivated with her energy and persistence. The project kept as close to its timetable as was humanly possible, even when Heather took a few days off to get married. In the days leading up to the delivery of the many chapter manuscripts to the publisher, Heather doubled, then redoubled, her commitment to achieve accuracy and consistency in the text, tables, charts, and graphs. Any errors that may have crept into the book will have been due to the editor's meddling in the process and not Heather's careful reworking of every chapter.

The four other center directors, Gary Hart at the WWAMI Rural Health Research Center, Ira Moscovice at the University of Minnesota Rural Health Research Center, Andy Coburn at the Maine Rural Health Research Center, and Curt Mueller at the Project HOPE, William Walsh Center for Rural Health Analysis, each entered the project with a spirit of cooperation and a desire to create a useful product. They were able to involve key staff to the drafting and revision of chapters and the creation of special analyses to display new data.

Each chapter was reviewed by outside experts (listed below) from across the United States and they did so with a thoroughness that helped improve each chapter. We want to express our thanks, once again, for their help with this project.

Reviewers

Calvin L. Beale, M.S.
Senior Demographer
Economic Research Service
U.S. Department of Agriculture
Washington, D.C.

David E. Berry, DrPH
Professor and Chair, Health Care Administration
University of Nevada at Las Vegas
Las Vegas, Nevada

Richard J. Bogue, Ph.D.
Senior Director of Governance Programs
Division of Trustee and Community Leadership
American Hospital Association
Chicago, Illinois

David L. Brown, Ph.D.
Professor and Chair, Rural Sociology
Cornell University
Ithaca, New York

Leslie L. Clarke, Ph.D.
Assistant Research Professor, Health Policy and Epidemiology
University of Florida
Gainsville, Florida

Denise Denton, M.S.
Director, Colorado Rural Health Center
Denver, Colorado

R. Paul Duncan, Ph.D
Professor, Health Services Administration
University of Florida
Gainsville, Florida

Suzanne Felt-Lisk, MPA
Senior Health Researcher
Mathematica Policy Research, Inc.
Washington, D.C.

Gerry Gairola, Ph.D
Chair, Department of Health Services
University of Kentucky Medical Center
Lexington, Kentucky

Tim Henderson, MSPH
Director, Primary Care Resource Center
National Conference of State Legislatures
Washington, D.C.

Doris A. Henson, M.S., M.P.H., R.N.
Assistant Professor of Nursing
Montana State University at Bozeman
Bozeman, Montana

Robert E. Hurley, MHA, Ph.D.
Associate Professor of Health Administration
School of Allied Health Professions
Medical College of Virginia
Richmond, Virginia

John A. Krout, Ph.D.
Director, Gerontology Institute
Ithaca College
Ithaca, New York

Joseph P. Morrissey, Ph.D.
Director, Mental Health Research Program
Cecil G. Sheps Center for Health Services Research
University of North Carolina at Chapel Hill
Chapel Hill, North Carolina

Keith J. Mueller, Ph.D.
Director, Nebraska Center for Rural Health Research
Department of Preventive and Societal Medicine
University of Nebraska Medical Center
Omaha, Nebraska

Tracey M. Orloff, MPH
Senior Policy Analyst, Health Policies Studies Division
National Governors Association
Washington, D.C.

Robert E. Schlenker, Ph.D.
Associate Director, Center for Health Services Research
University of Colorado
Denver, Colorado

Val Schott, MPH
Director
National Organization of State Offices of Rural Health
Oklahoma City, Oklahoma

John W. Seavey, Ph.D.
Professor of Health Management and Policy
University of New Hampshire
Durham, New Hampshire

LaVonne A. Straub, Ph.D.
Professor of Economics
Western Illinois University
Macomb, Illinois

Morton O. Wagenfeld, Ph.D.
Professor of Sociology
Western Michigan University
Kalamazoo, Michigan

Mary Wakefield, Ph.D.
Director, Capitol Area Rural Health Round Table
The Center for Health Policy
George Mason University
Fairfax, Virginia

Sheldon Weisgrau, M.H.S.
Senior Consultant
Rural Health Consultants
Lawrence, Kansas

Contents

Contributors

CONTRIBUTING CENTERS

North Carolina Rural Health Research Program
Cecil G. Sheps Center for Health Services Research, University of North Carolina at Chápel Hill
Chapel Hill, North Carolina

Maine Rural Health Research Center
Muskie Institute for Public Affiars, University of Southern Maine
Portland, Maine

Minnesota Rural Health Research Center
Institute for Health Services Research, University of Minnesota
Minneapolis, Minnesota

William Walsh Center for Rural Health Analysis
Project Hope
Bethesda, Maryland

WWAMI Rural Health Research Center
Department of Family Medicine, University of Washington
Seattle, Washington

U.S. Office of Rural Health Policy
U.S. Health Resources and Services Administration
Rockville, Maryland

CONTRIBUTING AUTHORS

JOHANNA R. AMES, BA
North Carolina Rural Health Research Program
Cecil G. Sheps Center for Health Services Research
University of North Carolina at Chapel Hill
Chapel Hill, North Carolina

LEONARD D. BAER, MS
North Carolina Rural Health Research Program
Cecil G. Sheps Center for Health Services Research
University of North Carolina at Chapel Hill
Chapel Hill, North Carolina

DONNA C. BIRD, MA
Maine Rural Health Research Center
Edmund S. Muskie School of Public Service
University of Southern Maine
Portland, Maine

ELISE J. BOLDA, PhD
Maine Rural Health Research Center
Edmund S. Muskie School of Public Service
University of Southern Maine
Portland, Maine

MICHELLE M. CASEY, MS
Rural Health Research Center
Institute for Health Services Research
University of Minnesota
Minneapolis, Minnesota

SARAH J. CLARK, MPH
Division of General Pediatrics
University of Michigan Medical Center
Ann Arbor, Michigan

Andrew F. Coburn, PhD
Maine Rural Health Research Center
Edmund S. Muskie School of Public Service
University of Southern Maine
Portland, Maine

Patricia Dempsey, RN
Maine Rural Health Research Center
Edmund S. Muskie School of Public Service
University of Southern Maine
Portland, Maine

Elizabeth Dorosh, BA
William Walsh Center for Rural Health Analysis
Project HOPE
Bethesda, Maryland

Heather McCary Edin, BA
North Carolina Rural Health Research Program
Cecil G. Sheps Center for Health Services Research
University of North Carolina at Chapel Hill
Chapel Hill, North Carolina

Sheila J. Franco, MS
William Walsh Center for Rural Health Analysis
Project Hope
Bethesda, Maryland

L. Gary Hart, PhD
WWAMI Rural Health Research Center
University of Washington
Seattle, Washington

David Hartley, PhD, MHA
Division of Rural Health
Maine Rural Health Research Center
Edmund S. Muskie School of Public Service
University of Southern Maine
Portland, Maine

Paige E. Heaphy, MSPH
North Carolina Rural Health Research Program
Cecil G. Sheps Center for Health Services Research
University of North Carolina at Chapel Hill
Chapel Hill, North Carolina

Eric H. Larson, PhD
WWAMI Rural Health Research Center
University of Washington
Seattle, Washington

Denise M. Lishner, MSW
WWAMI Rural Health Research Center
University of Washington
Seattle, Washington

Curt D. Mueller, PhD
William Walsh Center for Rural Health Analysis
Project HOPE
Bethesda, Maryland

Randy K. Randolph, MRP
North Carolina Rural Health Research Program
Cecil G. Sheps Center for Health Services Research
University of North Carolina at Chapel Hill
Chapel Hill, North Carolina

Thomas C. Ricketts, III, PhD, MPH
North Carolina Rural Health Research Program
Cecil G. Sheps Center for Health Services Research
University of North Carolina at Chapel Hill
Chapel Hill, North Carolina

Roger A. Rosenblatt, MD, MPH
Co-Principal Investigator
WWAMI Rural Health Research Center
University of Washington
Seattle, Washington

Lucy A. Savitz, MBA, PhD
Department of Health Policy and Administration
School of Public Health
University of North Carolina at Chapel Hill
Chapel Hill, North Carolina

Julie A. Schoenman, PhD
William Walsh Center for Rural Health Analysis
Project HOPE
Bethesda, Maryland

Claudia L. Schur, PhD
William Walsh Center for Rural Health Analysis
Project HOPE
Bethesda, Maryland

Rebecca T. Slifkin, PhD
North Carolina Rural Health Research Program
Cecil G. Sheps Center for Health Services Research
University of North Carolina at Chapel Hill
Chapel Hill, North Carolina

Laura M. Smith, BS
North Carolina Rural Health Research Program
Cecil G. Sheps Center for Health Services Research
University of North Carolina at Chapel Hill
Chapel Hill, North Carolina

Patricia Taylor, PhD
Office of Rural Health Policy
Health Resources and Services Administration
U.S. Department of Health and Human Services
Rockville, Maryland

Karen D. Johnson-Webb, MA
Department of Geography
University of North Carolina at Chapel Hill
Chapel Hill, North Carolina

Anthony Wellever, MPA
Rural Health Research Center
Institute for Health Services Research
University of Minnesota
Minneapolis, Minnesota

Rural Health in the United States

Introduction

THOMAS C. RICKETTS

Rural health policy has taken an important place on the American political agenda due to changes within the health care system and the policy environment that affects rural America. The demographic, social, cultural and economic changes in rural and urban populations are different in many respects, yet policy does not always recognize those differences and sometimes causes harm when policies that do recognize a difference are implemented. The financing and delivery of health care in this nation has undergone a revolution in the past decade. This is apparent to even the most casual observer as well as to people directly involved in health policy making. The changes of the past 10 years have been almost overwhelming in their scope and impact. Concerns for the costs of care have prompted the financing of medical and public health services to create new forms of organizations—managed care organizations, provider networks, and "plans" of all types—that have dominated the urban health care environment but have been slower to develop in rural places. Technological changes, including the development of drugs that are effective for many more diseases and rapid advances in telecommunications and its use, have brought new tools into the hands of the rural practitioner, making them less isolated on the one hand. On the other hand, the very high costs of many new technologies have concentrated them into fewer, more urban areas. Patients, especially inpatients, are finding their way into larger, more specialized, and typically urban facilities.

The rural environment has changed dramatically through economic and demographic transitions that affect rural, urban, and suburban places differently. Rural America is growing more slowly and its population is older than that of the rest of the nation. These economic and demographic changes have put the health status and health care resources of rural America at risk. The nation's population has grown because of births, longer life spans, the immigration of many new citizens from abroad, and the relatively faster growth of minority population groups. Many rural areas have shared in the economic growth and adapted to the demographic shifts but for a very substantial portion of rural America, change elsewhere has meant stagnation at home. The uneven growth of the economy has caused many rural places to suffer. Although technology in health care may bring more to rural patients and professionals, the ownership and control of those technologies is often in hands far from the communities they affect.

The demographic shifts in many rural areas have not been limited to the departure of working-age adults, although that is a very real problem in many rural areas, especially in the central heartland. Other rural places are experiencing very rapid growth due to natural resource exploitation and the expansion of recreational activities. Other rural areas are seeing population changes due to the immigration of workers from other countries who fill low-wage jobs or labor shortages.

Health and health care are linked closely to the economy and demography of a place (Evans, Barer et al., 1994). Where the economy is stagnant or contracting, health status suffers; where the population ages, the need for health care rises. Where there is a rapid change in the primary employer of a place, long-term residents feel dislocated and are likely to suffer behavioral and somatic problems; where the culture of a population changes, health care professionals may not be able to communicate effectively. These patterns of change have become very evident in rural America over the past 10 years. The changes that are evident have been identified and highlighted by a growing group of analysts and researchers whose work this book is intended to support. How this group has emerged and how they affect policy is discussed later in this introduction, however, the initial task is to describe the context of rural health and how it might be different and unique.

This degree of change should create apparent differences between the health status of the rural population and the rest of the nation. However, when considering all of the people we classify as rural, that is not the case. There are very healthy and well-served rural communities all across America. Indeed, when looking at summary data that combine all nonmetropolitan counties and adjust for differences in age and gender, the data do not show a dramatic difference in health status indicators such as mortality between the nonmetropolitan population and the metropolitan population (Miller, Stokes et al., 1987; Miller, Farmer et al., 1994). It is easy to see the disparity in access to health care resources by comparing, say, nonmetropolitan to metropolitan counties—nonmetropolitan counties have far fewer physicians, less available technology, and clearly lower payment for the same services provided in metropolitan counties. Despite all these differences, the overall health status indicators for all rural versus all urban populations remain very close together. Why is this?

Two important explanations account for the apparently weak national evidence of a rural health crisis. The first is that we do not effectively account for the characteristics of rurality that have the greatest effect on access to care when we classify counties as nonmetropolitan. The relative isolation from health services of a population is not captured in national categories used to report health statistics. The second is that there is a very wide range of variation in health status within rural places and among population groups that is related to poverty, race, and ethnicity. Within the nonmetropolitan classification of counties, counties in certain regions of the country have consistently higher rates of illness and death than urban counties, and that gradient is due to income, education, race, and ethnicity and is made worse by the geographic inaccessibility of care. There are important health status disparities between urban and rural places when region and remoteness are considered. These differences are ones of scale. Effective measures of unacceptability for thresholds of access and rates for mortality and morbidity do not exist.

Rural health policy has become an important issue on the national agenda. However, for many good reasons, the American system resists the creation of national policy that depends on identifying a group by a scale of relative need. The complexity of the use of federal poverty guidelines in Medicaid eligibility is an example. To effectively target efforts to address differences in health status and alleviate lack of access to health care, we would have to means test individuals. Again, the political difficulties of Medicaid and national welfare policy illustrate how difficult this is. We are far more comfortable identifying geographically defined populations or economically identifiable groups whom we can support with public programs than we are with letting a bureaucracy admit or reject people based on individual characteristics, like health, which are subject to wide variations in interpretation. To focus on just one component of the rural population—those who are more likely to have poor health—is very difficult because of this general reluctance to create special classes. It has been possible to have focused *rural* health policies, in general, because we have agreed there are general differences between urban and rural places that do not reflect a value judgement on whether rural or urban people are more or less deserving of assistance.

There are many example of policies that both positively and negatively affect rural people. The Congress created a series of policies that directly affect the volume and quality of health care delivered to people because of their geographic residence. In the Prospective Payment System (PPS) as it applies to the Medicare program, payments for medical care are calculated from locally applicable costs. The payments for hospital services through the PPS system are higher to urban areas. This is due to the perception that labor costs for rural hospitals are lower than for urban ones. However, the differences in payments have strained rural hospitals and, in turn, the supply of rural health care professionals for the most obvious economic reasons (Commission, 1991; Connor, Hillson et al., 1994; Connor, Hillson et al., 1995; Miller, Holahan et al., 1995; Buto, 1996). The secondary effects of discriminatory payment systems on health care are less evident, but we know that the wealth of a community has a direct relationships to its health status (Evans, Barer et al., 1994; Amick, Levine et al., 1995), perhaps even more so than the effects of the relative supply of health care providers (Bindman, Keane et al., 1990; Millman, 1993; Bindman, Grumbach et al., 1995) or of the extent of health insurance coverage (Miller, Holahan et al., 1995).

The factors that affect the health status of rural Americans are not limited to problems of the macro economy, or to demographic changes or national policy decisions. We also know that factors of geographic isolation, the culture of rural life, and the slower spread of technology and newer, more effective medical care into smaller, rural towns and places have very important effects on health status (Hogan, 1986; Horner and Chirikos, 1987; Patrick, Stein et al., 1988; Bindman, Keane et al., 1990; Park, Brook et al., 1990; Doll, 1991; Liff, Chow et al., 1991; Howe, Katterhagen et al., 1992; Monroe, Ricketts et al., 1992; Chen, Maio et al., 1995; Esposito, Sanddal et al., 1995; Charlton, 1996; Gerberich, Robertson et al., 1996; Amey, Miller et al., 1997; Grossman, Kim et al., 1997; Young, Bassam et al., 1998). These characteristics of isolation, culture, and small size are essential characteristics of rural life and are the specific descriptors of the rural experience that need special attention when we speak about creating, through policy, a health system that has equitable distributions of resources and equal chances for a healthy life for all Americans.

Unfortunately, the policy structure that we have built in health care has a tight link to the governmental structure of the republic. The regulation of health care delivery and its public financing are tied to the many levels of government in our federal, essentially decentralized, system (Steinmo and Watts, 1995). This applies to the private sector as well as the public. The nature of practice laws in one state will mean a distribution of primary care providers very different from the distribution in the next state. One state's historical tax policy will have cultivated a favored industry whose decline has resulted in a region of dying small towns once dependent on that industry. The latitude a state gives to local government to levy taxes for schools means that poorer communities have poorer schools. The result is that children in smaller communities won't have the same opportunities that other children will have, making it harder and harder to break patterns of poverty and economic isolation. Of these state policy choices, only one is labelled as health policy—the professional licensing laws—but that type of policy is only indirectly related to health status while the decision to allow poorer communities to have to support their own schools may have much more direct health consequences.

In a rural context it is not hard to imagine the case where a licensing policy that makes it hard for nonphysician primary care professionals to practice in small towns due to rigid supervision rules is combined with economic changes that result in a decline in a once important rural industry and policies that make it difficult for rural school systems to educate children, then the conditions are ripe for a "rural health" problem to appear. Layer on this the cultural and social problems of race or language, and the emergence of a difference in health status for a population is inevitable.

This gap between the structure of health policy and the realities of health needs is not restricted to rural communities—it is a problem that affects the entire health "system." American health policy must reconcile the awkward balance of health care as an economic activity with its social and cultural imperatives that tie us together as humans (Beauchamp, 1988). We have a great deal of attention paid to payment policies for hospitals divided by metropolitan-nonmetropolitan distinctions but less attention paid to the specific effects that distance to a primary care professional has on health. This is not necessarily irrational; it is precisely because health is tied closely to economics that we can make the argument that hospital payment policies affect health care needs and health status. It is not necessarily satisfying to succeed in changing those payment policies when you want to change the very poor health status of the rural poor in a neglected corner of a southeastern state, but it may be that reforming payment policies is the only way to progress toward that goal at that particular time. Nevertheless, it is imperative that we also recognize when the more direct approach is feasible and effective.

THE RURAL HEALTH POLICY WORLD AND INFORMATION NEEDS

Keith Mueller, former President of the National Rural Health Association and a political scientist at the University of Nebraska Medical Center, has outlined the structure of the rural health policy field (Mueller 1997). He sees rural health policy being motivated by a set of "relative needs." These needs apply to rural areas in general and include a relative shortage of health professionals, lower payment levels for health care services, and slower uptake of medical innovations. These needs are then translated into programs that address a specific need. This system of justifying policies by identifying specific needs reflects the realities of the public policy world that has left the United States without a general rural policy (Bonnen, 1992), much less a comprehensive rural health policy, but rather with many problem-specific policies and special programs.

Broad agreement exists that the nation continues to face challenges in creating an equitable system of health care for all but especially for the elderly, children, migrant workers, and those otherwise classified as the "underserved." To create policies that address the needs of these groups, the political system is sensitive to the effectiveness of the representatives who speak for each "faction" to argue for the priority of their need. This is called "the politics of representation" or interest group politics. The politics of representation of rural interests rests on a set of basic arguments that its constituents make on behalf of programs meant to benefit rural health systems or provide relief from regulation. These arguments depend largely on the description of differences in access to care for rural people and those arguments are usually separated into specific classes or components of the health care system such as hospitals, physicians, nurse practitioners, or mental health services.

Rural Health in the United States takes the same approach for its structure, the chapters describing particular elements of the rural health system that parallel the important sets of stakeholders in the overall system. Each group of stakeholders, whether providers (hospitals, physicians, managed care companies) or clients (children, mothers, the elderly) are then subject to comparison with the rest of the nation. This division of the policy world into stakeholder issues reflects the relative strength of a group's representation in the political sphere and is as old as the Republic (Madison, 1993). The use of factions to develop arguments for rural programs is more a characteristic of national policy making than of the rural condition. Because the rural stakeholders have joined across more traditional issue boundaries, there is, perhaps, more cohesiveness in rural health policy than is found in other areas of general policy or policy linked to geography. While it is perhaps difficult outside of the sphere of rural advocacy to speak of overall rural health policy, it is far more common to hear in the general policy field about the rural implications of Medicare hospital payment policy, or how graduate medical education payments will affect rural practitioner supply, or the impact on rural clinics of new regulations for clinical laboratories.

The salient rural health policy issues that are the subjects of this book's chapters address many basic questions often heard from policy makers, such as: "How big is the disparity between rural and urban places in physician supply?" and "What is the likely effects of changes in Medicare managed care payment rates?" These questions produce a need for information and analysis resources dedicated to rural issues. These are spread thinly across the agencies or organizations that are charged with creating, influencing, or applying those policies. Mueller (1997, p. 408) recounts how witnesses from the Medicare Prospective Payment Assessment Commission (ProPAC) and the Medicare Physician Payment Review Commission (PPRC) did not include rural issues in their prepared testimony but were able to discuss their rural relevant analyses when asked by a rural representative. This reveals the low salience of the rural issues but at the same time shows that someone is paying attention. Since the early 1980s, largely stimulated by the payment differential between urban and rural areas in the Medicare PPS, a "policy network" has emerged of analysts and researchers who share a common interest in rural health issues. In contrast to more traditional interest groups, policy networks are seen as the more effective vehicle for marshalling information and constructing arguments for or against policies affecting a wide range of interests (Peterson, 1994). The rural health policy network that has emerged includes those who have primary responsibility for general rural policy as well as those who must concern themselves with the specific rural effects of broader health policies. For example, ORHP in HRSA has a general charge to coordinate federal rural health policy and support all policies that benefit rural communities. However, an office within the Health Care Financing Administration (HCFA) (which manages Medicare) supporting Rural Health Clinics may be expected to report on rural issues and compile information concerning rural-focused polices and their effects as they affect overall HCFA policy, while an office in the US Department of Agriculture (USDA) may be expected to advocate for general rural interests due to a specific Congressional mandate. The overall policies of the larger organizations may, at times, conflict with the specific policies that benefit rural areas and these conflicted members of a policy network may have to play opposition roles at certain times. This mix of roles and expectations for various groups is not uncommon in policy networks. However, what remains is the common demand across the network for information to either understand program effects and options or to bolster a case for new or revised policies.

THE POLITICS OF RURAL HEALTH AND INFORMATION

The rural voice in health policy is more effective when the various interests speak through a unified association. The National Rural Health Association (NRHA), which emerged in 1978 from the combination of once-fractious smaller groups, has given rural interests an effective voice at the national level. That association and its constituency groups represent the diverse components of the rural health system, which have been drawn together by a common perception of their potential marginalization. A second organization, the National Organization of State Offices of Rural Health (NOSORH), has recently developed as a national association that speaks from the perspective of state rural policy needs.

Structural opportunities offered by omnibus appropriations bills and the energy of policy entrepreneurs (Oliver and Paul-Shaheen, 1997) resulted in the passage of many policies and programs helpful to rural communities in the 1980s and 1990s including the establishment of an office in the federal government charged with expressing the views of rural constituents within the Executive Branch and advising the Secretary of HHS on the effects of departmental policies and regulations on rural communities. It is important to contrast the roles of the federal agency and the grass roots organizations with the responsibility for creating a comprehensive rural health policy, that, so far, remains a Congressional responsibility.

The successes of rural advocates in the political arena have been substantial in one sense but have also driven home the reality of the inferior political position of a segment of the population that can be as large as one quarter of the nation but enjoys little direct representation within the legislative branch. Many representatives in Congress do serve from predominantly rural districts and a substantial portion of the Senate can be said to represent essentially rural states, especially those states in the intermountain West, the Plains and parts of the Midwest. This has allowed rural health caucuses to emerge in both houses and for the informal rural health policy network to more effectively provide expert advice to the Congress. The Rural Health Panel of the Rural Policy Research Institute (RUPRI) links university and institution-based analysts and researchers with the staff and members of Congress. The panel has circulated brief assessments of various legislative and administrative proposals as side-by-side analyses and summaries as well as more lengthy, analytical pieces that estimate small area effects of national policy shifts. The intention of this panel of rural health policy experts is to avoid the mistakes that Mueller perceived were committed by the administration in the debate over national health reform in 1992–1994. He (Mueller, 1997, p. 412) describes the principles that were learned as: "argue from principles, find strength in numbers, use information and analysis, find effective champions and strategic allies, articulate concerns in a manner consistent with the dominant policy direction being taken, and be persistent." The political process demands accurate information sufficient to understand options and futures. This book is a response to the admonition to use information and analysis to argue for rural health policies.

It is because of this need for reliable and timely information that this book was created. The structure of the book reflects the relative emphasis some sectors of the rural health domain hold in current politics. However, a review of the issues of the past 20 years shows that there is a degree of constancy and the expressed needs of rural communities for their health care revolves around the issues that are presented in each of the following chapters.

REFERENCES

Amey CH, Miller MK, et al. 1997. The role of race and residence in determining stage at diagnosis of breast cancer. The Journal of Rural Health 13(2): 99–108.

Amick BC, Levine S, et al., eds. 1995. Society and Health. New York: Oxford University Press.

Beauchamp DE. 1988. The Health of the Republic. Epidemics, Medicine, and Moralism as Challenges to Democracy. Philadelphia: Temple University Press.

Bindman A, Grumbach K, et al. 1995. Preventable hospitalizations and access to health care. JAMA 264(4): 305–311.

Bindman AB, Keane D, et al. 1990. A public hospital closes: impact on patients' access to care and health status. JAMA 264: 2899–2904.

Bonnen JT. 1992. Why Is There No Coherent U.S. Rural Policy? Policy Studies Journal 20(2): 190–201.

Buto K. 1996. Rural Health Care Issues. Statement before the Subcommittee on Health of the House Ways and Means Committee. Baltimore, Health Care Financing Administration.

Charlton J. 1996. Which areas are healthiest? Population Trends 83: 17–24.

Chen B, Maio RF, et al. 1995. Geographic variation in preventable deaths from motor vehicle crashes. Journal of Trauma 38(2): 228–232.

Commission PPA. 1991. Rural Hospitals under Medicare's Prospective Payment System. Washington, DC: Prospective Payment Assessment Commission.

Connor RA, Hillson SD, et al. 1994. Association between rural hospitals' residencies and recruitment and retention of physicians. Acad Med 69(6): 483–488.

Connor RA, Hillson SD, et al. 1995. An analysis of physician recruitment strategies in rural hospitals. Health Care Manage Rev 20(1): 7–18.

Doll R. 1991. Urban and rural factors in the aetiology of cancer. International Journal of Cancer 47: 803–810.

Esposito TJ, Sanddal ND, et al. 1995. Analysis of preventable trauma deaths and inappropriate trauma care in a rural state. Journal of Trauma 39(5): 955–962.

Evans RG, Barer ML, et al., eds. 1994. Why Are Some People Healthy and Others Not? The Determinants of Health of Populations. Social Institutions and Social Change. New York: Aldine de Gruyter.

Gerberich SG, Robertson LS, et al. 1996. An epidemiological study of roadway fatalities related to farm vehicles: United States, 1988 to 1993. Journal of Occupational and Environmental Medicine 38(11): 1135–1140.

Grossman DC, Kim A, et al. 1997. Urban-rural differences in prehospital care of major trauma. Journal of Trauma 42(4): 723–729.

Hogan C. 1986. Patterns of travel for rural individuals hospitalized in New York State: relationships between distance, destination, and case mix. Journal of Rural Health 4(2): 29–41.

Horner RD, Chirikos TN. 1987. Survivorship differences in geographical comparisons of cancer mortality: an urban-rural analysis. International Journal of Epidemiology 16(2): 184–189.

Howe HL, Katterhagen JG, et al. 1992. Urban-rural differences in the management of breast cancer. Cancer Causes and Control 3: 533–539.

Liff JM, Chow W-H, et al. 1991. Rural-urban differences in stage at diagnosis: possible relation to cancer screening. Cancer 67(5): 1454–1459.

Madison J. 1993. Federalist Paper, Number 10. The American Polity Reader. Serow AG, Shannon WW, and Ladd EC. New York: W.W. Norton: 48–55.

Miller ME, Holohan J, et al. 1995. Geographic variations in physician service utilization. Medical Care Research and Review 52(2): 252–278.

Miller MK, Farmer FL, et al. 1994. Rural Populations and Their Health. Rural Health Services. A Management Perspective. In: Beaulieu JE, Berry DE, eds. Ann Arbor, MI: AUPHA Press/Health Administration Press: 3–26.

Miller MK, Stokes CS, et al. 1987. A comparison of the rural-urban mortality differential for deaths from all causes, cardiovascular disease and cancer. Journal of Rural Health 3(2): 23–34.

Millman M, ed. 1993. Access to Health Care in America. Washington, DC: National Academy Press, Institute of Medicine.

Monroe AC, Ricketts TC, et al. 1992. Cancer in rural versus urban populations: a review. J Rural Health 8(3): 212–220.

Mueller KJ. 1997. Rural Health Delivery and Finance: Policy and Politics. In: Litman TJ, Robins LS, eds. Health Politics and Policy. Albany, NY: Delmar: 402–418.

Oliver TR, Paul-Shaheen P. 1997. Translating ideas into actions: entrepreneurial leadership in state health care reforms [see comments]. Journal of Health Politics, Policy and Law 22(3): 721–788.

Park RE, Brook RH, et al. 1990. Explaining variations in hospital death rates: randomness, severity of illness, quality of care. JAMA 264(4): 484–490.

Patrick DL, Stein JS, et al. 1988. Poverty, use of health services, and health status in rural America. Milbank Quarterly 66(1): 105–136.

Peterson MA. 1994. Congress in the 1990s: From Iron Triangles to Policy Networks. In: Morone JA, Belkin GS, eds. The Politics of Health Care Reform. Lessons From the Past, Prospects for the Future. Durham, NC: Duke University Press: 103–147.

Steinmo S, Watts J. 1995. It's the institutions, stupid. Why comprehensive national health insurance always fails in America. Journal of Health Politics, Policy and Law 20(2): 329–372.

Young JS, Bassam D, et al. 1998. Interhospital versus direct scene transfer of major trauma patients in a rural trauma system. American Surgeon 64(1): 88–91; discussion 91–92.

1

Populations and Places in Rural America

THOMAS C. RICKETTS III, KAREN D. JOHNSON-WEBB, AND RANDY K. RANDOLPH

The United States is a continental nation; it covers 3,787,319 square miles and is the third largest nation in the world. Its size and physical characteristics have meant that this single nation could accommodate thriving cities built on the trade from sheltered ports as well as vast farm, ranch, and wilderness areas distant from urban growth. The great land area and generally moderate climate of the United States offer conditions for successful rural habitation. Even as the country's population has become proportionally more urban, its rural population has continued to grow. The 1990 census counted 61,658,330 "rural" people. That total is greater than the 1996 population of the United Kingdom (58 million), Spain (39 million), Italy (57 million), or France (58 million). It is more than the combined populations of Canada, Australia, and New Zealand. Rural America alone would be the second largest western European nation—behind only Germany (83 million)—and the sixteenth largest nation in the world. The rural people and resources of the United States have shaped the nation's economy, stimulated its development, and played an important role in its politics, social structure, and character. However, rural America presents as many challenges as opportunities. One particularly challenging issue for rural America is its access to health services. This chapter statistically describes rural America and its people. It points out not only how rural persons use health care and how health care resources are made available to them but also how and where rural people live, how long they live, and who they are.

DEFINING RURALITY

The two most common designations of rurality are those of the U.S. Bureau of the Census and the U.S. Office of Management and Budget (OMB). The Census Bureau designation classifies persons according to the population size and residential population density of the places where they live. The Census Bureau (1993) defines urban as "all territory, population and housing units in urbanized areas and in places of 2,500 or more persons outside urbanized areas." Rural areas are all "territory, population and housing units not classified as urban." The rural designation is also subdivided into "rural farm" and "rural non-farm" populations. Plate 1.1 shows U.S. counties and the percentage of their 1990 population defined as rural by the Census Bureau.

The OMB designation classifies counties as metropolitan or nonmetropolitan, based on whether the county has a large city and suburbs, and has a functional element that measures how economically integrated peripheral counties are with their surrounding metropolitan counties (Ricketts and Johnson-Webb, 1997). Plate 1.2 identifies the counties and county equivalents classified as nonmetropolitan by the OMB as of April 1, 1998.

The OMB definition of metropolitan areas is based on census data and census definitions of urban and rural, commuting patterns, and business activity. A metropolitan area (MA) is defined as a core area (usually a county) containing a large population (densely settled) along with a set of adjacent communities that exhibit a high degree of economic and social integration with that core. An MA must contain either a place with a population of at least 50,000 or a census-defined urbanized area and a total MA population of at least 100,000 (U.S. Bureau of the Census, 1990). The most commonly known designation of an MA is the Metropolitan Statistical Area (MSA). MSAs may include one or more central counties, and one or more outlying counties that are economically and socially integrated with the central area. New England has two versions of MAs, one comprising counties, cities, and towns and another whole counties. Except in the Northeast and southern California, MAs are bounded by nonmetropolitan counties and are not closely integrated with other MAs. All territory, population, and housing units within MAs are considered metropolitan. (For more detailed discussions, see U.S. Bureau of the Census, 1993; Ricketts and Johnson-Webb, 1997; Johnson-Webb, Baer, and Gesler, 1997).

Using these designation systems, populations may be classified into two different categories. In 1990, 47.5% of people classified by the Census Bureau as rural lived in OMB-defined metropolitan areas, and 14.8% of metropolitan residents lived in census-defined rural areas (Table 1.1). Table 1.1 also shows the 1990 census population data for counties classified as metropolitan and nonmetropolitan.

Other county-based classifications are also in use. Some of the most commonly known are the "frontier counties" classification, the urban influence codes, and the rural-urban continuum codes. Frontier county status is based on population densities within counties. Although there is no universally agreed-upon threshold, counties with fewer than seven persons per square mile are most often classified as "frontier" (Fig. 1.1). The urban influence codes were created by Linda Ghelfi and Tim Parker at the U.S. Department of Agriculture Economic Research Service (ERS) (Ghelfi and Parker, 1996; Baer et al., 1997). In this classification, nonmetropolitan counties, as determined by the OMB, are divided into seven classifications according to their adjacency to metropolitan counties and the size of their largest town. The adjacency factor is an indicator of urban influence and economic integration with metropolitan counties (Plate 1.3).

Rural-urban continuum codes (RUCCs; also developed at the USDA in the 1970s by David Brown and Fred Hines and updated by Calvin Beale), which are much like the urban influence codes, are also based on the OMB methodology used to classify metropolitan or nonmetropolitan counties. RUCCs are 10 codes that differ in significant ways from the urban influence codes in terms of size of population breakdowns and for fringe and central counties (Plate 1.4).

The designation of counties as metropolitan versus nonmetropolitan is a constant process controlled by the OMB; it responds to changes in population reflected in the decennial censuses and in special intercensal enumerations and estimates. In all, 116 counties have been designated metropolitan by the OMB since 1983. The changing status of counties can be problematic for health services research in that it impedes replicability of studies over time, or makes comparisons of certain counties from one time period to another difficult (Hewitt, 1992). In the past decade, several counties have changed status from metropolitan to nonmetropolitan and back again to metropolitan (e.g., Brunswick County, NC). Also, counties may be transferred from one metropolitan area to another (e.g., Shiawassee County, Mich., added to Flint, Mich., MSA in 1973, deleted from Flint, Mich., MSA in 1983, and added to Detroit–Ann Arbor–Flint, Mich., CMSA in 1992) (OMB, 1994).

Many policy decisions are based on county classification, so inconsistent and conflicting definitions and classifications can have important implications. Federal funds are often allocated to areas based on their rural/nonmetropolitan or urban/metropolitan status. These types of issues may impede the ability of policy makers to determine where health personnel shortages actually exist. Recommendations for opening or closing such crucial services as hospitals and clinics are often based on how an area is classified. Replicability of studies may be called into question. The effectiveness of strategies

Table 1.1 Comparison of Rural–Urban and Metropolitan–Nonmetropolitan Residence Patterns, 1990

		Percent of Total	Percent Rural	Percent Urban
Nonmetro	50,985,524	20.5	63.6	36.4
Metro	197,724,349	79.5	14.8	85.2
Total	248,709,873	100		
		Percent of Total	**Percent Nonmetro**	**Percent Metro**
Rural	61,680,049	24.8	52.5	47.5
Urban	187,029,824	75.2	9.9	90.1
Total	248,709,873	100		

Source: United States Department of Agriculture, Economic Research Service calculation from 1990 census data.

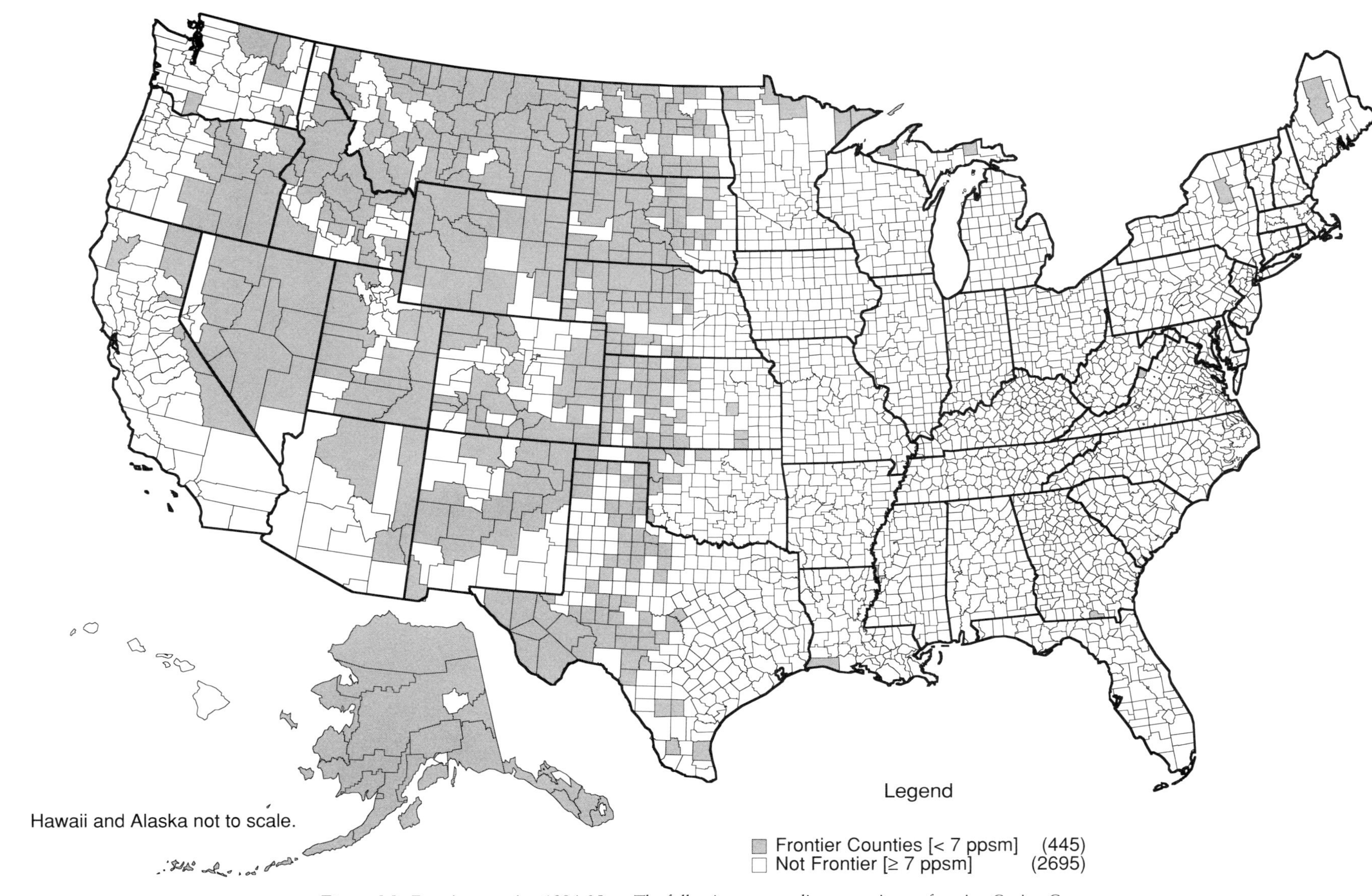

Figure 1.1. Frontier counties, 1994. Note: The following metropolitan counties are frontier: Cocino Co., AZ; Nye Co., NV; and Kane Co., UT. Source: Area Resource File, OHPAR, BHPr, HRSA, PHS, US DHHS, February 1997. Produced by North Carolina Rural Health Ressearch and Policy Analysis Center, Cecil G. Sheps Center for Health Services Research, University of North Carolina at Chapel Hill.

An Alternative to County-based Classifications: The Goldsmith Modification

Another definition of rural, developed specifically for policy purposes, is the Goldsmith modification, which was developed in the early 1990s for the Office of Rural Health Policy's grant programs and later used to facilitate the implementation of the universal access provisions of the Telecommunications Act of 1996 (Fig. 1.2). Table 1.1 showed that significant populations within OMB-designated metropolitan areas are considered rural by the census definition and that many census-defined urban populations fall within OMB-designated nonmetropolitan areas. The Goldsmith strategy was developed in partial response to this problem in order to permit a more equitable eligibility for federal rural health services grants than is the case using existing county-based classification schemes. Rural populations residing in metropolitan counties that have a very large land area, and thus have no easy access to health services, are better identified through the Goldsmith strategy (Goldsmith, Puskin, and Stiles, 1993). Using census data, large metropolitan counties are identified and then rural populations are further identified within large metropolitan areas using census tract data. Next, isolated rural census tracts are identified using commuting data. The Goldsmith methodology better designates isolated rural populations so that they may be targeted for federal government assistance to their health services programs.

to address the health problems of people in rural areas, the effectiveness of community efforts to recruit and retain health personnel in programs geared specifically toward rural or nonmetropolitan areas, and the ability of government programs to coordinate health policy strategies can all be affected by use of these classifications (Johnson-Webb, Baer, and Gesler, 1997).

RURALITY VERSUS ISOLATION

The OMB definition of nonmetropolitan assumes that some areas are not large enough to be metropolitan centers and not integrated enough with a metropolitan center to be part of a metropolitan region. The disadvantages of rurality are often expressed as a lack of access to or isolation from urban/metropolitan services. This isolation often can be bridged by travel between city or suburb and isolated rural areas. The transportation system available to a community determines its degree of isolation. Rural areas served by high-quality transportation corridors will typically have better access to health services. Even rural residents without easy access to automobiles benefit from highways because the modest rural transit that is available almost always depends on roads and vehicles.

Interstate highways and other limited-access highways create relatively rapid automobile transportation corridors to services not found easily or quickly in a local community. Approximately the same number of metropolitan and nonmetropolitan counties have any interstate highways passing somewhere within their area: 692 nonmetropolitan and 665 metropolitan counties; only 30% of nonmetropolitan counties, compared to 78% of metropolitan counties, are touched by the interstate system (Fig. 1.3) (Claritas, 1996; Department of Helth and Human Services [DHHS], 1997). The distribution of the interstate highway system makes a western county less likely to be crossed by an interstate and more likely to be a long distance from an interstate.

A well-developed highway system creates access for patients to local services and facilitates a referral system that links clinics to hospitals, and small hospitals to larger, tertiary care centers. However, the locations of rural hospitals were largely determined before the construction of the interstate highway system. Nonmetropolitan counties with no interstate connections have more hospitals and beds per resident than do nonmetropolitan counties with interstates, as well as metropolitan counties. Nonmetropolitan counties with no interstate highway have 53.7 nonfederal general hospitals per million people and 40.2 total beds per 10,000 residents, which is considerably higher than the rates of 37.0 and 35.6, respectively, for nonmetropolitan counties with interstates and 12.9 and 31.6 for metropolitan areas (Table 1.2) (Ameican Hospital Association, 1997; Claritas, 1996).

Physician supply is essentially the same for counties with and without interstate highways, with 4.7 primary care physicians per 10,000 residents in rural areas with interstate highways and 4.5 per 10,000 in rural counties without direct interstate access (Claritas, 1996; DHHS, 1997). A nonmetropolitan county with no interstate access is more likely to be designated as a whole-county Health Professional Shortage Area (HPSA). Over 37% of nonmetropolitan counties that are isolated from interstates are designated as full-county HPSAs compared with 30% that are crossed by an interstate (Claritas, 1996; Federal Register, 1997).

Access to the interstate highway system provides a framework within which differences between rurality

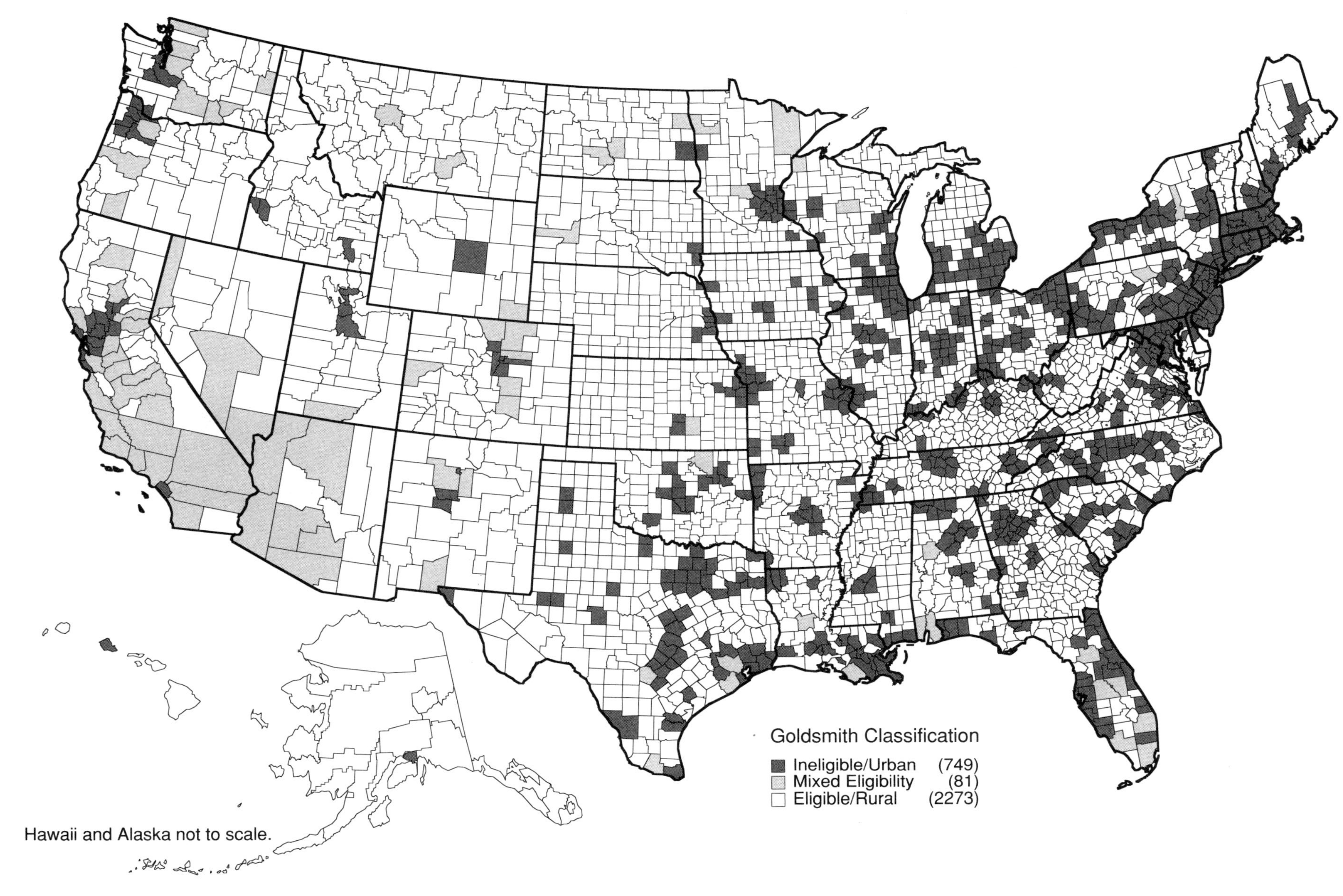

Figure 1.2. Goldsmith modifications, 1997. Source: Federal Office of Rural Health Policy, HRSA, U.S. DHHS, 1997; Office of Management and Budget, 1997. Produced by North Carolina Rural Health Research and Policy Analysis Center, Cecil G. Sheps Center for Health Services Research, University of North Carolina at Chapel Hill with support from the Federal Office of Rural Health Policy, HRSA, US DHHS.

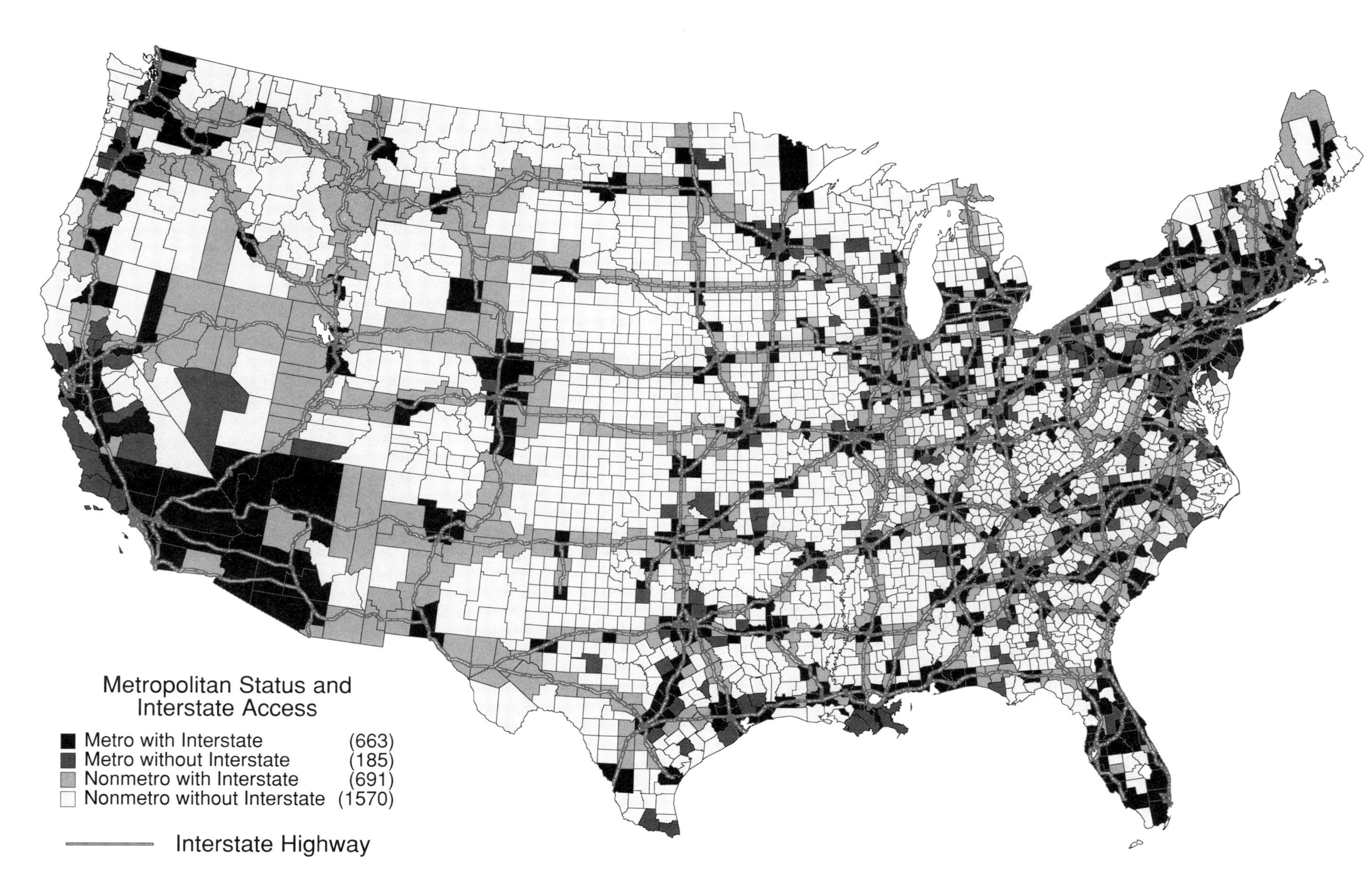

Figure 1.3. US interstate highway access, 1996: metropolitan and nonmetropolitan counties, 1998. Source: Claritas, 1996; Office of Management and Budget, 1998. Produced by North Carolina Rural Health Research and Policy Analysis Center, Cecil G. Sheps Center for Health Services Research, University of North Carolina at Chapel Hill with support from the Federal Office of Rural Health Policy, HRSA, U.S. DHHS.

Table 1.2 Health Care Resources and Interstate Highway Access

	Interstate, Nonmetro	*Non-Interstate, Nonmetro*	*Metro Counties*
Number of Counties	691	1570	858
Number of Hospitals/million population	37.03	53.71	12.92
Number of Hospital beds/10,000	35.56	40.19	31.59
Primary care physicians per 10,000 population	4.69	4.52	7.12
Percent Whole County Health Professional Shortage Areas	29.93%	37.28%	8.52%

Source: U.S. Bureau of Health Professions. Area Resource File, March 1998. American Hospital Association, 1997; Claritas, 1996.

and isolation can be studied, but other factors also affect transportation issues in access to health care. The U.S. landscape provides a variety of physical obstacles to travel. Mountainous terrain, bodies of water, and difficult climates can complicate the relationship between physical, straight-line distance and transportation access. The willingness to travel is also considered to vary regionally in the United States. Residents of western and Plains states are more likely to be willing to travel great distances, because most services are dispersed and there are few physical obstacles to travel.

DISTRIBUTION DEMOGRAPHY, AND INCOME CHARACTERISTICS OF RURAL POPULATIONS

The rural population of the United States is different from the urban part in more ways than location. There are important regional patterns of concentration and dispersion, the age and income structures are different, and access to health care services is considerably different. These patterns and tendencies have important implications for health status and how policies and markets can provide rural communities with needed health care.

The rural population is distributed unevenly across regions of the United States. According to the 1990 census, the South census region has the largest proportion of rural population (29.1%) followed by the Midwest region (28.5%). The Northeast region has the smallest proportion of rural population (11.8%). For 1992 (estimated) data, both the proportion of nonmetropolitan population at the national level and in census regions decreased across the board (Table 1.3) (Bureau of the Census, 1994). Over 33% of counties and county equivalents have 80% of their population classified as rural, 56.8% over 60%, and 23.7% have 40% or less classified as rural. Counties with relatively high proportions of rural population are concentrated in the South, in Appalachia, and in the Great Plains.

One useful way to compare populations is through population pyramids. The 1996 (estimated) metropolitan and nonmetropolitan county population pyramid shapes are fairly typical for the population of a highly developed country like the United States (Fig. 1.4) (U.S. Bureau of the Census, 1990, 1996). Higher levels of economic development are characterized by declining birth and declining death rates and the pyramid begins to resemble a rectangle more than a pyramid.

The median age of the U.S. nonmetropolitan population was 35.6 years in 1996 compared with 33.8 for the metropolitan population. Within census regions, nonmetropolitan residents are older than their respective metropolitan counterparts with the exception of the Northeast region. The elderly use more health care services and are an important component of any estimation of health care resources needs for a community. In 1996, the Census Bureau estimated that the nonmetropolitan population over the age of 65 was 7,912,537, having grown by 7.3% from 1990 (Table 1.4). The proportion of the population that is 65 years or older is higher in rural counties—15.03% versus 12.77%. From the population pyramids it is possible to calculate the relative growth of certain age cohorts. Nonmetropolitan persons 85 years and older increased by 20.63% from 1990 to 1996 compared to a slight drop among those aged 65 to 69. This rapid aging of the nonmetropolitan population is highlighted by the population pyramid in Figure 1.5, which depicts the nonmetropolitan population by age group in the year 2020 as projected by Woods and Poole, Inc. (1997).

The proportion of the population aged 25 to 44 years is also an important component of the rural population and its growth. This is the age group in which childbearing is most concentrated. Population growth due to births, also called natural increase, has historically been an important element of rural population growth, and this segment of the population is a critical element in

Table 1.3 Metropolitan-Nonmetropolitan Population Characteristics by Census Region, 1990[a]

	United States	*Northeast*	*MidWest*	*South*	*West*
TOTAL POPULATION					
Nonmetro	55,983,543	6,017,411	16,980,129	24,857,852	8,128,151
Metro	192,726,330	44,791,818	42,688,503	60,588,078	44,657,931
PERCENT OF POPULATION (1992)					
Nonmetro	20.3%	10.6%	26.6%	25.8%	13.9%
Metro	79.7%	89.4%	73.4%	74.2%	86.1%
MEDIAN AGE (IN YEARS)					
Nonmetro	35.1yr	34.1yr	34.3yr	33.8yr	32.9yr
Metro	33.8yr	34.2yr	32.5yr	32.4yr	31.6yr
PERCENT BELOW 18 YEARS OF AGE					
Nonmetro	26.7%	24.8%	26.6%	26.4%	28.9%
Metro	25.3%	23.3%	26.0%	25.5%	26.2%
PERCENT 25–44 YEARS OF AGE					
Nonmetro	29.3%	30.8%	28.7%	28.9%	30.5%
Metro	33.4%	32.7%	32.8%	33.4%	34.6%
PERCENT > 65 YEARS OF AGE					
Nonmetro	14.7%	14.4%	15.8%	14.6%	12.9%
Metro	11.9%	13.7%	11.9%	11.7%	10.6%
PERCENT WHITE					
Nonmetro	89.0%	97.2%	96.5%	79.2%	85.2%
Metro	78.3%	80.9%	83.5%	75.8%	74.2%
PERCENT BLACK					
Nonmetro	8.7%	1.4%	1.5%	17.8%	1.0%
Metro	13.0%	12.3%	12.7%	18.8%	6.1%
PERCENT ASIAN					
Nonmetro	0.8%	0.6%	0.4%	0.4%	3.0%
Metro	3.5%	2.9%	1.6%	1.7%	8.5%
PERCENT HISPANIC					
Nonmetro	3.8%	1.1%	1.2%	3.6%	11.5%
Metro	10.3%	8.0%	3.4%	9.5%	20.2%
PERCENT FEMALE-HEADED HOUSEHOLDS					
Nonmetro	9.7%	8.9%	7.6%	10.6%	8.8%
Metro	11.7%	12.4%	11.7%	12.1%	10.6%
PERCENT CHILDREN LIVING WITH 2 PARENTS					
Nonmetro	73.3%	76.4%	79.2%	68.4%	73.7%
Metro	69.2%	69.5%	70.6%	67.7%	69.6%

[a]All data are 1990 unless otherwise noted.

Sources: U.S. Department of Commerce, Bureau of the Census, Census of Population, 1990; Day and Curry, 1996; (U.S.) Bureau of the Census, 1996; Baugher and Lamison-White, 1996; Economic Research Service, 1993; 1997.

the natural increase in nonmetropolitan counties. Over 32% of the U.S. population are between the ages of 25 and 44. Nonmetropolitan areas had a smaller proportion from this age group in 1990 (29.3%). Within census regions, the Midwest region nonmetropolitan population has the smallest proportion of population aged 25 to 44 (28.7%). Of all the regions, the Northeast region's nonmetropolitan population had the largest proportion of those aged 25 to 44 in 1990 (30.8%). This proportion is also greater than that of the U.S. nonmetropolitan population for this age group. The West region, at 30.5%, also has a proportion greater than the national nonmetropolitan population of this age group (Bureau of the Census, 1990).

Race and ethnic groups are also distributed differently in the nonmetropolitan population and within census regions. The South region had the largest proportion of black population in 1990. The Northeast had the largest

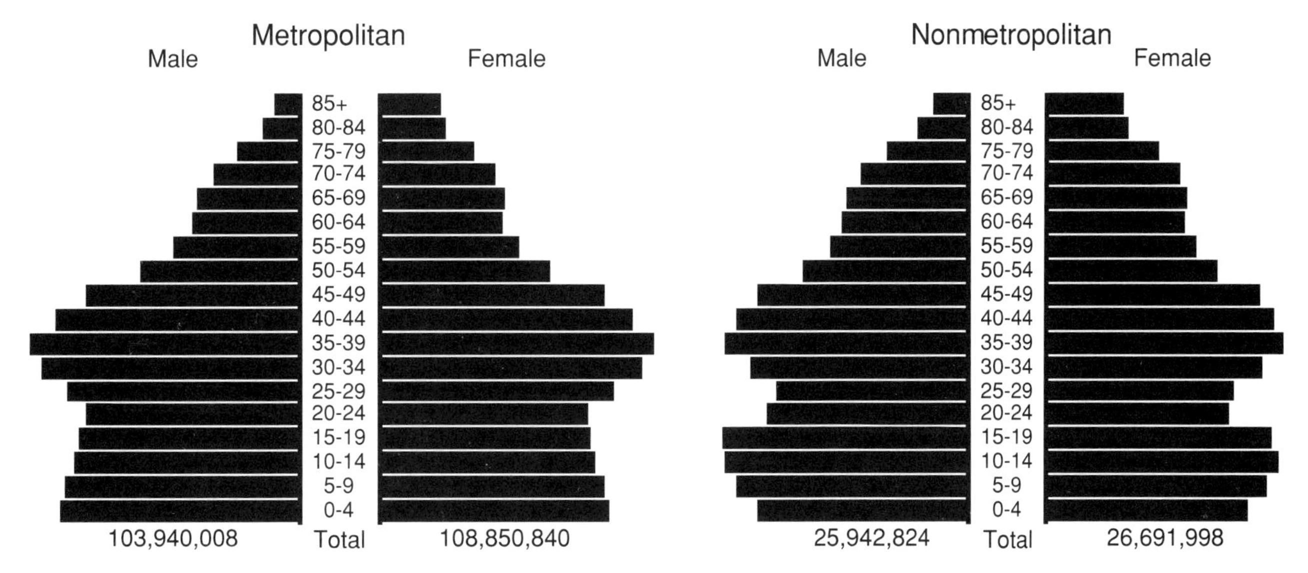

Figure 1.4. Metro and nonmetro population by age and gender, 1996. Source: U.S. Bureau of the Census, 1996.

proportion of white population. The Native American population is present in relatively high proportions in the West region. The Asian and Pacific Islander population is largely metropolitan and concentrated in the West region, as is the Hispanic population (of any race) (Bureau of the Census, 1990).

Income and employment opportunities are distributed differentially between metropolitan and nonmetropolitan populations (Table 1.5). According to the Census Bureau, 1995 median income for nonmetropolitan households was $27,766 in comparison with $36,079 for metropolitan households. Median income also varies within each group by race of family, with nonmetropolitan black households being the worst off. Female-headed households also have relatively low median incomes in both nonmetropolitan and metropolitan areas (Bureau of the Census, 1996).

Table 1.5 also shows that nationally, nonmetropolitan populations are generally poorer, have higher unemployment rates, and are less educated than metropolitan populations (Baugher and Lamison-White, 1996; ERS, 1997a; Day and Curry, 1996).

TRENDS IN NONMETROPOLITAN POPULATION GROWTH

Since its inception, the U.S. population has changed from overwhelmingly rural (95% in 1790 and 60% in 1900) to predominantly urban (75% in 1990) (Bureau of the Census, 1993) (Fig. 1.6).

Historically, population change in nonmetropolitan areas has been dominated by (1) natural increase, accounting for almost all of the growth, and (2) net out-migration from nonmetropolitan areas to metropolitan areas. The pattern of excess natural increase over net out-migration was the rule of thumb for the gradual increase in nonmetropolitan growth during the 19th century (Johnson and Beale, 1993).

These long-standing population trends changed quite suddenly in the 1970s. This period is now well-known as the nonmetropolitan turnaround or "rural renaissance" (Frey, 1987; Johnson and Beale, 1993). This period was characterized by a dramatic increase in population gains fueled primarily by net in-migration to nonmetropolitan counties from metropolitan counties. In addition, the role of natural increase was far less important to population gains in nonmetropolitan areas during this period. In fact, there occurred a sharp reduction in natural population increase in nonmetropolitan areas that paralleled a fertility drop across the nation.

In the 1980s, nonmetropolitan population trends again shifted. A majority of nonmetropolitan areas lost population during this decade (Johnson and Beale, 1994). Additionally, any gains in nonmetropolitan areas due to natural increase continued to be small relative to the largest national natural increase since the post–World War II baby boom. However, since the early 1990s, many nonmetropolitan counties have experi-

Table 1.4 Nonmetropolitan Population Change, 5-Year Cohorts 65 Years of Age and Older

Age Group (years)	*1990 Nonmetro Population (Census)*	*1996 Population (Census Bureau Estimates)*	*Population Change 1990–1996*
85–89	763,679	921,240	20.63%
80–84	973,885	1,103,199	13.28%
75–79	1,493,965	1,633,057	9.31%
70–74	1,879,924	2,029,378	7.95%
65–69	2,260,930	2,223,667	−1.65%
Total	7,374,373	7,912,537	7.30%

Source: U.S. Bureau of the Census, Population Division, Release PPL-91 United State Population Estimates, by Age, Sex, Race, and Hispanic Origin.

enced a population growth, indicating that another turnabout appears on the horizon (Frey and Liaw, 1998; Edmondson and Klein, 1997; Johnson and Beale, 1994). Nonmetropolitan job growth also has grown at a faster rate than in metropolitan areas annually since 1988.

These trends also have policy implications. An understanding of population trends in nonmetropolitan areas is crucial for health services policy makers. Such information is critical in determining the size, distribution, and composition of the rural population in order to design and implement programs that are relevant to rural needs in different counties and regions now as well as over time. In addition, the underlying causes of these changes must be understood in order to formulate theoretical models of rural/nonmetropolitan population change. This will further facilitate planning and implementation in rural health policy.

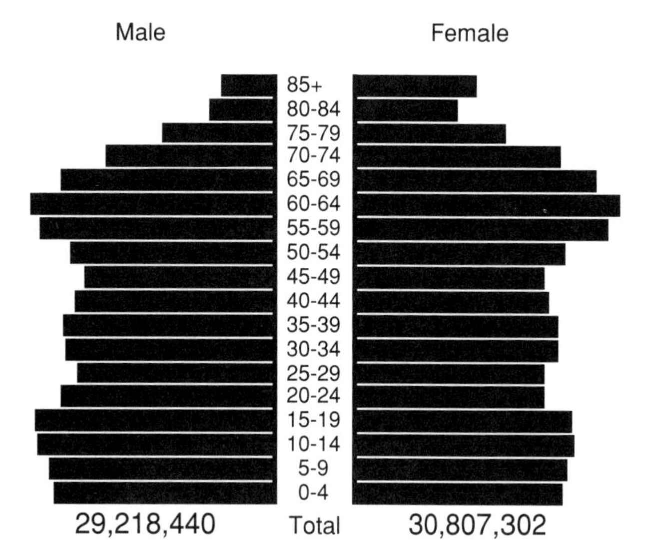

Figure 1.5. Projected nonmetropolitan population by age and gender, 2020. Source: Woods and Poole, Inc., 1997.

THE RURAL ECONOMIC ENVIRONMENT

The prevailing impression of rural America may be that of an agrarian countryside, but agriculture in reality represents a small proportion of U.S. rural employment. The proportion of people working and living on farms in the United States has continued to decrease since World War II. During the 1980s and 1990s the rural farm proportion of the population fell to less than 2% of the total. Although many rural counties rely on a few industrial sectors for their economic base, the rural employment base usually needs to be described as a mixed system of characteristic economies instead of using a single model.

The proportion of nonmetropolitan populations engaged in agriculture, forestry, and fishing sectors is much greater than that in metropolitan areas, but has nevertheless declined from 11% in 1980 to 6.5% in the 1990s. In addition to this, employment in manufacturing and services has begun to predominate over agriculture in nonmetropolitan areas (Bureau of the Census, 1982, 1992; Bureau of the Census & Bureau of Labor Statistics, 1997).

During the second half of the twentieth century, rural areas of the United States experienced significant decreases in agricultural employment. Figure 1.7 shows the declining employment in agriculture from nearly 8 million workers at the end of the 1940s to little more than 3 million in 1991 (U.S. Department of Agriculture [USDA], 1991). Technological innovations and related economic changes have contributed to the decline in agricultural employment but have not replaced those jobs in rural areas. Farm productivity has increased with improvements in farm machinery, livestock and crop sci-

Table 1.5 Characteristics of Nonmetropolitan and Metropolitan Population in the United States

	NonMetro	*Metro*
Population density, persons per square mile (1993)	18	202
Median income of households (1995)	$27,776	$36,079
Non-Hispanic, white	$29,392	$40,342
Black	$16,530	$23,348
Hispanic	$21,322	$23,090
Two-parent family	$37,075	$51,023
Female-headed family	$17,182	$22,478
Percent of families below poverty (1995)	15.6%	13.4%
Educational of those older than 25 yrs (1995)		
High school graduation	76.9%	82.9%
Some college	37.8%	50.3%
B.A. and higher	14.8%	25.0%
Percent Foreign-Born (1996)	2.0%	11.0%

Sources: U.S. Department of Commerce, Bureau of the Census, Census of Population, 1990; Statistical Abstract of the United States, 114th ed., 1994; 117th ed., 1997. Day J, Curry, A. March 1995. Educational Attainment in the US. Washington, DC Department of Commerce (U.S.) Bureau of the Census; August 1996. Current Population Reports, Series P20–489; Money Income in the US: 1995. Washington DC: Department of Commerce (U.S.), Bureau of Census; March 1997. Current Population Reports, Series P60–193. Baugher E, Lamison-White, L. Poverty in the US; 1995. Washington D.C.: Department of Commerce (U.S.), Bureau of the Census; 1996. Current Population Reports, Series P60–194. Department of Agriculture (U.S.). Rural Conditions and Trends September 1997:8(20);Spring 1995:6(1).

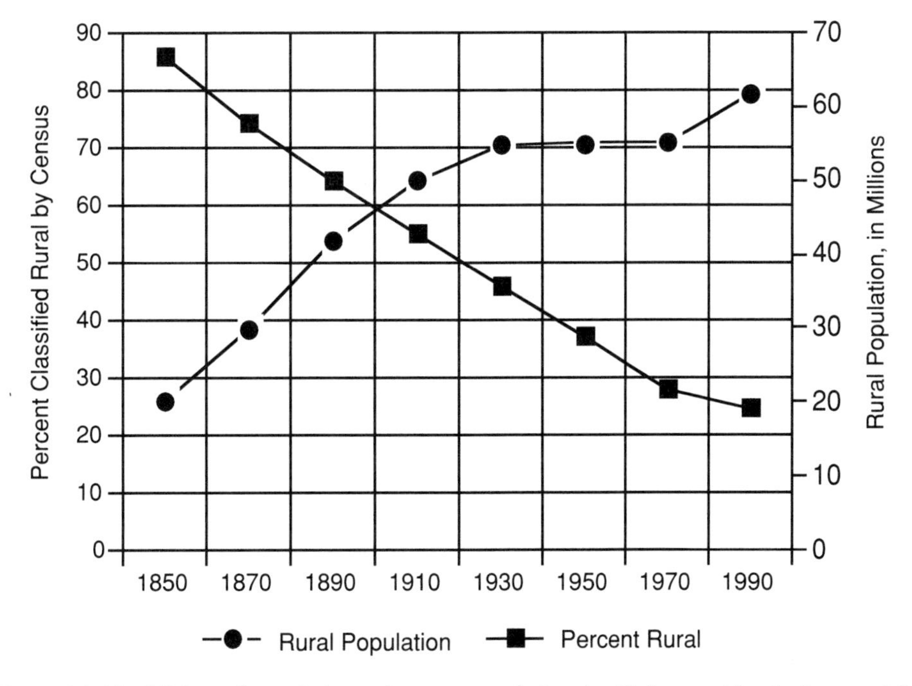

Figure 1.6. Total U.S. rural population and percent population classified as rural by the Bureau of the Census, from 1850 to 1990. Source: U.S. Bureau of the Census, 1994.

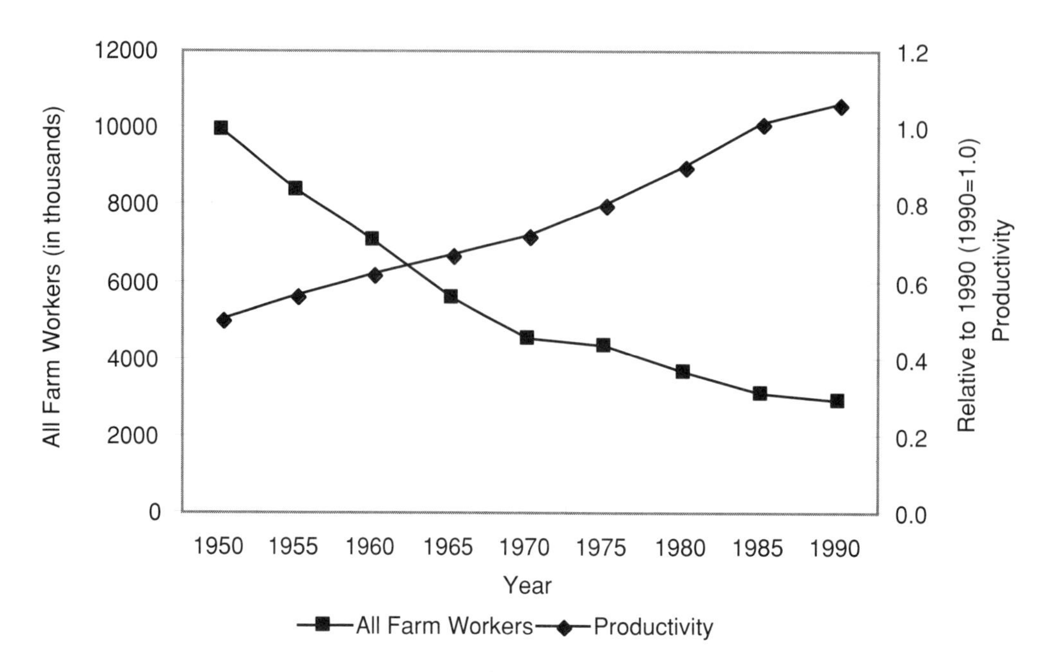

Figure 1.7. Trends in number of farm workers and productivity, from 1948 to 1990. Source: United States Department of Agriculture. Farm Employment and Wage Rates 1910–1990. Washington, DC: USDA, March 1991.

ence, and transportation (USDA, 1998). The transformation of land from agriculture to other uses is proceeding at a slower rate than the decline in agricultural employment because, with the exception of land bordering on rapidly developing areas, agriculture remains the most efficient use of the land.

Increased productivity and the increased burden of regulation and overhead has led to farm consolidation. From the late 1950s to the late 1980s, the size of farms grew from an average of about 240 acres to about 460 acres, but the number of farms diminished from about 4.8 million to about 2 million. This combination of factors meant that 20% of the 1950s farmland was removed from production by the late 1980s (Reimund and Gale, 1992). Farm households that do remain in agriculture are likely to seek financial support from non-agricultural sources; 58% of rural-farm households reported receiving some income from non-agricultural sectors in 1993 (USDA, 1995).

The manufacturing and industrial sectors have maintained a larger share of the rural employment base than metropolitan areas. A variety of factors support the rural manufacturing base. Improvements in rural highway systems and the decline of rail freight systems have taken many of the access advantages away from the cities. International competition has driven down wages in many manufacturing and fabrication industries, leading domestic competitors to seek the lower wage labor found in rural America (USDA, 1995). When building new factories, which tend to be spread-out, single-story facilities, companies prefer to develop on clear tracts of land rather than to redevelop sites. Building in less developed, less expensive rural areas allows a company to build accommodating structures with recreation amenities on the grounds while maintaining reserve land for expansion. Rural manufacturing often develops along transportation corridors and adjacent to metropolitan areas. In addition to the attraction of rural amenities, local rural governments, especially in the South, have recruited business with enticements of bond financing, tax credits and breaks, and employee training. Nonmetropolitan manufacturing has been strong in the southeastern United States, where the scattered medium-sized cities found in these areas combine rural, but accessible, areas with suppliers and the relative density of population means a workforce is close at hand. Some rural manufacturing is agriculture-related, about 13% nationally, but the majority of rural industry is not related to food or fiber production.

Some nonmetropolitan areas became characterized by relatively new economic forces in the 1980s and 1990s: the shift to service sector employment and the growth of retirement centers. These represent a departure from the production of tangible products that have traditionally been associated with the rural economy. Service sector activity in nonmetropolitan areas can serve regional or national demand through communications—the growth of mail order firms, the internet, and centralized telephone contact systems for national businesses allows these services to be provided in rural places. Regional service providers are located in population centers that can be distant from any metropolitan area. These centers function as mini-metropolises providing trade and health services to the sparsely populated areas surrounding them and often benefit from being at the intersection of several transportation corridors or railroad and trucking terminals or river ports.

Rural services that serve a national base include tourism and recreational facilities. The location of these areas is often determined by the presence of a natural, historic, or climatic amenity, though the amenity can occasionally be created by designing a local theme park or initiating an annual festival. Trade or tourism services can serve as the main export base of nonmetropolitan areas that have the geographic or amenity advantages.

Many rural communities have experienced in-migration of retirees. This is not restricted to movement from the North and Midwest to the South and Southwest; however, the largest component of retirement immigration is from colder northern climates among people who wish to retire to areas where the cost of living is lower, the weather is milder, and the pace of life is generally slower. This migration parallels the recent rapid growth of the Sunbelt (Abbott, 1990). Beginning in the 1970s, the Sunbelt, which includes the South and West regions, has emerged as a major growth center in terms of manufacturing and services employment and population growth. The two trends have combined to create economic engines for the region, retirees bringing in incomes based on pensions earned elsewhere and industry contributing investments and payrolls. There are significant "destination retirement" counties in the Northwest, Midwest, and Northeast. The Upper Peninsula of Michigan is an example of a rural area that has seen sharp increases in the number of retiree immigrants.

Rural retirement communities spark a need for shopping and health care facilities, and many military retirees often meet those needs by locating near military bases, which are now located disproportionately in the south (USDA, 1995b). Many rural communities seek retirees for the injection of income that is brought to the area, supporting the service and retail sectors. Other areas with low real estate prices will advertise for properties in national newspapers with the goal of attracting urban workers planning their retirement. Additionally, the southeastern United States is experiencing a return migration of retirement-age African Americans, who left the South to go North and West during the Great Migration (1910–1920) (Johnson and Roseman, 1990). Descendants of these migrants are returning to the South, as well, to take advantage of the job growth and quality of life.

HEALTH STATUS OF RURAL POPULATIONS

The health status of rural populations is a very important issue in provision of and access to health care. As we have seen, rural populations tend to be poorer than urban populations and therefore many of the ills associated with poverty are magnified in rural areas. Rural areas report higher rates of chronic disease and infant mortality. Injuries related to use of farm machinery and rural occupational hazards associated with mining, forestry, and fishing are unique problems for rural health care systems. Trauma mortality, especially for motor vehicle crashes and gun-related reasons, is disproportionately higher in rural areas (Chen et al., 1995). In the following section, we will discuss how health status varies regionally and by rural and urban status using mortality as the key indicator.

MORTALITY RATES

When overall mortality rates are compared between rural and urban areas for the nation, the crude death rates are generally higher in the rural or nonmetropolitan areas. However, when the rates are standardized by gender and age, the differences all but disappear (Miller, Farmer, and Clarke, 1994). Tracing trends in mortality across county types, from the most urban to the most rural (Fig. 1.8) illustrates how mortality rates appear to increase as the population is more rural. However, after adjusting the rates to reflect the differences in age and gender between groups of counties, the trend is no longer apparent. Although the underlying or comparative rate may not be different, the per-population rate that health care providers must cope with does increase; therefore, rural areas similar in population size to urban places will have more actual end-of-life-related need for health services.

Plate 1.5 shows age-adjusted mortality rates for all causes for nonmetropolitan counties for 1990 through 1994. High mortality is concentrated in the South, throughout Appalachia, and in certain pockets in the Midwest and Southwest. In contrast, Alaska and Hawaii

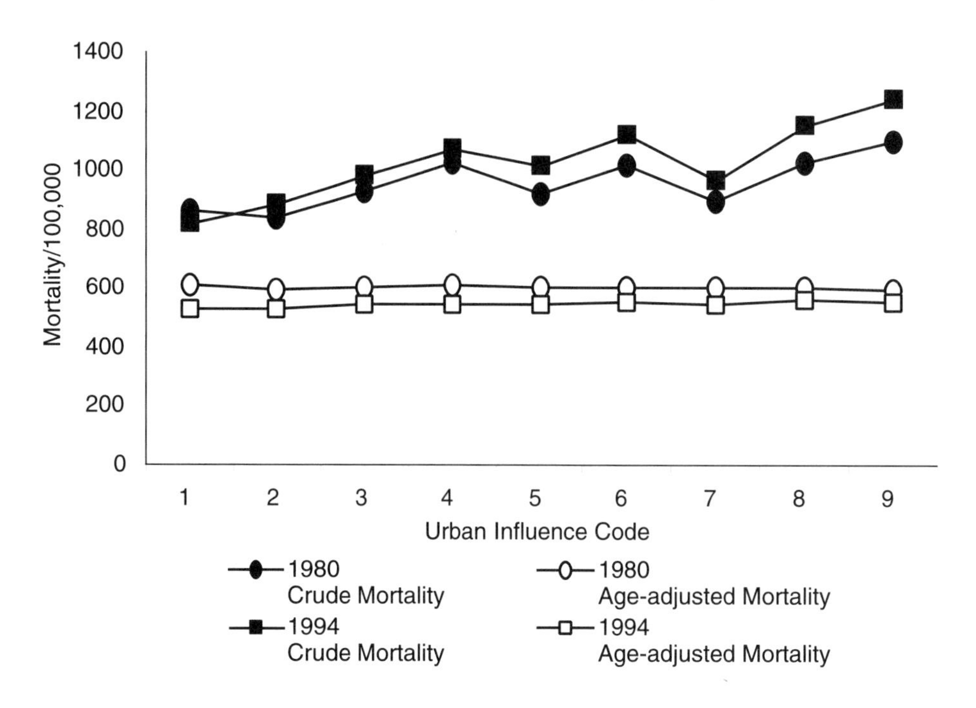

Figure 1.8. Crude and age-adjusted mortality rates per 100,000, all causes, by urban influence codes, 1980 and 1994. Source: National Center for Health Statistics, 1998.

have relatively lower mortality rates than the northeastern part of the United States extending westward to the Great Plains. Data on infant mortality is described in Chapter 12, Rural Maternal and Perinatal Health. In general, infant mortality is highly concentrated in many southern counties, especially along the Mississippi River along the borders of Arkansas, Louisiana, and Mississippi. Alaska also has high infant mortality in its sparsely populated western county equivalents.

RACE AND ETHNICITY AND RURAL URBAN DIFFERENCES IN MORTALITY

In early 1998 President Clinton described a national goal to reduce and eventually eliminate race and ethnic disparities in mortality and morbidity rates for six areas of health status. Those areas include infant mortality, cancer screening and management, cardiovascular disease, diabetes, HIV infection, and child and adult immunizations. There are serious differences between races in access and outcome measures, nationally, and there are even wider gaps when rural and urban comparisons are made at the regional level. For example, the ratio of national rates of infant mortality of whites (6.3 infant deaths per 1,00 live births in 1995) to African Americans (14.6/1,000) is 1.31. African-American infant death rates are 131% higher than that of whites.

Data from the National Center for Health Statistics Compressed Mortality Files show that there are some clear patterns of rural disadvantage that emerge across race and ethnic descriptions. Figure 1.9 shows the persistence of these differences over time for rural and urban white, African-American, and other race groups.

For other diseases, these rate differences do not reveal a consistent geographic disadvantage for the rural population. Figure 1.10 shows the same mortality trend for diabetes. Black nonmetro and metro mortality exceeds that of white mortality in every year.

MORBIDITY RATES—HIV/AIDS IN RURAL AREAS

One relatively recent trend in morbidity rates in rural areas is the increase in rates of human immunodeficiency virus (HIV) infection and acquired immunodeficiency syndrome (AIDS) (CDC, 1995; Graham et al., 1995; Lam and Liu, 1994). The HIV/AIDS epidemic was first identified in large urban centers in the United States largely among homosexual white males (Gould, 1989; Gardner et al., 1989). Between 1991 and 1992, AIDS in-

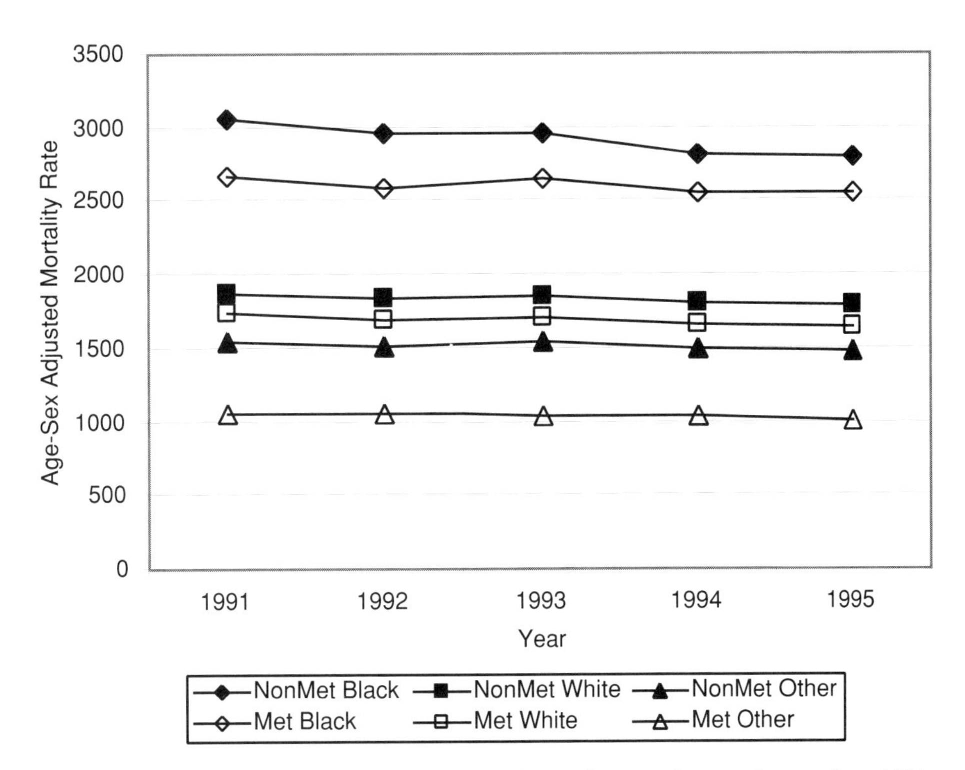

Figure 1.9. Metro versus nonmetro differences in cardiovascular mortality rates by race from 1991 to 1995.

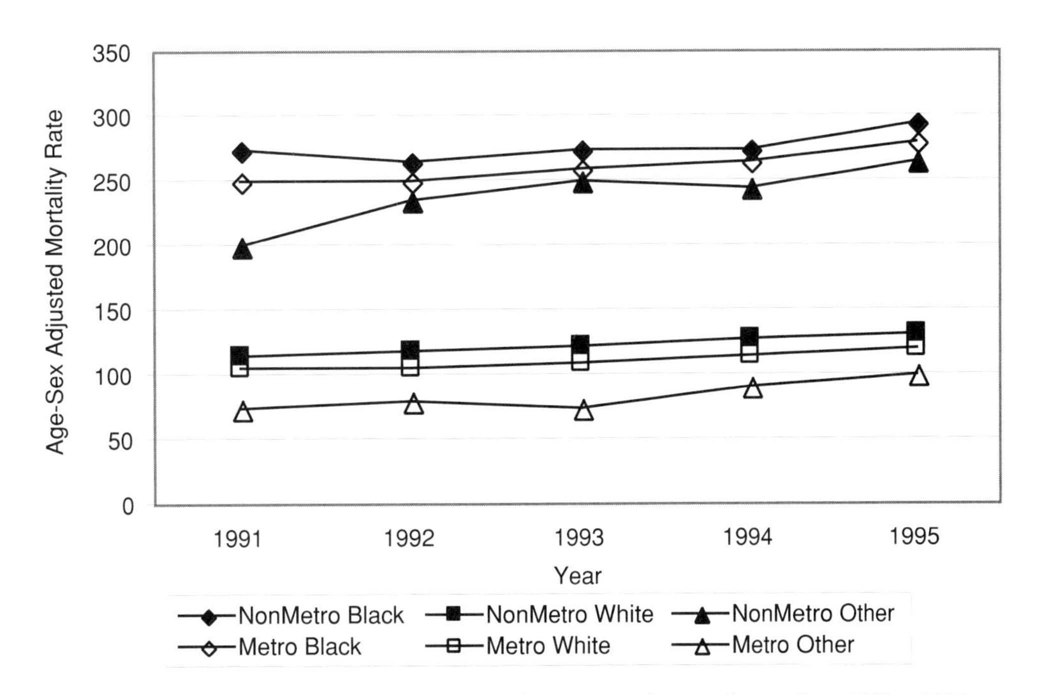

Figure 1.10. Metro versus nonmetro differences in diabetic mortality rates by race from 1991 to 1995.

cidence as well as the rate per 100,000 in nonmetropolitan areas increased by 9.4% as opposed to metropolitan areas with less than 500,000 population (3.1%) and those with between 50,000 and 500,000 population (3.3%) (CDC, 1993; Berry, 1993).

Although the total number of rural HIV/AIDS cases constitutes a relatively modest percent (5.5%) of the total reported in the United States, there is a rapid increase in the number of cases being reported from the South and Midwest regions of the United States (Brownlea et al., 1997; CDC, 1995, 1996). The South also contains a high proportion of rural and black population (see Table 1.3). In addition, the epidemiology of AIDS is also changing. In recent years, the face of HIV/AIDS is becoming increasingly rural, female, black, and heterosexual (Voelker, 1998; CDC, 1995; Berry, 1993).

Because the U.S. HIV/AIDS epidemic was first identified in large metropolitan centers, many rural physicians and residents see HIV/AIDS as an urban problem (Voelker, 1998; Cohn, 1997). Evidence exists that patients who are diagnosed in major urban centers often return home to rural areas for family support (Cohn et al., 1994). Although the absolute numbers of cases in rural areas may be small, these cases can have a great impact on communities already stressed by lack of access to health care for basic health needs. Also, much of the funding for HIV/AIDS treatment is distributed based on where a patient was diagnosed. Therefore, many rural areas that are experiencing return-migration of HIV/AIDS patients may not be receiving the funding designated to treat AIDS patients.

Additionally, in rural communities (as well as across the United States), HIV/AIDS is still stigmatized as a disease that results from socially unacceptable behaviors and lifestyles. Physicians in rural areas may not have the experience or expertise to treat HIV/AIDS, and anonymity in many rural areas is nonexistent (e.g., a patient may attend church with the only pharmacist in town) (Voelker, 1998; Cohn, 1997; Brownlea et al, 1997).

IMMIGRATION: IMPLICATIONS FOR RURAL AREAS

Immigrants in Rural Towns

The Census Bureau estimates that in 1996, 24.6 million of the general population were foreign-born (9% of the total). Most foreign-born persons reside in metropolitan areas and make up 11% of that population. Foreign-born persons made up 2% of the nonmetropolitan population in 1996 (see Table 1.4).

Nonmetropolitan immigrants are concentrated in the South and the West regions of the United States. Since 1990, these immigrants have been predominantly of Mexican or other Latin American origin. Nonmetropolitan immigrants are more likely to be naturalized than their metropolitan counterparts. And among nonmetropolitan immigrants, 38% of those naturalized and 24% of noncitizens were under the age of 18 (compared to 28% of the native nonmetropolitan population) (ERS, 1997b).

In recent years, immigration patterns have changed in response to employment opportunities in rural areas, and foreign-born persons, especially Hispanic and Asian immigrants, are increasingly settling in nontraditional locations in the rural United States (Gouveia and Stull, 1995; Griffith, 1995; Grey, 1995; Johnson, Johnson-Webb, and Farrell, forthcoming). The fact that many of these immigrants are responding to increased demand for workers in the agribusiness sector, especially in meat processing, raises a range of issues surrounding workplace conditions, injuries, and employer-provided health insurance coverage. Health and social services are often inadequate to meet the needs of the native population, let alone those of newcomers who may have limited English as well as cultural practices that may act as barriers to seeking health care. The Immigrant Reform and Immigration Responsibility Act of 1996 also may limit options for workers, both documented and undocumented, who have been recruited by employers to their respective communities.

Migrant Farm Workers

Farm workers, found mostly in rural, agriculturally based areas, are estimated to number 1.5 to 2.5 million and make up less than 1% of all workers (ERS, 1997b; GAO, 1992). Migrant and seasonal farm workers are a sub-population of this group and are estimated to total 750,000 to 850,000 (Rural Migration News, 1995). Farm workers are subject to poor working conditions including substandard housing, exposure to pesticides and other chemicals, poor sanitation, and few or nonexistent medical services (GAO, 1992). In addition, farm work is often seasonal, is usually performed out of doors, and involves lifting and carrying heavy objects as well as frequent bending and stooping (ERS, 1997c).

Findings from the 1990 National Agricultural Workers Survey show that over 70% of farm workers are foreign-born and are of Mexican or other Latin American ancestry (Mines et al., 1997). Over 60% of farm workers live below the poverty level and this proportion has increased over time. Most farm workers are married and have children, but they live and work separately from their families. Farm workers use few social services, and many who were once eligible for services are now excluded from access to food stamps, Medicaid, and WIC because of recent immigration legislation passed by the 104th Congress (Mines et al., 1997).

CONCLUSION

We have outlined and described the size as well as the geographic and demographic distribution of the rural population and how these may affect access to and provision of health care. These factors will continue to have important ramifications in the future of rural health policy and planning, especially in the light of the demographic changes occurring in the rural population in the next three decades. The declining role of agriculture coupled with the growth of low-wage employment without benefits all over the nation, and especially in the South, is sure to make it harder for rural people to pay health care costs, notwithstanding the booming economies in growing Sunbelt communities.

The health status of rural Americans does not differ substantially from that of the remainder of the nation when we control for age and sex distribution. However, the indicators that are used to compare health status by geography are end events, mortality or severe morbidity. The quality of life of rural versus urban people is seldom considered. Rural people more often describe their health as poor or fair, and there are indications that the types of care they receive and its timeliness compare unfavorably with those of urban dwellers.

Many challenges face rural America. The continuing overall urbanization of the U.S. population, population shifts, the aging of the rural population, as well as the serious challenges presented by the growing presence of immigrants in many rural areas, will require that health policy makers be creative and innovative in their health policy formulation. In the coming millennium, health policy will increasingly have to be tailored to local and regional characteristics and needs for it to be effective in improving the health of rural populations.

REFERENCES

Abbott C. 1990. New West, new South, new region. In: Mohl R, ed. Searching for the Sunbelt: Historical Perspectives on a Region. Knoxville, Tenn: University of Tennessee Press, pp. 7–25.

American Hospital Association. 1997. Annual Survey of Hospitals 1996, American Hospital Association, Chicago, Ill.

Baer LD, Johnson-Webb KD, Gesler WM. 1997. What is rural? A focus on urban influence codes. Journal of Rural Health 13(4): 329–333.

Baugher E, Lamison-White L. 1996. Poverty in the United States: 1995. Washington, D.C.: Department of Commerce (U.S.), Bureau of the Census.

Berry DE. 1993. The emerging epidemiology of rural AIDS. Journal of Rural Health 9(4): 293–304.

Brownlea S, McDonald M, Ackerman E. 1997. AIDS Comes to small-town America. US News & World Report 123(18): 52–55.

Bureau of the Census (U.S.) and Bureau of Labor Statistics. 1997. Current Population Survey, March 1997. Washington, DC: Department of Commerce and Bureau of Labor Statistics.

Bureau of the Census (U.S.). 1990. Census of Population and Housing, 1990: Table 4 Population 1790 to 1990.

Bureau of the Census (U.S.). 1994. Statistical Abstract of the United States: 1994, 114th ed. Washington, DC: Department of Commerce.

Bureau of the Census (U.S.). 1993. Census of Population and Housing, 1990: Public Use Microdata Samples, Technical Documentation. Washington, DC: Department of Commerce.

Bureau of the Census (U.S.). 1996. Money Income in the United States: 1995/With Separate Data on Valuation of Noncash Benefits/. Washington, DC: Government Printing Office (U.S.).

Bureau of the Census (U.S.). 1997. Statistical Abstract of the United States: 1997, 117th ed. Washington, DC: Department of Commerce.

Bureau of the Census (U.S.). 1982. Census of Population and Housing, 1980: Standard Tape File 3C. Washington, DC: Department of Commerce.

Bureau of the Census, (U.S.). 1992. Census of Population and Housing, 1990: Standard Tape File 3C. Washington, DC: Department of Commerce.

Centers for Disease Control and Prevention (CDC). 1995. First 500,000 cases—United States, 1995. JAMA 274(23): 1827–1829.

Centers for Disease Control and Prevention (CDC). 1993. HIV/AIDS Surveillance: Year End Edition. Washington, DC: CDC.

Centers for Disease Control and Prevention (CDC). HIV/AIDS Surveillance Report. 1996; 8: 7–35.

Chen B, Maio RF, Green PE, Burney RE. 1995. Geographical variation in mortality from motor vehiclee crashes. Journal of Trauma 38(2): 228–232.

Claritas Inc. 1996. [Interstate Highway MapInfo Data Table], Claritas Inc.

Cohn SE, Klein JD, Mohr JE, van der Horst CM, Weber DJ. 1994. The geography of AIDS: patterns of urban and rural migration. Southern Medical Journal 87(6): 599–606.

Cohn SE. 1997. AIDS in rural America. Journal of Rural Health 13(4): 237–239.

Day J, Curry A. 1996. Educational Attainment in the United States: March 1995. Washington, DC Department of Commerce (U.S.) Bureau of the Census; Current Populations Reports, Series P20–489.

Department of Health and Human Services. 1997. Area Resource File, 1997. Washington, DC: Office of Research and Planning, Bureau of Health Professions, Health Resources and Services Administration, Department of Health and Human Services.

Economic Research Service (ERS) U.S. Department of Agriculture. 1997a. Employment growth rates converge for metro and nonmetro areas. Rural Conditions and Trends. 8(2): 9–13.

Economic Research Service (ERS) U.S. Department of Agriculture. 1997b. Fewer immigrants settle in nonmetro areas and most fare less well then metro immigrants. Rural Conditions and Trends. 8(2): 60–65.

Economic Research Service (ERS) U.S. Department of Agriculture. 1997c. Number of hired farm workers increases, but their median weekly earnings show little improvement. Rural Conditions and Trends. 8(2):75–78.

Edmondson B, Klein M. 1997. A new era for rural America. American Demographics Sept: 30–31.

Federal Register. 1997. List of Designated Primary Medical Care, Mental Health, and Dental Health Professional Shortage Areas, 1997. Federal Register (Vol. 62, no. 104, p. 29395), Washington, DC.

Frey WH, Liaw K-L. 1998. Immigrant concentration and domestic migrant dispersal: is movement to nonmetropolitan areas "white flight"? Professional Geographer 50(2): 215–232.

Frey WH. 1987. Migration and depopulation of the metropolis: regional restructuring or rural renaissance? American Sociological Review 52: 240–257.

Gardner LI, Brundage JF, Burke DS, McNeil JG, Visintine R, Miller RN. 1989. Spatial diffusion of the human immunodeficiency virus infection epidemic in the United States, 1985–87. Annals of the Association of American Geographers 79(1): 25–43.

General Accounting Office (U.S.). 1992. Hired Farm Workers: Health and Well-being at Risk. Washington, DC: GAO; Report No. HRD-92–46.

Ghelfi LM, Parker TS. 1996. A county-level measure of urban influence: what metro adjacency and cities do for nonmetro county economics. Presented at Regional Science Association International Meeting.

Goldsmith HF, Puskin DS, Stiles DJ. 1993. Improving the operational definition of "rural areas" for federal programs. Federal Office of Rural Health Policy [monograph online] 1993. Available from URL: http://www.nal.usda.gov/ric/richs/goldsmit.htm.

Gould PR. 1989. Geographic dimensions of the AIDS epidemic. Professional Geographer 41: 71–78.

Gouveia l, Stull D. 1995. Dances with cows: beef packing's impact on Garden City, KS and Lexington, NE. In: Stull D, Broadway M, Griffith D, eds. Any Way You Cut It: Meat Processing and Small-Town America. Lawrence, Kan: University of Kansas Press; 85–107.

Graham RP, Forrester ML, Wysong JA, Rosenthal TC, James PA. 1995. HIV/AIDS in the rural United States: epidemiology and health services delivery. Medical Care Research Review 52(4): 435–452.

Grey M. 1995. Pork, poultry and newcomers in Storm Lake, Iowa. In: Stull D, Broadway M, Griffith D, eds. Any Way You Cut It: Meat Processing and Small-Town America. Lawrence, Kan: University of Kansas Press, 109–127.

Griffith D. 1995. Hay trabado. In: Stull D, Broadway M, Griffith D, eds. Any Way You Cut It: Meat Processing and Small-Town America. Lawrence, Kan: University of Kansas Press; 129–151.

Hewitt M. 1992. Defining "rural" areas: impact on health care policy and research. In: Gesler W, Ricketts TC, eds. Health in Rural North America. New Brunswick, NJ: Rutgers University Press.

Johnson JH, Johnson-Webb KD, Farrell WC. Newly emerging Hispanic communities in the US: a spatial analysis of settlement patterns, in-migration fields, and social receptivity. In: Socio-demographic Aspects of Immigration. New York: Russel Sage Foundation. Forthcoming.

Johnson JH, Roseman CC. 1990. Increasing black out-migration from Los Angeles: the role of household dynamics and kinship systems. Annals of the Association of American Geographers 80: 205–222.

Johnson KM, Beale CL. 1993. Demographic change in nonmetropolitan America, 1980 to 1990. Rural Sociology 58(3): 347–365.

Johnson KM, Beale CL. 1994. The recent revival of widespread population growth in nonmetropolitan areas of the United States. Rural Sociology 59(4): 655–667.

Johnson-Webb KD, Baer LD, Gesler WM. 1997. What is rural? Issues and considerations. Journal of Rural Health 13(3): 253–256.

Lam NS-N, Liu K. 1994. Spread of AIDS in rural America, 1982–1990. Journal of Acquired Immune Deficiency Syndromes 7(5): 485–490.

Miller MK, Farmer FL, Clarke LL. 1994. Rural populations and their health. In: Beaulieu JE, Berry DE, eds. Rural Health Services. Ann Arbor, Mich: AUPHA Press/Health Adminsitration Press.

Mines R, Gabard S, Steirman A. 1997. A Profile of US Farm Workers: Demographics, Household Composition, Income and Use of Services. Washington, DC: Department of Labor (U.S.) Research Report No. 6.

Office of Management and Budget. Metropolitan areas, 1994. In: Changes in Metropolitan Areas: 1950–1994. Washington, DC: Statistical Policy Office, Office of Information and Regulatory Affairs.

Reimund DA, Gale F. 1992. Structural Change for the U.S. Farm Sector, 1974–87, 13th Annual Family Farm Report to Congress, Agriculture Information Bulletin No. 647. Washington, DC: United States Department of Agriculture.

Ricketts TC, Johnson-Webb KD. 1997. What is "rural" and how to measure "rurality": a focus on health care delivery and health policy. Technical Issues Paper. Chapel Hill, NC: North Carolina Rural Health Research and Policy Analysis Center, Cecil G. Sheps Center for Health Services Research. Contract No.: HRSA 93–857(P). Sponsored by the Federal Office of Rural Health Policy, HRSA, U.S. DHHS.

Rural Migration News. Farm Worker Assistance Programs. Author [serial online] 1995 June; Available from URL: http://128.36.171/RMN-Archive/jun__95-05.html.

United States Department of Agriculture. 1998. Agricultural Productivity in the U.S. Washington, DC: United States Department of Agriculture.

United States Department of Agriculture. 1991. Farm Employment and Wage Rates 1910–1990. Washington, DC: United States Department of Agriculture.

United States Department of Agriculture. 1995. Understanding Rural America, Agriculture Information Bulletin No. 710. Washington, DC: United States Department of Agriculture.

Voelker R. 1998. Rural communities struggle with AIDS. JAMA 279(1): 5–6.

Woods and Poole Economics, Inc. 1997. The Complete Economic and Demographic Data Source. Washington, DC: Woods and Poole, Inc.

2

Access to Health Care

CLAUDIA L. SCHUR AND SHEILA J. FRANCO

Ensuring equitable access to health care is an important public policy goal for the nation. A significant body of research and policy analysis has been focused on documenting access problems for vulnerable populations and suggesting policy options to eliminate access barriers (Aday, 1993; Aday et al., 1998). Rural populations have often been viewed as especially vulnerable with respect to access to health care because of poorly developed and fragile health infrastructures, high prevalence rates of chronic illness and disability, socioeconomic hardships, and physical barriers such as distance and availability of transportation, including a lack of public transportation (Rowland and Lyons, 1989).

This chapter examines access to health care services for rural Americans in the 1990s using a variety of access indicators. Differences in access to care among demographic subgroups are explored with a primary focus on variations in access across rural and urban areas. Wherever possible, a more disaggregated definition of rural is used instead of the usual urban-rural dichotomy in an attempt to account for the wide variations found across communities. The data presented are drawn primarily from the 1994 Access to Care supplement of the National Health Interview Survey, the 1996 Medical Expenditure Panel Survey, and the 1994 Robert Wood Johnson Foundation National Access to Care Survey.

DEFINING AND MEASURING ACCESS

In providing information on access to health care in rural areas, widely accepted measures of access are employed that were developed in the 1970s as part of a framework for studying access to care (Aday, Andersen, and Fleming, 1980). Where possible, this is supplemented with indicators from an Institute of Medicine (IOM) study emphasizing both the receipt of services and the effect on health status or outcomes (IOM, 1993).

Access measures are examined by a variety of individual sociodemographic characteristics known to influence the use of health care (Berk, Schur, and Cantor, 1995; Mueller, Patil, and Boilesen, 1997; Cornelius, Beauregard, and Cohen, 1991). Health insurance coverage is examined because, controlling for other characteristics, persons with third-party coverage for health care are more likely to have a usual source of care and have more physician visits, and are less likely to report problems obtaining care (Berk, Schur, and Cantor, 1995; Mueller, Patil, and Boilesen, 1997; Weissman and Epstein, 1994; Spillman, 1992). Data on usual source of care, site of care, travel and waiting times are also provided. A usual source of care—a regular place at which an individual seeks medical care when sick or in need of advice about health—is viewed as an entry point to the health care system and is seen as increasing continuity of care. Because of concern about differences in quality or continuity across sites of care, only variation reported in regular care sites is presented. Other dimensions of the usual care site that may be related to access are travel and waiting times: the time associated with making a physician contact may be viewed as one of the resources necessary to obtain care.

Actual use of health care services and its converse—the inability to obtain needed care—are also examined.

The mean number of physician visits and the percentage of the population with a hospitalization in the previous year are used in this instance. For some people, however, lack of utilization may indicate lack of need rather than inability to access services. With the advent of managed care, utilization may be lowered without a concomitant decrease in access. For this reason, the percent of the population in fair or poor health with no visits in the prior year is also reported because it is believed that those in fair or poor health should have at least one visit per year (American College of Physicians, 1995).

The proportion of the population with a hospital admission has traditionally been seen as an indicator of access to care; however, more recent work suggests that many hospitalizations may result from insufficient ambulatory care and may be suggestive of poor access. The IOM found that hospital admissions for relatively controllable chronic conditions were almost five times higher in low-income neighborhoods compared with high-income neighborhoods (IOM, 1993). The same link between social and economic conditions has been demonstrated for rural populations but the correlation is not as strong (Ricketts, 1997; Schreiber and Zielinski, 1997; Silver, Babitz and Magill, 1997)

The effect of a barrier to access creates a "non-event"—failure to use services—so it is difficult to capture the extent to which people have access difficulties. An expressed inability to obtain medical care implies that a person identified a need for care (albeit from the individual's perspective) and was unable to obtain it. In many household surveys, respondents are asked if they were unable to obtain care that they believed they needed in a timely manner. Summary indices of access can be created from satisfaction measures, attitudes toward the effectiveness of the health care delivery system as well as toward its organization, and information on the proportion of office visits to regular providers, or to generalist and even specialist physicians, or primary care professionals. These measures are used in the National Health Interview Survey and the 1994 Robert Wood Johnson Foundation National Access to Care Survey and form the basis for the analysis described here.

ACCESS FROM A RURAL PERSPECTIVE

Access to health care services in rural versus urban areas has been explored by health services researchers for decades. Rural residents are, on average, poorer, older, and, for those under age 65, less insured than persons living in urban areas (Braden and Beauregard, 1994; American College of Physicians, 1995; Hartley, Quam, and Lurie, 1994). Rural Americans also report more chronic conditions and describe themselves in poorer health than urban residents (Braden and Beauregard, 1994). Further, injury-related mortality and the number of days of restricted activity are higher in nonurban areas (Braden and Beauregard, 1994).

It is possible that measures of access need to be expanded to address issues of particular concern in rural areas and to gain a better understanding of access problems that may be specific to rural areas. Access to health care in rural areas is complicated by different patterns of employment and insurance coverage among rural residents. Rural residents are more likely to be self-employed; if employed by a firm, those firms are smaller than those in urban areas. Consequently, employment-related insurance benefits may be less widespread and less generous (Frenzen, 1993). State-focused studies have found that urban families have more insurance coverage than their rural counterparts and that rural families pay a higher proportion of their income for insurance premiums (Hartley, Quam, and Lurie, 1994; Mueller, Patil and Boilsesen, 1997; Mueller, Patil and Ullrich, 1997). Previous research found that rural residents are no more likely than urban residents to lack a usual source of care. However, rural residents more commonly cite lack of local resources as the reason they do not have a usual source of care (Hayward et al., 1991). Issues of transportation and travel times also may have particular importance in rural areas. Evidence indicates that rural residents have greater transportation difficulties and often travel longer distances to receive health care (Cunningham and Cornelius, 1995; Seccombe, 1995; Edelman and Menz, 1996). Lack of adequate public transportation in rural areas also creates a barrier to receiving care: only 12% of communities with populations less than 2,500 have public transportation systems (Seccombe, 1995; Comer and Mueller, 1995; Birdwell and Calesaric, 1996).

Availability of specialist physicians or specialized equipment may also differentially affect rural residents. Overall, in 1996, there were 190 patient care specialists per 100,000 people in metropolitan counties versus 54.6 per 100,000 in nonmetro counties (see chapter 3 for a comprehensive discussion of these ratios). An analysis of services provided to Medicare beneficiaries found not only that the volume of physician services per beneficiary was 15% lower in rural areas than urban areas but also that this disparity was largest for technology-intensive specialties. For example, the volume of cardiology services was 40% lower for rural Medicare enrollees than for urban beneficiaries (Dor and Holahan, 1990).

ANALYSIS

Generally lower levels of availability of health care due to geographic factors is one important characteristic of rural populations. There are fewer health care professionals of all kinds in rural areas and distances to care are greater for more rural than urban people. The availability of health care varies; some rural communities may be close to urban centers whereas very remote villages and isolated towns may have few medical resources. In an attempt to gain more insight into differences in access for different types of rural populations, a measure of the comparative "rurality" of counties, the urban influence coding system, is used to classify the data (Ghelfi and Parker, 1997). The urban influence system divides counties into nine categories; metropolitan counties are classified into two categories and nonmetropolitan into seven. The nonmetropolitan categories are based on adjacency to a large or small metropolitan areas and the size of the largest city in the county. Because the surveys that are analyzed in this chapter have relatively small sample sizes, those categories were consolidated into five classes: (1) all metropolitan counties; (2) nonmetropolitan counties adjacent to any metropolitan county and having a city of 10,000 or more; (3) adjacent but with a city of fewer than 10,000; (4) nonadjacent with a city of 10,000 of more; or (5) nonadjacent with no large city. This classification does not represent a pure gradation of relative rurality but does reflect the relative isolation of populations from most tertiary care centers and the presence of general hospitals and more commonly encountered specialties. For some data items, this level of categorization was not possible and certain tables describe only metropolitan and nonmetropolitan comparisons. Throughout, the terms "rural" and "urban" are used interchangeably with metropolitan and nonmetropolitan.

Health Insurance Coverage

Past research has found that insurance coverage differs in metropolitan and nonmetropolitan areas. It has been suggested that residents in rural areas are less likely to have private insurance coverage through their employers because of the industries they work in and the larger share of part-time workers. An examination of the 1996 Medical Expenditure Panel Survey data on health insurance coverage supports these previous findings. Rural residents were less likely to have private health insurance through their employers or unions or through a self-owned business. Only 54% of rural residents had insurance coverage through their employers as compared to 63% for urban residents (Fig. 2.1). Twenty percent (20%) of rural respondents were uninsured, compared to 16% of urban residents.

When health insurance coverage is examined using the modified urban influence categories, not only do the differences between individuals in metropolitan and nonmetropolitan areas remain, but variations across the different types of nonmetropolitan areas emerge (Table 2.1).

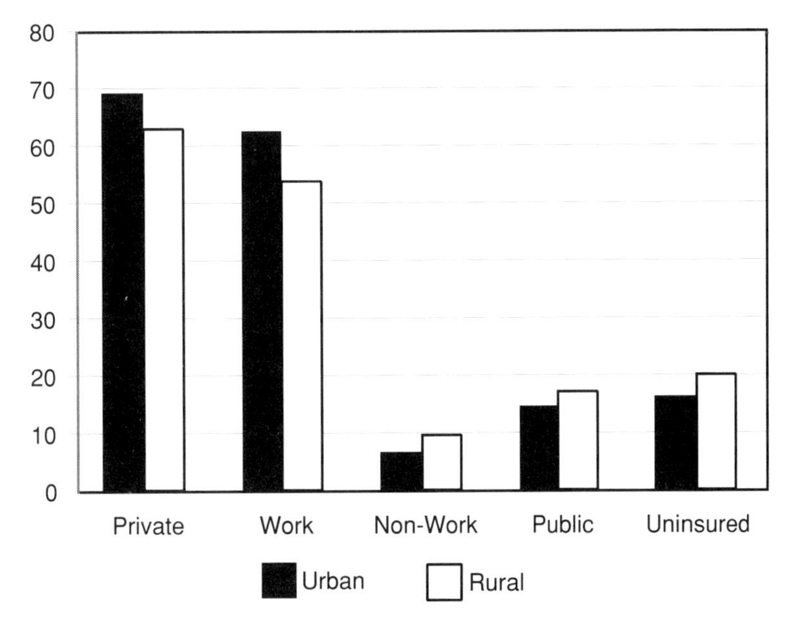

Figure 2.1. Source of Health insurance coverage, rural and urban populations. Source: AHCPR, 1996.

Table 2.1 Health Insurance Coverage of the Civilian Noninstitutionalized Population as Percentages of the Population

	Total Population (in thousands)	Private			Public Only	Uninsured
		Total Private	*Work Related*	*Non-Work Related*		
Total	263516	67.9	60.8	7.1	15.2	17.0
Metro	210687	69.1[ce]	62.5[cde]	6.5[de]	14.7[de]	16.3[c]
Nonmetro	52829	63.1[a]	53.7[a]	9.4[a]	17.1	19.8[a]
Adjacent to Metro Area						
City of 10,000+	15517	69.5[e]	61.2[de]	8.4	14.5[e]	16.0[c]
No City	12996	60.5[a]	52.9[a]	7.6	14.6	24.9[ab]
Not Adjacent to Metro Area						
City of 10,000+	10476	61.6	50.3[ab]	11.2[a]	19.2[a]	19.3
No City	13840	59.4[ab]	48.5[ab]	10.9[a]	20.8[ab]	19.8

[a]Statistically significantly different from metro counties at 0.05 level.
[b]Statistically significantly different from adjacent counties with cities.
[c]Statistically significantly different from adjacent counties without cities.
[d]Statistically significantly different from non-adjacent counties with cities.
[e]Statistically significantly different from non-adjacent counties without cities.
Source: Center for Cost and Financing Studies, Agency for Health Care Policy and Research: Medical Expenditure Panel Survey Household Component, 1996 (Round 1).

Insurance coverage in metropolitan areas and counties that are adjacent to metro areas and have a city of 10,000 or more is similar. People living in these places have more private coverage, more employment-related insurance, and less public coverage than those in the most rural counties. Examining insurance coverage for those under 65 provides further confirmation that differences in insurance coverage between rural and urban areas is related to employer-provided insurance (Table 2.2).

It is clear that insurance coverage of rural and urban residents is considerably different. The pattern is similar to that found above—inhabitants of rural areas, in general, have lower private insurance coverage and higher public insurance coverage than dwellers in more popu-

Table 2.2 Health Insurance Coverage of the Civilian Noninstitutionalized Population Under 65 Years of Age, Percentages of Respondents

	Total Population (in thousands)	Private			Public Only	Uninsured
		Total Private	*Work-Related*	*NonWork-Related*		
Total	231,676	68.7	64.1	4.6	12.1	19.2
Metro	186,200	70.2[cde]	65.9[cde]	4.3[e]	11.5[de]	18.3[ce]
Nonmetro	45,477	62.7[a]	57.0[a]	5.7[a]	14.3	23.0[a]
Adjacent to Metro						
City of 10,000+	13,525	70.0[ce]	66.0[cde]	4.1[e]	11.7	18.3[c]
No City	11,194	60.2[ab]	55.7[ab]	4.4[e]	10.9[de]	28.9[ab]
Not Adjacent to Metro						
City of 10,000+	9,081	60.5[a]	53.2[ab]	7.3[f]	17.3[ac]	22.2
No City	11,677	58.3[ab]	50.6[ab]	7.7[abc]	18.2[ac]	23.5[a]

[a]Statistically significantly different from metro counties at 0.05 level.
[b]Statistically significantly different from adjacent counties with cities.
[c]Statistically significantly different from adjacent counties without cities.
[d]Statistically significantly different from non-adjacent counties with cities.
[e]Statistically significantly different from non-adjacent counties without cities.
[f]Relative standard error is greater than or equal to 30%.
Source: Center for Cost and Financing Studies, Agency for Health Care Policy and Research: Medical Expenditure Panel Survey Household Component, 1996 (Round 1).

lated areas. The rural population of counties that are not adjacent to metropolitan areas and do not have a city have less private insurance coverage than those in metropolitan counties for all demographic variables for which reliable estimates can be made. This pattern is particularly strong for persons aged 18 to 44, who are also more likely to be uninsured in two of the four types of nonmetro areas.

Inability to Obtain Care

Several indicators of access include self-reports of having a usual source of care, of not receiving needed care, and of "delayed care due to cost" (Table 2.3). The 1994 National Health Interview Survey Access to Care supplement included a question on whether there was a time in the past 12 months when an individual needed care but was unable to obtain it. Only 3% of respondents indicated that they had needed care and could not obtain it. This did not vary by type of geographic area. However, there is a small difference in ability to obtain eyeglasses: 2.9% of residents in metro areas reported being unable to get eyeglasses compared to 4% or more of those in rural areas.

Although the data do not suggest that rural residents fail to obtain needed care, they are more likely than their urban counterparts to delay getting care because of financial barriers. Only 8.0% of urban residents reported delaying care due to cost; 11% of residents in rural counties adjacent to metro areas and including a city reported a delay in care, as did 10% of those in counties adjacent to a metro area but without a city of more than 10,000, 12% in counties not adjacent to a metro area but with a city, and 10% of residents in the most rural counties (not adjacent to a metro area and no city of more than 10,000).

Almost two thirds of respondents who indicated that they did not get needed care reported that the reason was that they could not afford it or they did not have insurance (Fig. 2.2). There were no significant differences between metropolitan and nonmetropolitan areas.

Usual Source of Care

The vast majority of persons had a usual source of care (USOC) (Table 2.3). Although there were differences by sociodemographic characteristics in the proportion of persons having a USOC, the distribution of those having a USOC was similar across the rural-urban continuum for those under 65 years of age (Table 2.4). The exception was those living in a county not adjacent to a metro area and including a city of 10,000 or more persons, who were frequently less likely than others to report having a USOC. Of those with a USOC, mroe than 85% saw a particular provider at that site of care.

Table 2.3 Selected Access Variables for Population

	Metro Counties (Percent of residents)	Adjacent to Metro Area		Not Adjacent to Metro Area		Total Nonmetro
		City of 10,000+	*No City*	*City of 10,000+*	*No City*	
Have usual source of care	87.0	88.0	89.1[d]	84.6[c]	88.7	87.7
Had at least one doctor visit in past 12 months	77.1[bcde]	74.6[a]	73.9[a]	72.3[ae]	75.2[ad]	74.2[a]
Mean number of visits	5.6	6.0	5.7	5.5	5.8	5.7
Were hospitalized in past 12 months	7.2[ce]	8.0[e]	9.0[ad]	7.7[ce]	9.8[abd]	8.6[a]
Did not get needed care	2.6	2.4	2.8	2.1	2.6	2.6
Delayed care due to cost	7.9[bcde]	10.5[a]	9.6[a]	12.4[a]	10.4[a] 1	0.4[a]
Did not get needed:						
Dental care	7.6	8.5	9.2	11.1	8.0	9.2[a]
Prescription drugs	2.3	2.3	2.3	3.0	3.0	2.7
Eyeglasses	2.9[bde]	4.0[a]	4.0	4.7[a]	4.2[a]	4.0[a]
Mental health care	0.5[c]	*0.5	0.3[a]	*0.7	0.6	0.5

[a]Statistically significantly different from metro counties at the 0.05 level.
[b]Statistically significantly different from adjacent counties with cities.
[c]Statistically significantly different from adjacent counties without cities.
[d]Statistically significantly different from non-adjacent counties with cities.
[e]Statistically significantly different from non-adjacent counties without cities.
[f]Relative standard error is greater than or equal to 30%.
Source: 1994 National Health Interview Survey, Access to Care Supplement; National Center for Health Statistics.

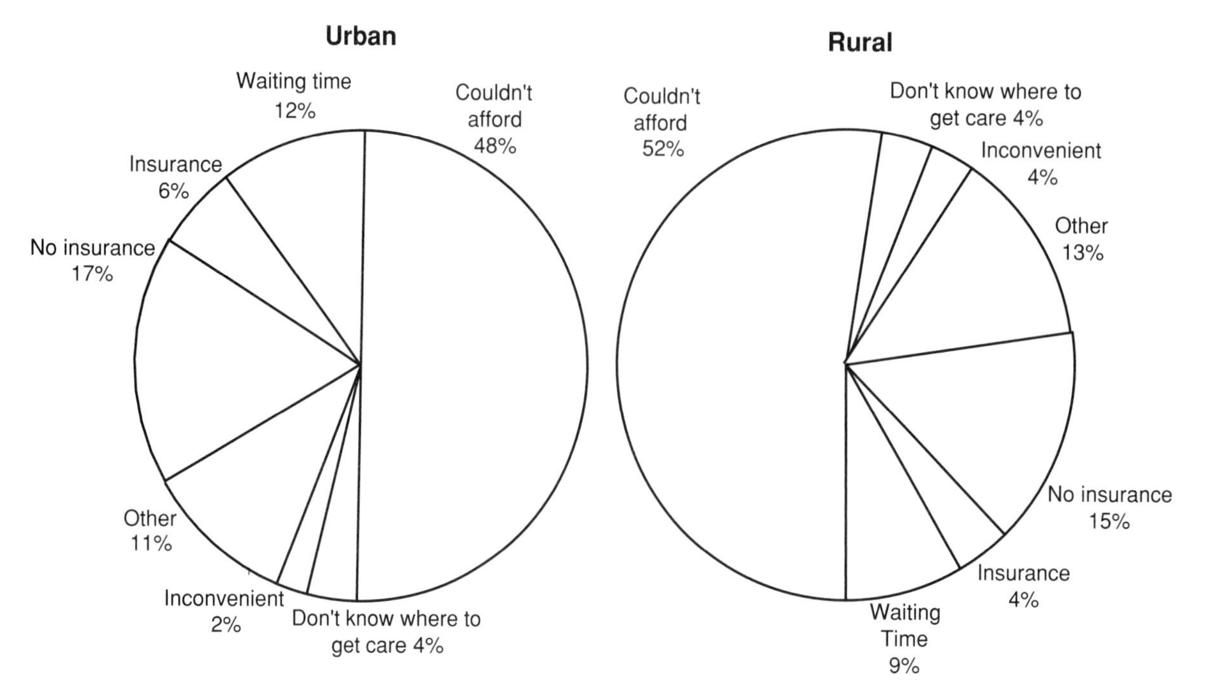

Figure 2.2. Reasons why people were unable to obtain care. Source: NCHS, 1994.

There were few significant differences across the rural-urban continuum for USOC for those over age 65. For almost all categories, over 90% of the elderly report a USOC regardless of place of residence; this reflects the importance of Medicare as a guarantor of access for rural elders as well as a greater need for physician visits among the elderly.

For those who have a USOC, the site at which residents of metro and nonmetro counties seek care differs somewhat (Table 2.5). Persons living in metro counties were more likely than those residing in nonmetro counties to obtain care in a community, school, or county clinic or from an HMO or prepaid group. For those who received care in the past year but did not have a usual source of care, doctors' offices remained the most common site of care for both metro and nonmetro residents, though the latter group were more likely to obtain care at this site. Nonmetro residents were again less likely to receive care in a community clinic or HMO than those in metro areas.

The reasons given for not having a usual source of care differed somewhat between urban and rural areas. More than half of both urban and rural respondents indicated that the main reason they did not have a primary source of care was because they did not need one. Urban residents, however, were more likely than rural residents to cite cost or lack of insurance as the reason for not having a USOC (23% vs. 14%). Rural residents were more likely to cite the provider having moved (14%) as the reason they did not have a USOC (compared to urban: 8%).

For the 8% who had changed their health care provider in the past year, reasons for the change differed significantly between rural and urban residents (Fig. 2.3). Rural residents were more likely than urban residents to state that moving or changing jobs was the reason they changed providers (46% vs. 34%). Rural residents more often indicated that they changed providers because their previous provider moved out of the area (10% compared with 4% for urban residents). On the other hand, employer-related insurance changes were more commonly cited by urban residents than rural respondents (16% vs. 3%).

As previous research has found, travel times to doctors' offices are longer for rural residents than for their urban counterparts (Fig. 2.4). The average travel time for metropolitan residents was 17 minutes, compared with 19 minutes for nonmetropolitan residents (median time 15 minutes for both groups). Although a greater percentage of urban residents reported traveling more than one hour to their usual source of care (2% vs. 1% for rural residents), more rural residents traveled between 30 and 60 minutes to obtain care (17% vs. 14% for urban residents).

Office waiting times to see the doctor were similar for urban respondents (mean 27 minutes; median 15 minutes) and rural respondents (mean 27 minutes; median 20 minutes). The distribution of waiting times was also

Table 2.4 Percent of People Younger than 65 Years of Age Having a Usual Source of Care, by Demographic Variables

		Adjacent to Metro Area		*Not Adjacent to Metro Area*		
	Metro Counties	*City of 10,000+*	*No City*	*City of 10,000+*	*No City*	*Total Nonmetro*
Total[f]	86.0	87.1	86.8	83.0[e]	88.2[d]	86.6
AGE IN YEARS						
under 18	93.3	93.7	91.4	93.0	95.3	93.0
18–44	80.1[d]	81.7[d]	82.7[d]	73.8[abce]	82.8[d]	80.9
45–64	88.7	89.6	87.9	87.9	88.8	89.0
EMPLOYMENT STATUS[g]						
Employed	82.8[d]	84.0[d]	84.7[d]	76.3[abce]	85.7[d]	83.8
Not Employed	71.7[bc]	82.9[ad]	82.0[ad]	60.2[bc]	65.9	71.6
SEX						
Male	82.6[e]	82.7	82.8	78.5[e]	86.3[ad]	83.2
Female	89.4	91.4	90.7	87.6	90.0	89.9
RACE/ETHNICITY						
Total Hispanic	77.4	72.8	73.8	66.0	75.8	71.9
Total black	87.4[ce]	81.2[ce]	93.3[ab]	83.8	93.5[ab]	90.1
Total white	87.7	88.1	86.6	83.7	87.2	86.9
CENSUS REGION						
Northeast	89.8[b]	86.7[a]	86.2	87.6	89.1	89.1
Midwest	88.2	90.7	89.7	85.1	88.8	90.0
South	83.1[e]	82.7[e]	85.8	85.2	89.4[ab]	85.5
West	84.1[cd]	88.3	78.9[a]	75.8[a]	84.0	81.3
HEALTH STATUS						
Excellent/very good/good	85.8	86.8	86.6[e]	82.2	87.8[c]	86.2
Fair/poor	87.8	91.3	88.7	91.9	90.8	89.9
INCOME						
Under $10,000	79.1	76.7	81.3	76.1	79.5	78.1
$10,000–34,999	81.3[be]	86.9[a]	84.9	81.5	88.0[a]	85.2[a]
$35,000–49,999	89.4[b]	93.6[ad]	92.0	85.5[b]	91.3	91.3[a]
$50,000 or more	92.6[e]	91.6	90.3[e]	92.3	95.9[ac]	92.2

[a]Statistically significantly different from metro counties at the 0.05 level.
[b]Statistically significantly different from adjacent counties with cities.
[c]Statistically significantly different from adjacent counties without cities.
[d]Statistically significantly different from non-adjacent counties with cities.
[e]Statistically significantly different from non-adjacent counties without cities.
[f]Excludes person younger than 18 years of age.
[g]Persons with unknown responses to any characteristics below were excluded.
Source: 1994 National Health Interview Survey, Access to Care Supplement; National Center for Health Statistics

similar, with over half of both urban and rural residents waiting less than 30 minutes to see their health care provider.

On average, rural residents (mean 3 days; median 1 day) had to wait fewer days for an appointment with their physician than urban residents (mean 6 days; median 1 day). Although 14% of both metropolitan and nonmetropolitan residents waited less than a day for an appointment, 14% of metropolitan residents, as compared with 8% of nonmetropolitan residents, waited more than a week for an appointment (Fig. 2.5).

Use of Services

There are several indicators of health care services utilization including doctor visits and hospitalization. Approximately three quarters of the population had at least one doctor's visit in the past 12 months (Table 2.3). Although the proportion with at least one visit is lower for residents of all types of nonmetropolitan counties compared with residents of metropolitan counties, the difference is small. And for persons with at least one visit in the past year, the average number of visits is uniform

Table 2.5 Site of Care (percent of respondents)

	No Usual Source of Care but had care in last year[c]		*Have Usual Source of Care*[b]	
	Metro Counties	*Nonmetro Counties*	*Metro Counties*	*Nonmetro Counties*
Doctor's office	59.1	64.6	80.7	88.8
Community clinic[c,d]	16.9	11.1	6.3	4.9
Hospital outpatient clinic[e]	5.2	3.7	2.4	1.6
Hospital ER	9.6	11.1	0.8	0.8
HMO/prepaid group[a]	2.6	1.1	7.3	1.2
Military/VA	2.0	4.9	1.7	1.9
Other	4.5	3.6	0.8	0.9

[a]The distribution of responses was statistically significantly different; chi-square 21.94, p-value 0.003.
[b]The distribution of responses was statistically significantly different; chi-square 212.33, p-value 0.000.
[c]Includes school and county clinics.
[d]Metro and nonmetro were statistically significant different at the 0.05 level.
[e]For private hospitals.
Source: 1994 National Health Interview Survey, Access to Care Supplement; National Center for Health Statistics.

across place of residence (approximately six visits). Thus, although rural residents report higher levels of chronic conditions, they do not visit the doctor more frequently than urban residents.

Residents in nonmetropolitan counties without a city of 10,000 or greater were more likely to have been hospitalized in the past year (9% for rural counties adjacent to metropolitan areas; 10% for rural areas not adjacent to metropolitan counties). This higher rate may reflect any number of factors, including higher accident rates, underlying characteristics such as age or health status, or inadequate ambulatory care.

The mean numbers of physician visits in the past year reported by urban and rural residents were compared according to selected demographic groupings. For those under age 65, few statistically significant differences were found although the general trend was for rural people to report fewer doctors' visits. Where significant differences exist across the rural-urban continuum, it was often those living in counties not adjacent to metro areas and with a city of 10,000 or more who have fewer visits than those in metro areas. In particular, those who were employed, Hispanic, residing in the Midwest or West, or persons in the middle income range

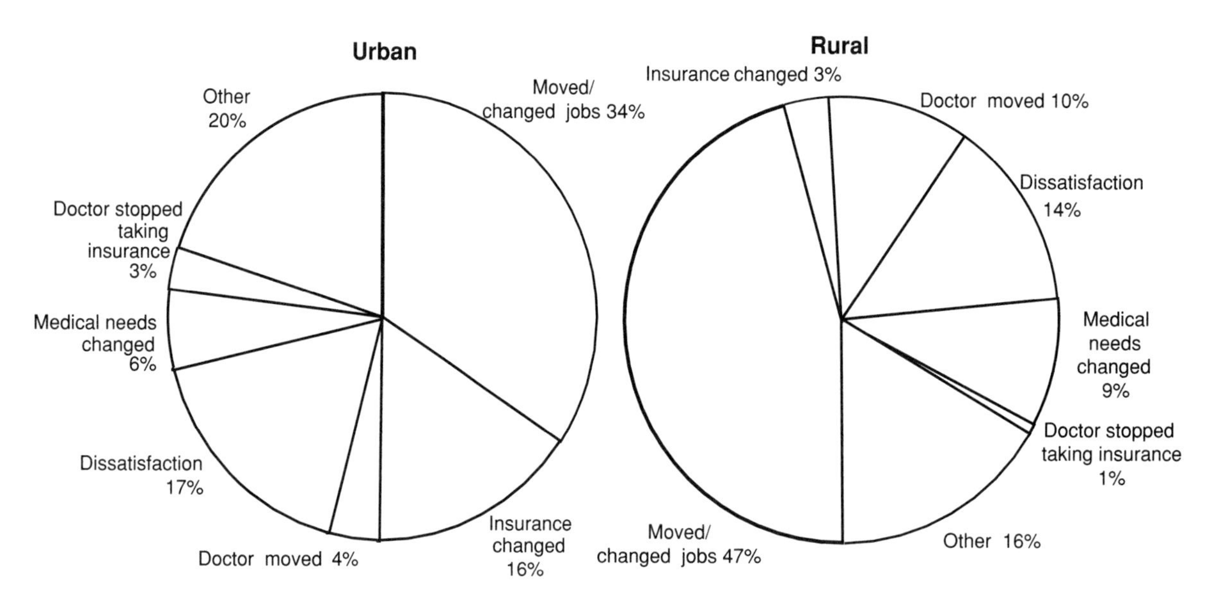

Figure 2.3. Reasons why people changed provider. Source: NCHS, 1994.

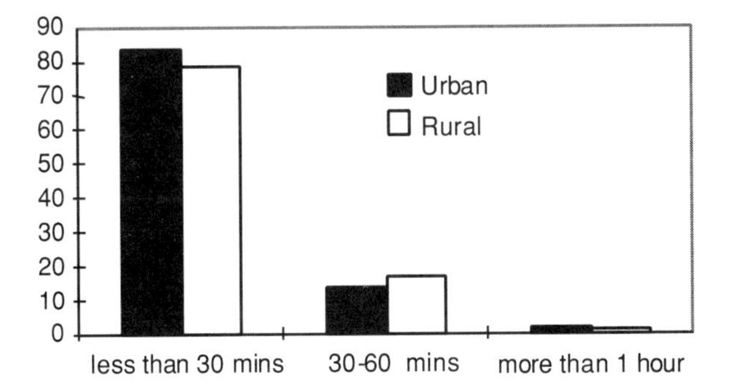

Figure 2.4. Travel time to usual source of care. Source: NCHS, 1994.

($35,000–49,999) had fewer visits than their counterparts in metropolitan areas.

The elderly have more visits, on average, than the nonelderly, but the patterns for both populations appear similar. Among those residing in nonmetro counties, people in counties not adjacent to metro areas and with cities of 10,000 or more most often were different from those living in metro counties. Of the former group, males, those in the Northeast and the West, and those in good health had fewer visits than those in urban counties.

As mentioned earlier, examining the use of physician visits by those in fair or poor health is used as an access indicator in order to control for differences in health care need. Approximately 10% of those in fair or poor health did not have any physician visits in the last year (Table 2.6). These persons may have critical access problems, but there were no statistically significant differences between urban and rural areas.

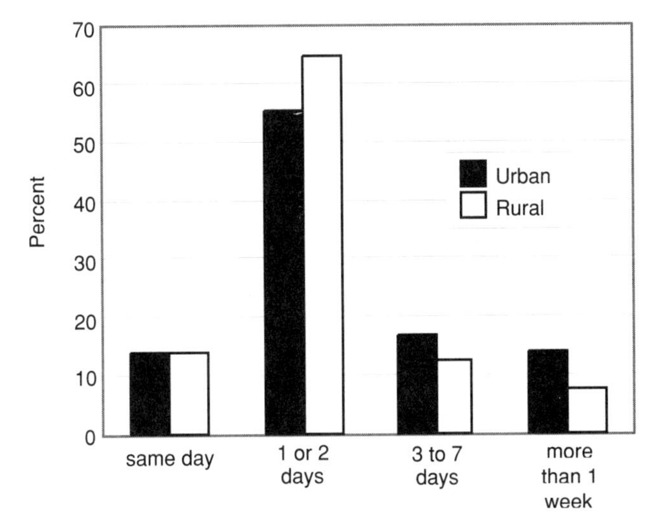

Figure 2.5. Wait time for an appointment. Source RWJF, 1994.

Use of Specialist versus Primary Care Physicians

Past research has found that rural areas have fewer specialist physicians and, consequently, one would expect that rural residents have less access to specialists. Data from the 1996 National Ambulatory Medical Care Survey (NAMCS) are used to show the distribution of visits to specialist versus non-specialist physicians in rural and urban areas. Because NAMCS is a survey of physicians about their patient visits, statistics reported here are based on physician practice location rather than patient place of residence.

Almost three quarters (72%) of total visits to physicians in nonmetropolitan counties were to primary care physicians (general internal medicine, family practice, general practice, and general pediatrics) compared with 63% of visits to physicians in metropolitan counties (Fig. 2.6). The remaining visits were to physicians specializing in cardiology, dermatology, ophthalmology, otolaryngology, urology, neurology, and other specialties. Given research indicating that rural residents are more likely to suffer from chronic diseases, the lower proportion of specialist visits may present a particular area of concern in terms of access to care. It should be noted that those rural residents who travel to urban areas to obtain specialty care are included in the count of metropolitan physician visits. The data, therefore, are limited in their utility in assessing the problem of access to specialists in rural areas. When visits to all specialty types are examined, the difference between rural and urban visits remains (Fig. 2.7). Not only are specialist visits fewer in rural areas, but visits to obstetricians and gynecologists (9% for urban areas compared to 3% for rural areas) and psychiatrists (5% in urban areas versus 1% in rural areas) are also fewer.

Satisfaction

Data from the Medical Expenditure Panel Survey (MEPS) are presented in order to provide information on satisfaction with medical care. More than three quarters of respondents reported being 'very satisfied' with the quality of care they receive. Satisfaction levels did not differ between metropolitan and nonmetropolitan areas. Less than 3% of respondents reported being "not too satisfied" or "not at all satisfied" with their care.

This high level of satisfaction with care is further supported by respondents' confidence in the ability of their provider. More than 95% of respondents indicated they are confident in their provider's ability to care for them.

Table 2.6 Percent of Respondents in Fair or Poor Health Status with No Physician Visits in Past 12 Months

	Adjacent to Metro Area		*Not Adjacent to Metro Area*		
Metro Counties	*City of 10,000+*	*No City*	*City of 10,000+*	*No City*	*Total Nonmetro*
10.2%	10.1%	10.6%	10.8%	12.5%	10.9%

Source: 1994 National Health Interview Survey, Access to Care Supplement; National Center for Health Statistics.

Ninety-seven percent (97%) of both urban and rural residents believed that their providers listened to their concerns.

Urban residents were slightly less satisfied with the staff at their usual source of care than their rural counterparts. Although the differences were statistically significant, they are small. More than 70% of respondents in both urban (73%) and rural (77%) areas were very satisfied with their provider's staff. More urban respondents (3%) reported being "not too satisfied" with the staff, compared to rural respondents (2%).

Slightly less than three quarters of respondents, overall, were "very satisfied" that their families could get the medical care they need (urban 75%; rural 73%). When "very satisfied" and "somewhat satisfied" were combined, the satisfaction level increased to more than 90% for both urban (93%) and rural (93%) residents, indicating a very high overall level of satisfaction.

Health Beliefs

Individual beliefs about the effectiveness of health care and feelings of trust toward medical professionals may affect use of (and therefore observed access to) health care services. Information from the Robert Wood Johnson Foundation 1994 National Access to Care Survey looked at three specific health beliefs: ability to recover from illness without medical care, effectiveness of home remedies compared with prescription drugs, and whether physicians recommend surgery only when there are no other options.

There were no differences between urban and rural residents in terms of these health beliefs. Metropolitan residents (62%) and nonmetropolitan residents (59%) had similar responses to the statement, "If you wait long enough, you can get over most any illness without medical care," with the majority disagreeing. Slightly more than

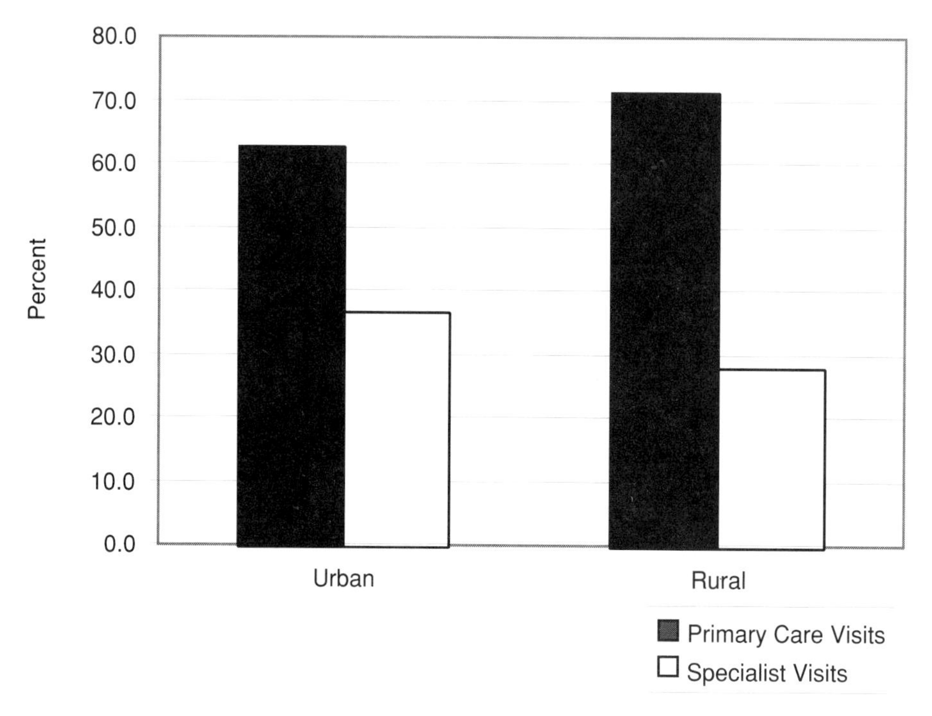

Figure 2.6. Specialist versus primary care visits. Source: NCHS, 1996.

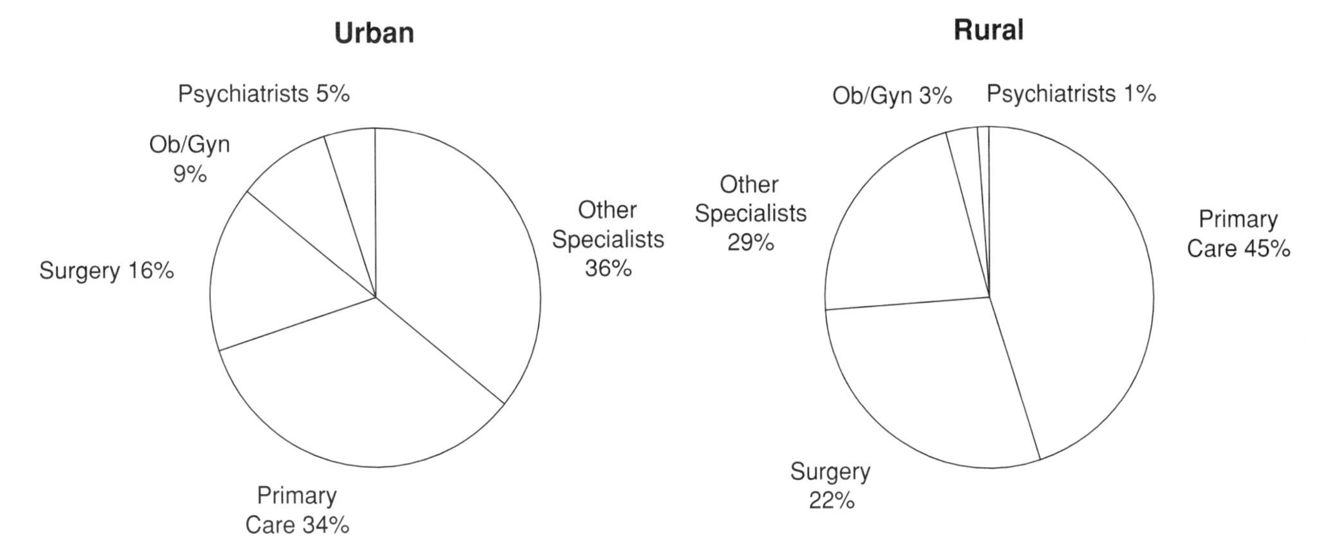

Figure 2.7. Ambulatory care visits to specialists. Source: NCHS, 1996.

half (53%) of urban and rural respondents agreed that home cures were sometimes better than prescribed medicines, and rural and urban respondents were equally split on whether doctors recommend surgery as a last resort, with 46% of respondents disagreeing and 48% agreeing.

Attitudes Toward Change in the Delivery System

The Robert Wood Johnson Foundation Access to Care Survey also included questions about changes in the health care system that respondents would be willing to accept if it meant they would pay significantly less for their health care. Almost 70% of respondents indicated that they would mind if they had to obtain a referral from their regular doctor to see a specialist, with about 35% saying they would mind a lot and 35% minding a little. The overwhelming opposition to a gatekeeper system did not differ between metropolitan and nonmetropolitan areas. Over 70% also reported that they would mind selecting a doctor from a list provided by the insurance carrier. Residents of metropolitan areas differed somewhat from those living in nonmetropolitan areas in their attitude toward choosing a doctor from a list: 72% of urban respondents would object to this restriction on choice, whereas 78% of rural residents were opposed to such a limitation. This stronger opposition among rural residents to restricted choice may reflect the fact that those in rural areas initially have fewer providers from which to choose; thus, choosing a doctor from a list might require them to travel farther to obtain medical care. This might also reflect stronger physician-patient relationships in rural areas and/or less managed care penetration and therefore less familiarity with (and less acceptance of) this concept.

Two thirds of respondents would mind if they occasionally had to see a nurse instead of a physician, and the responses of urban and rural residents were similar, with 39% of urban and 38% of rural residents minding a lot if this change in medical care delivery were imposed.

Paid Sick Leave

Previous research suggested that although insurance levels may be similar between rural and urban areas, rural residents are more likely to be underinsured than their urban counterparts (Hartley, Quam, and Lurie, 1994). Insured rural residents may have fewer benefits and higher coinsurance and deductibles. This underinsurance is due in part to the size (small) and nature of the industries in which rural residents work. Employees in rural firms are also less likely to have other benefits like extended sick leave or time off for doctor visits.

The Robert Wood Johnson Foundation 1994 Access to Care Survey asked employed participants about paid sick leave and time off to visit the doctor. It is important to note that the survey does not distinguish between respondents employed full-time and those employed part-time, which may be an important component in provided benefits. Employed persons in metropolitan areas were no more likely to have paid sick leave than their nonmetropolitan counterparts (65% compared with 60%).

In contrast, rural residents were less likely to have paid leave to visit their doctors. Fifty percent (50%) of urban residents have paid leave but only 43% of rural residents do. Rural residents, therefore, may have greater difficulty in affording the time off from work to obtain preventive care.

CONCLUSION

This chapter has used a number of national data sets to explore access to care in rural areas of the United States. Using many of the traditional access indicators from two nationally representative sample surveys provides evidence that people living in rural communities face many serious barriers to obtaining health care services. One in five rural residents has no health insurance to assist in paying for health care. In some types of rural communities (those adjacent to metro areas with no city of 10,000 persons or more), almost 30% of the population under 65 years of age is without such coverage. In these same types of communities, as well as in the most rural areas—those not adjacent to a metropolitan area and with no city as large as 10,000 persons—one third of those aged 18 to 44 years are uninsured.

Approximately one quarter of rural residents did not have a physician visit in the past year. Of greater concern, between 10% and 13% of rural residents (depending on the type of community) who reported being in fair or poor health had not seen a physician in the previous 12-month period. Approximately 3% of persons reported being unable to obtain medical care they thought they needed. In rural areas not adjacent to a metropolitan area and with a city of 10,000 or more persons, 5% were unable to obtain eyeglasses and 11% were unable to obtain dental care. Approximately two thirds of those who said they were unable to obtain needed care said it was because they could not afford the care or had no insurance.

Although many of the barriers to care faced by rural residents are similar to those experienced in more urbanized areas, the nature of rural and urban access problems differ along many dimensions. In terms of insurance coverage, rural residents are less likely to have employment-related private insurance than persons living in urban areas. Although the level of benefits provided could not be explored, those who have individual rather than employment-related insurance policies generally have less comprehensive benefits and less generous coverage. Between 10% and 12% of the population in different types of rural areas reported that they delayed care due to cost, compared to 8% in metropolitan counties. Those living in metropolitan areas were more likely than those outside of metro areas to have at least one physician visit annually, though the mean number of visits for those with at least one visit was similar across the different types of communities. Differences also were found with respect to visits to specialists (lower in rural areas), likelihood of hospitalization (higher in rural areas), the proportion with paid sick leave from work for doctor visit (lower in rural areas), and the reasons for not having a usual source of care (rural residents are more likely to cite the provider having moved). Travel times to usual providers were also somewhat longer for rural residents.

These data paint a picture of overall levels of reduced access to health care for rural populations. These general indicators may obscure specific areas or subpopulations that are seriously affected and whose health suffers. A large number of nonmetro areas are critical health professional shortage areas (HPSAs). In 1997, 20,689,000 nonmetropolitan residents (approximately 40%) lived in 1,742 primary care HPSAs designated by the federal government (Bureau of Primary Health Care, 1998) versus only about 12% of the nonmetropolitan population. In addition, almost 75% of U.S. nonmetro counties are designated as whole- or part-county Medically Underserved Areas (MUAs). These issues are discussed in greater detail in various chapters throughout this volume.

These indices of underservice are used to direct capacity building resources to communities but also reflect the very great gaps in resource distribution in health services and health status. Efforts to enhance access to care must recognize that rural places face substantially different conditions that clearly affect their ability to use services and that reflect cultural, social, and economic factors that make it more or less possible for people to use services effectively.

REFERENCES

Aday, LA. 1993. At Risk in America. San Francisco: Jossey-Bass.
Aday LA, Begley CE, Lairson DR, Slater CH. 1998. Evaluating the Healthcare System: Effectiveness, Efficiency and Equity. Chicago, Ill: AHSR/Health Administration Press.
Aday LA, Andersen R, Fleming GV. 1980. Health Care in the US: Equitable for Whom? Beverly Hills, Calif: Sage Publications.
Aday LA, Fleming GV, Andersen R. 1984. Access to Medicare Care in the US: Who has it, Who Doesn't. Chicago, Ill: Pluribus Press.
American College of Physicians. 1995. Rural primary care. Annals of Internal Medicine 122: 380–390.
Berk ML, Schur CL, Cantor JC. 1995. Ability to obtain health care: recent estimates from the Robert Wood Johnson Foundation National Access to Care Survey. Health Affairs 14: 139–146.
Birdwell SW, Calesaric H. 1996. Identifying health care needs of rural Ohio citizens: an evaluation of a two-stage methodology. Journal of Rural Health 12: 130–136.
Braden JJ, Beauregard K. 1994. Health status and access to care of rural and urban populations. National Medical Expenditure Survey

Research Findings 18, Agency for Health Care Policy and Research. Rockville, MD: Public Health Services.
Cafferata GL. 1983. Private health insurance: premium expenditures and sources of payment. National Health Care Expenditures Data Preview 17. National Center for Health Services Research. Rockville, MD: Public Health Service.
Comer J, Mueller K. 1995. Access to health care: urban-rural comparisons from a midwestern agricultural state. Journal of Rural Health 11: 128–136.
Cornelius L, Beauregard K, Cohen J. 1991. Usual sources of medical care and their characteristics. National Medical Expenditure Survey Research Findings 11, Agency for Health Care Policy and Research. Rockville, MD: Public Health Services.
Cunningham PJ, Cornelius LJ. 1995. Access to ambulatory care for American Indians and Alaska Natives: the relative importance of personal and community resources. Social Science and Medicine 40: 393–407.
Dor A, Holahan J. 1990. Urban-rural differences in medicare physician expenditures. Inquiry 27: 307–318.
Edelman MA, Menz BL. 1996. Selected comparisons and implications of a national rural and urban survey on health care access, demographics, and policy issues. Journal of Rural Health 12: 197–205.
Estrada A, Trevino FM, Ray L. 1990. Health care utilization barriers among Mexican Americans: evidence from HHANES 1982–84. American Journal of Public Health 80(suppl): 27–31.
Freeman HE, Blendon RJ, Aiken LH, Sudman S, Mullinix CF, Corey CR. 1987. Americans report on their access to health care. Health Affairs 6: 6–18.
Frenzen PD. 1991. The increasing supply of physicians in US urban and rural areas, 1975 to 1988. American Journal of Public Health 81: 1141–1147.
Frenzen PD. 1993. Health insurance coverage in U.S. urban and rural areas. Journal of Rural Health 9(3): 204–214.
Ghelfi LM, Parker TS. 1997. A County-Level Measure of Urban Influence. Washington, DC: Economic Research Service, Rural Economy Division.
Hartley D, Quam L, Lurie N. 1994. Urban and rural differences in health insurance and access to care. Journal of Rural Health 10: 98–108.
Hayward RA, Beynard AM, Freeman HE, Corey CR. 1991. Regular source of ambulatory care and access to health services. American Journal of Public Health 81: 434–438.
Hewitt M. 1989. Defining "Rural" Areas: Impact on Health Care Policy and Research. Washington, DC: Office of Technology Assessment.
Hicks LL. 1990. Availability and accessibility of rural health care. Journal of Rural Health 6: 485–505.
Institute of Medicine. 1993. Access to Health Care in America. Washington, DC: National Academy Press.
Kasper JA, Walden DC, Wilensky GR. 1978. Who are the uninsured? National Health Care Expenditures Study Data Preview 1. National Center for Health Services Research. Hyattsville, MD: Public Health Service.
Kindig DA, Movassaghi H. 1989. The adequacy of physician supply in small rural counties. Health Affairs 8(2): 63–76.
Mueller KJ, Patil K, Boilsesen E. 1997. The Role of Uninsurance and Race in Health Care Utilization by Rural Minorities. Omaha, NE: University of Nebraska Medical Center, Department of Preventive and Societal Medicine.
Mueller KJ, Patil K, Ulrich F. 1997. Lengthening spells of uninsurance and their consequences. Journal of Rural Health 13(4): 29–37.
Patton L. 1989. Setting the Rural Health Services research agenda: the congressional perspective. Health Services Research 23: 1005–1051.
Ricketts TC. 1997. Access and ambulatory care sensitive conditions. Journal of Rural Health 13(4): 275–276.
Ricketts TC, Johnson-Webb KD. 1997. What is "rural" and how to measure "rurality": a focus on health care delivery and health policy. Working Paper of the Rural Health Research Center, University of North Carolina at Chapel Hill.
Rowland D, Lyons B. 1989. Triple jeopardy: rural, poor, and uninsured. Health Services Research 23(6): 975–1004.
Schreiber S, Zielinski T. 1997. The meaning of ambulatory care sensitive admissions: urban and rural perspective. Journal of Rural Health 13(4): 276–284.
Seccombe K. 1995. Health insurance coverage and use of services among low-income elders: does residence influence the relationship? Journal of Rural Health 11: 86–97.
Silver MP, Babitz ME, Magill MK. 1997. Ambulatory care sensitive hospitalization rates in the aged medicare population in Utah, 1990 to 1994: a rural-urban comparison. Journal of Rural Health 13(4): 285–294.
Spillman BC. 1992. The impact of being uninsured on utilization of basic health care services. Inquiry 29: 457–466.
Weinick RM, Zuvekas SH, Drilea SK. 1997. Access to health care—sources and barriers, 1996. Medical Expenditure Panel Survey Research Findings 3, Agency for Health Care and Research. Rockville, MD: Public Health Services.
Weissman JS, Epstein AM. 1994. Falling through the Safety Net: Insurance Status and Access to Health Care. Baltimore, MD: The Johns Hopkins University Press.

3

Physicians and Rural America

ROGER A. ROSENBLATT AND L. GARY HART

RURAL PROVIDER SHORTAGES IN RURAL AMERICA

Large numbers of rural Americans have limited access to health care. This problem stems from two defining and interrelated characteristics of the health care system: the large number of Americans without health care insurance and the tendency of health care professionals to locate and practice in relatively affluent urban and suburban areas. Although the problem of health insurance exists in both urban and rural areas, the problem of an inadequate number of health professionals is concentrated in rural areas.

The relative shortage of health professionals in rural areas of the United States is one of the few constants in any description of the U.S. medical care system. About 20% of the U.S. population—over 50 million people—live in rural areas, but only 9% of the nation's physicians practice in rural communities (Bureau of Health Professions, 1992). Severe rural physician shortages were the primary stimulus behind the development of many of the federal health care workforce programs described in Chapter 5, Federal Programs and Rural Health, and the persistence of the rural-urban disparity continues to prompt federal and state educational and service efforts designed to address the residual inequities.

Historically, perceptions of physician shortages date back to the late eighteenth century (Council on Graduate Medical Education [COGME], 1992). The first national effort to remedy these shortages was the rapid increase in the number and size of medical schools in the United States starting in the late 1960s. As a result, the absolute number of physicians in rural areas has increased, as has the physician-to-population ratio, although the relative differences between rural and urban areas has changed little.

It is critical to make a distinction between the adequacy of health professional supply in rural areas and the disparity between the supply in rural and urban areas. Crude comparisons of the physician-to-population ratio in rural versus urban areas can be extremely misleading and provide almost no information about whether shortages or surpluses exist in either location (Center for the Evaluative Clinical Sciences, 1996). In 1996—the latest year for which data are available—gaps existed between the supply of active physicians in counties of different size (Fig. 3.1). As can be seen in this figure, major differences persist between the aggregate supply in urban and rural areas, with the larger counties having many more physicians per 100,000 population.

But this information obscures the fact that the physician supply has grown in rural areas over the past 20 years, although the growth has not been uniform. The supply of rural physicians has increased modestly in the past few decades, with most of the increase in the larger rural communities adjacent to metropolitan areas (Fig. 3.2).

Rural supply lags far behind the current urban supply of physicians, but the urban supply of physicians is, in the opinion of many experts, excessive. It is likely that some of the larger rural areas are now approaching optimal physician-to-population ratios, both as a result of the expansion of the overall physician supply and because of the educational interventions that have increased the number of physicians with the willingness and ability to practice in rural areas.

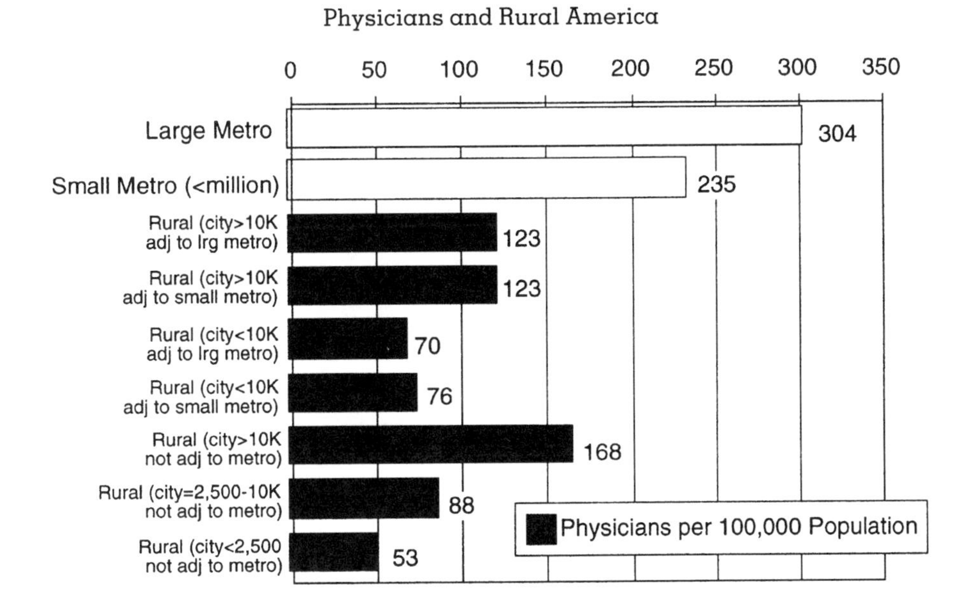

Figure 3.1. Active physicians per 100,000 population by location, 1996. Source: AMA data from BHPr, 1998.

Physician supply in rural areas is closely tied to the specialty mix of American physicians. Specialty has a powerful impact on physician location choice for each of the major specialty groups (Fig. 3.3). Family physicians distribute themselves in proportion to the population in both rural and urban locations and are the largest single source of physicians in rural areas. All other specialties are much more likely to settle in urban areas, even the other generalist disciplines.

Given the expansion of the rural physician supply, it is important to distinguish between rural areas that have definite shortages of critical health professionals and those that have fewer health professionals relative to oversupplied urban areas. Historically, the government has designated areas as seriously underserved based on the physician-to-population ratio within a specific health service area. Populations with too few physicians have been categorized as health professional shortage ar-

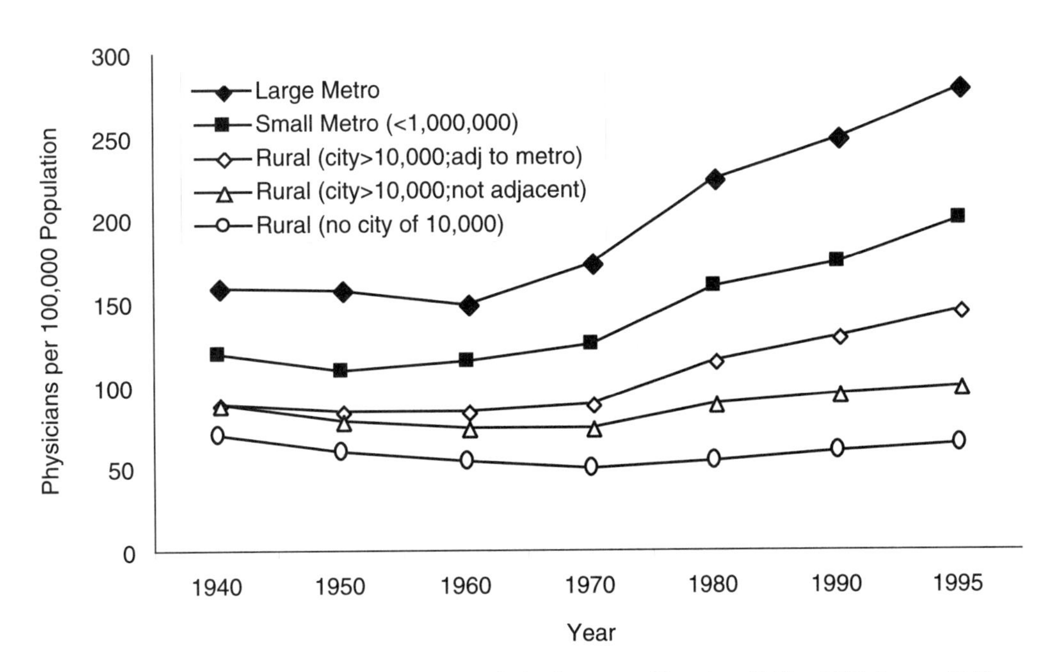

Figure 3.2. Active physicians per 100,000 population by year and location, 1940 to 1995. Source: AMA data from BHPr, 1997.

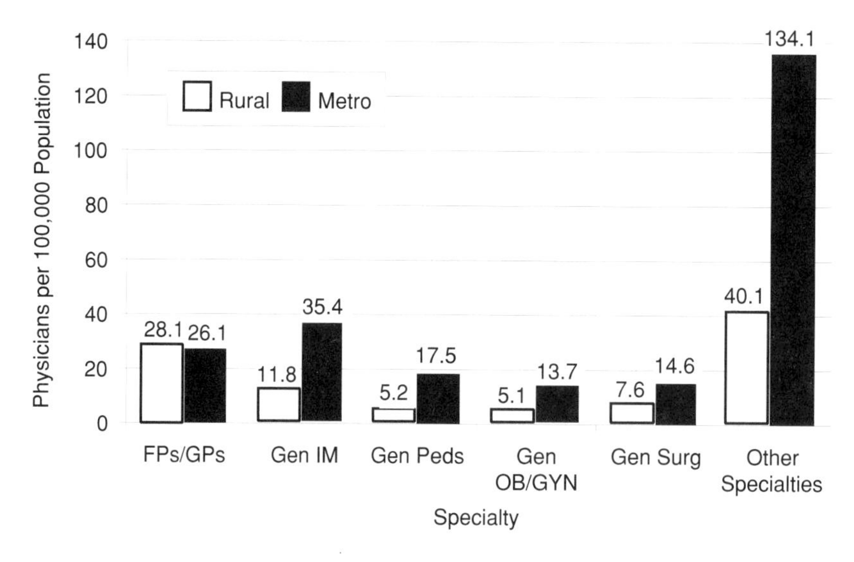

Figure 3.3. Patient care physicians per 100,000 population by location and specialty, 1995. Source: AMA data from BHPr, 1997.

eas (HPSAs), thus becoming eligible for a broad array of governmental assistance (Plate 3.1). In order to remove the designation, a number of physicians would have to be deployed into rural health profession shortage areas (Fig. 3.4).

As the figure shows, the number of rural HPSAs and the number of primary care physicians needed to remedy the designated shortages have increased in recent years. The process of designating HPSAs has long been a contentious process and the General Accounting Office, in 1995, issued a report that suggested that the current method of designating underserved areas was neither precise nor accurate (GAO, 1995). The Health Resources and Services Administration and the Bureau of Primary Health Care responded to that criticism and a prior call from a congressional committee by issuing proposed regulations to combine the HPSA designation process with the Medically Underserved Area process and use a new system of Medically Underserved Populations (MUPs) as the basis for identifying areas with health professional shortages (Federal Register, 1998). The original measure of shortage, called the Health Manpower Shortage Areas, relied strictly on physician-to-population ratios, but currently states can request

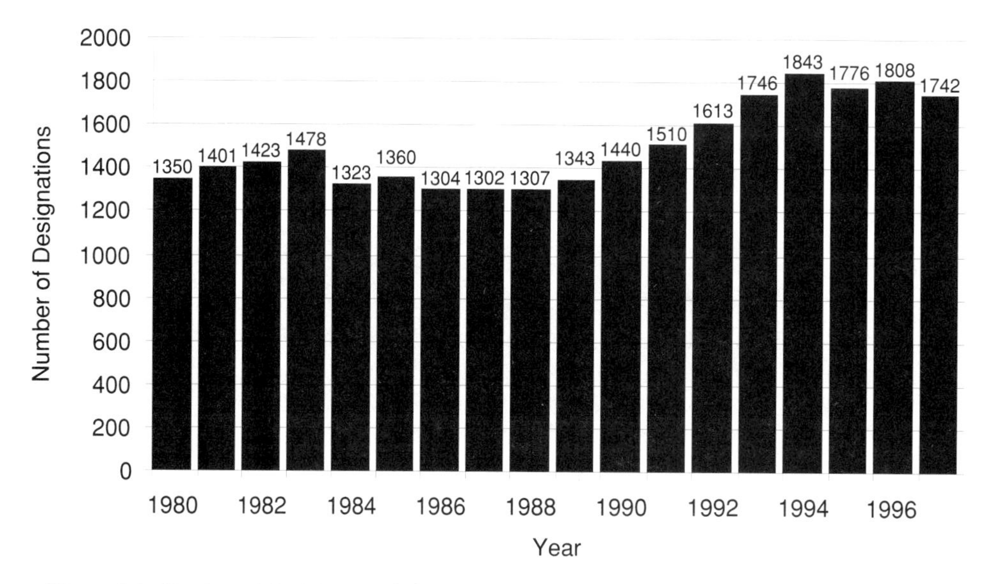

Figure 3.4. Number of physicians needed to remove current HPSA designation. Source: BPHC, 1997.

designation for specific populations or institutions even if they exist in a area with an adequate number of physicians; that state-by-state flexibility will remain in the proposed regulation. The increase in the number of rural HPSAs may have been a function of an increase in the rate at which designations have been requested—possibly because of declining rates of health insurance rather than because of a deterioration in physician supply in rural areas. The revitalization of the National Health Services Corps (NHSC) and the Medicare bonus payment program that give rural organizations and communities an incentive to apply for designation, may also have influenced the number of designations more than changes in the relative supply of health professionals.

The Effect of Specialty Choice and Distribution

Nothing affects the location decision of physicians more than specialty. The more highly specialized the physician, the less likely he or she will settle in a rural area. As a consequence, the growth of specialization is a major contributor to the geographic maldistribution of physicians. Many of the shortages in communities with fewer than 10,000 residents could have been reduced or eliminated if even a small fraction of subspecialists produced over the past 15 years had chosen to become primary care physicians in rural or underserved areas (Konrad, 1997).

The decision of specialists to settle in cities is neither random nor capricious: specialists require a large population base, sophisticated hospitals and laboratories, and specialty colleagues to be able to pursue their expertise. The average family physician may serve 2,000 people; the typical neurosurgeon requires a population base of 100,000 people to achieve professional and economic equilibrium. When specialists are in oversupply, they can reduce the amount of time they work, practice outside the traditional domain of their specialty, or generate demand by increasing the rate at which they perform investigations or procedures. Only at the margin will they migrate to smaller places, and there is a population threshold below which it is not feasible for them to continue to pursue the specialty in which they trained.

In addition to the technical requirements of the specialty, there are also important behavioral and philosophical differences that cause specialty imbalances to be translated into geographic maldistribution. Family physicians—the quintessential generalists—are the only specialty group as likely to locate in a small rural as in a large urban area (Bureau of Health Professions, 1992). Part of the reason is that their practice breadth permits flexibility. In addition, family medicine has always had strong roots in rural practice and many of the educational programs in this new discipline reinforce those roots. Some specialists have migrated to rural areas, but rural medicine remains highly dependent on the supply of family practitioners.

The recent revived interest in family medicine and the other generalist disciplines is a major factor in addressing rural geographic maldistribution. The decreasing proportion of generalist physicians leveled off in the 1980s (Fig. 3.5). (Despite recent increased interest in primary care, the percentage in generalist disciplines has not yet shown a substantial increase.) An improvement in the balance of generalists and specialists is a necessary precondition for eliminating rural physician shortages.

Specialty-Specific Issues—Internal Medicine, Pediatrics, Obstetrics and Gynecology, and General Surgery

The previous discussion has focused on generalists—in particular, family physicians—because the supply of rural doctors is so closely tied to the supply of both allopathic and osteopathic family doctors. The supply of the other two generalist disciplines—general internists and pediatricians—is directly proportional to the size of the communities in which they are located (Fig. 3.6)

Because of the necessity to provide 24-hour on-call coverage in rural communities—and because of the difficulties that internists and pediatricians have in covering each other's practices or the practices of family physicians—internists and pediatricians are unlikely to settle in communities where they will be the only member of their discipline. In practice groups with fewer than five physicians, it becomes very difficult to incorporate internists and pediatricians into the call schedule. Once the catchment area is large enough to support five or more physicians—populations above 10,000—it becomes more feasible to add internists and pediatricians to the practice mix. This phenomenon is reflected in the patterns seen in Figure 3.6.

Obstetrician-gynecologists work on the borderline between specialty and primary care, and the discipline is increasing its emphasis on primary care. The provision of high-quality local obstetrical care is a critical component of the scope of service of rural communities; loss of local services imposes significant economic and travel burdens on rural residents and may have an impact on perinatal outcomes, as discussed in Chapter 12, Rural Maternal and Perinatal Health. Although family physicians can provide excellent-quality obstetric care in rural areas, they require the ready availability of obstetric consultation and the ability to refer their patients expeditiously to their consulting physicians.

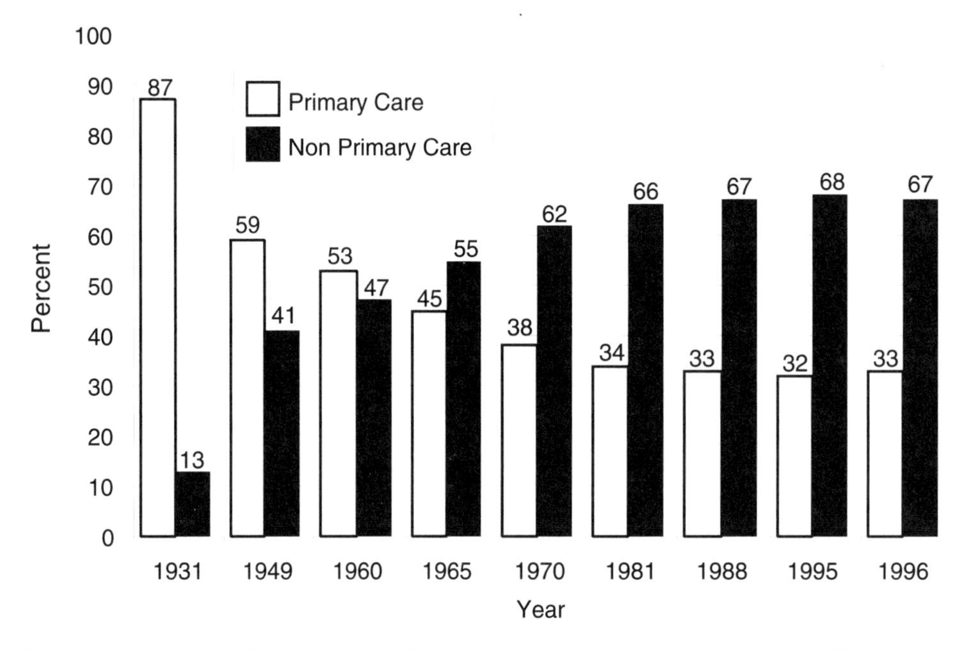

Figure 3.5. Percentage of primary care and non-primary care physicians, selected years, 1931 to 1996. *Primary care includes family physicians, general internists, and general pediatricians. Source: AMA, 1997.

Obstetricians are heavily concentrated in urban areas and almost nonexistent in the smaller rural communities. In rural counties whose largest city has fewer than 10,000 people, there are fewer than three obstetrician-gynecologists per 100,000 residents. Given these patterns, it is likely that smaller rural communities will need to continue to depend on family physicians for basic obstetric and gynecologic care, with defined links with obstetric specialists providing referral and consultation.

General surgeons represent a special case because at one time they were a very important source of care for rural areas. There has been a modest but steady decline in the number and proportion of general surgeons

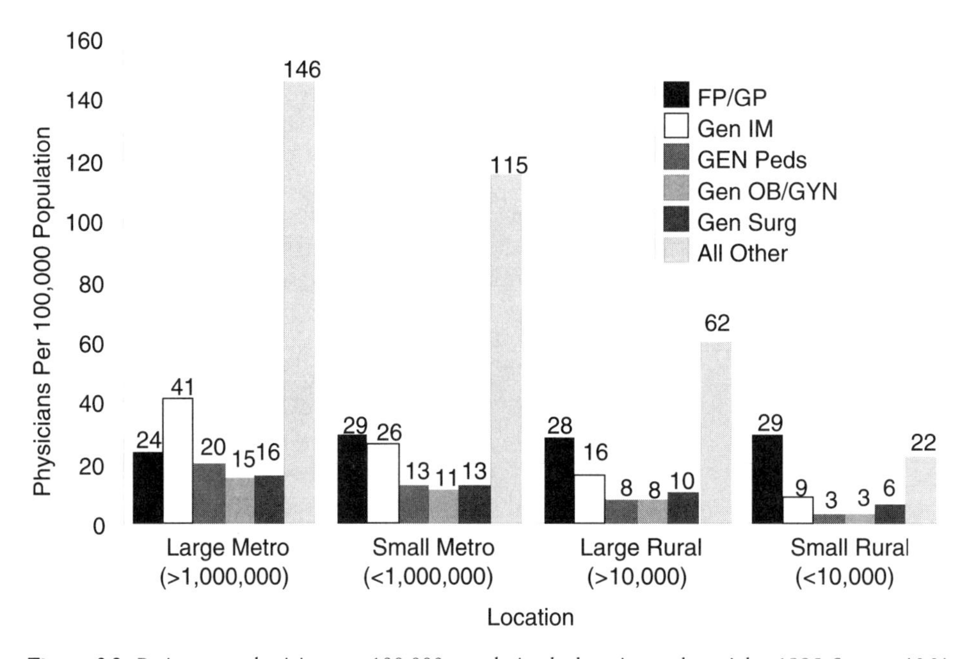

Figure 3.6. Patient care physicians per 100,000 population by location and specialty, 1995. Source: AMA data from BHPr, 1997.

in smaller rural communities (Fig. 3.7). Part of this is caused by the evolution of surgery as a discipline. As surgery has become more and more specialized, the domain of the general surgeon has shrunk and the number of general surgeons being trained has decreased. The result is that there are fewer general surgeons produced, and those who do finish the arduous residency have a more narrow breadth of practice and feel less comfortable practicing alone in smaller rural areas.

The rapid changes in technology make it difficult to set a standard or target for the supply of general surgeons in rural communities. Circuit-riding and itinerant surgery by surgeons based in larger rural or nearby metropolitan areas is common and may be increasing. Improving telecommunications and the advent of telemedicine make it possible for these itinerant surgeons to better manage surgical patients at a distance, with the help of local rural family physicians and general internists. The evolution of vertically organized networks increases the contact and interdependence of physicians living in different locations, with regionally based organizations employing physicians who are located centrally and who back up family physicians practicing in more remote rural areas.

Despite organizational and telecommunication innovations, there are still important benefits to having broadly trained general surgeons available to rural communities. It is certainly worth exploring whether residency programs can be designed that will train competent rural general surgeons who are willing to settle in smaller areas and work collaboratively with local generalists. This may be an area where educational experimentation is possible. Rural fellowships have been very successful within the context of family medicine; they might be replicated in surgical programs as well (Norris and Acosta, 1997).

The Impact of Gender on Choice of Practice Location

Until very recently, medicine was a largely male profession. Starting a decade ago, the proportion of women attending medical school increased rapidly. The number of allopathic women physicians in the United States more than quadrupled between 1970 and 1991 and has continued to rise (COGME, 1995).

Historically, rural medical care was almost exclusive-

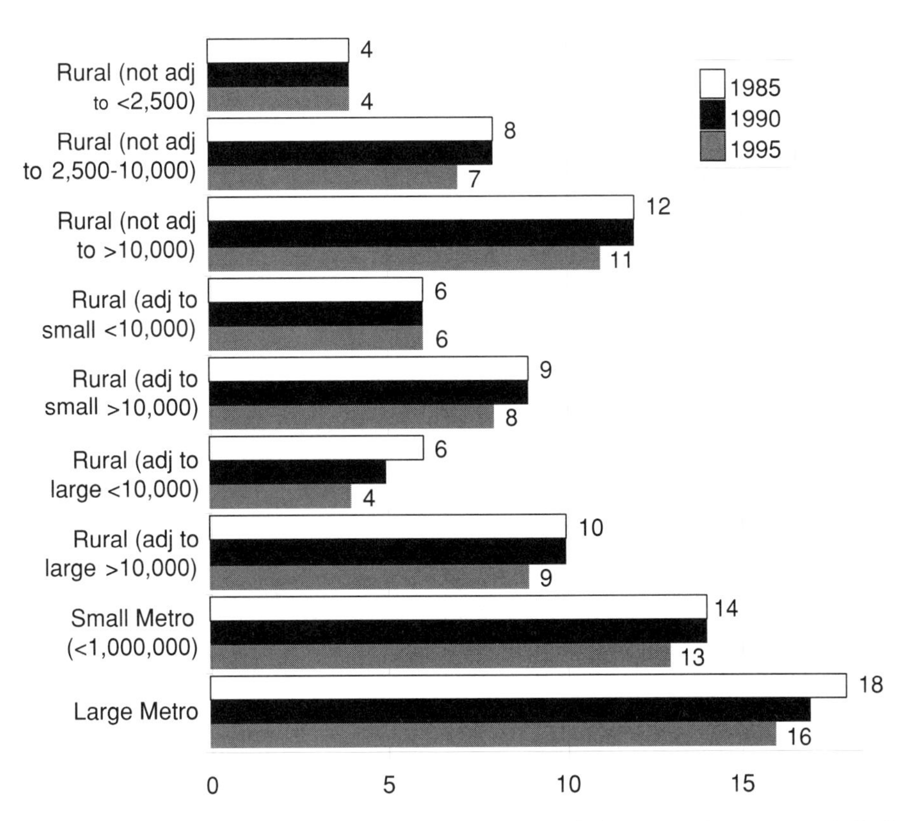

Figure 3.7. Patient care general surgeons per 100,000 population by location and year. Source: AMA data from BHPr, 1997.

ly provided by male physicians as well. This was a product of the paucity of women in medicine and the tendency of the few female graduates to locate in urban areas. Male generalist physicians far outnumber their female counterparts in rural areas across the United States. As the proportion of women in medical schools has increased, there have been concerns that the supply of rural physicians might dwindle if women continued to settle almost exclusively in urban areas.

Recent work suggests that the disparity between male and female physicians may be growing less acute with time. The gap between male and female family physicians has narrowed dramatically for more recent graduates (Fig. 3.8). Still, even women in the most recent graduate cohort are much less likely than their male counterparts to locate in rural areas, and the disparity is greatest for the smaller and more remote communities. The continuing preference of women for urban practice—even though less pronounced than in earlier years—may still pose a problem for the future recruitment of rural physicians. Further research must be done in this area, and programs that support women who have the potential for practicing in underserved rural areas should be encouraged and supported.

The Role of International Medical Graduates in Rural Areas

The role of international medical graduates (IMGs) in the American workforce is highly controversial. At one time, most IMGs who came to the United States to obtain specialized training subsequently returned to their home countries to practice. The original intent of the federal Physician Exchange Visitor Program was to strengthen international relations and further mutual understanding through educational and cultural exchange; the program was not intended to add physicians to the U.S. physician workforce.

This is no longer the case. Today a large proportion of exchange visitor IMGs eventually settle permanently in the United States. IMGs are drawn to the United States by multiple training opportunities, relatively high salaries, and the opportunity to establish themselves in practice here. Training opportunities for IMGs have expanded rapidly since 1988. The number of foreign-born IMGs currently working as allopathic residents in the United States has increased from 7,227 in 1988–89 to 22,565 in 1995–96, an increase of 321% in 7 years (Fig. 3.9). Foreign-born IMGs now constitute 21.6% of all

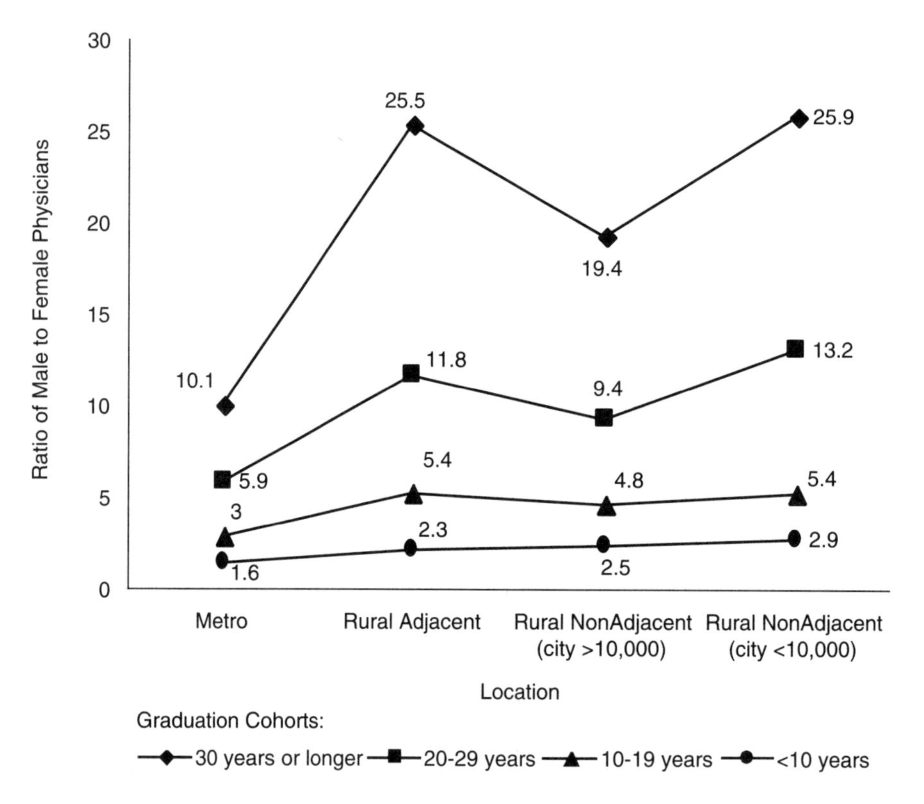

Figure 3.8. Ratio of male to female family practice/general practice by graduation cohort and location of practice, 1997. Source: Doescher, et al. 1998.

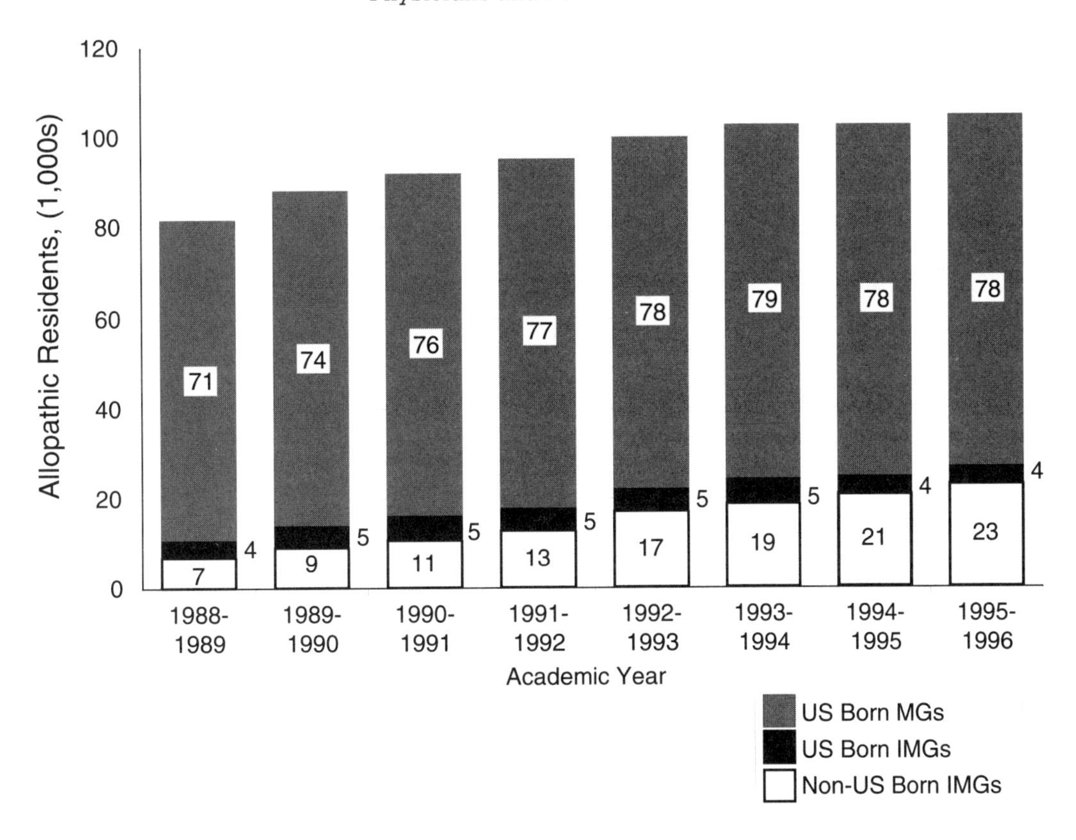

Figure 3.9. Total U.S. allopathic residents by birthplace and medical school location, 1988 to 1996. Source: Bureau of Health Professions, 1998.

residents in training in the United States (COGME, 1997).

One of the major reasons for the significant expansion in the number of exchange visitor physicians has been physician maldistribution. IMGs go where the jobs are, and more jobs are available in areas where U.S. graduates do not locate. In selected urban areas, large metropolitan hospitals have become extremely dependent on the services rendered by IMGs and on the substantial subsidies received from Medicare for both direct (DME) and indirect medical education (IME). In addition, interested government agencies have had wide latitude in requesting visa waivers: the J-1 Visa WaiverProgram is one vehicle enabling IMGs to work in underserved rural areas. Nationally the number of J-1 visas processed has increased from 70 in 1990 to 1,374 in 1995 (GAO, 1996a) . Although it has been proposed to limit the J-1 waivers to officially designated areas, the process of designation is currently so malleable that most rural areas with programs that service the underserved can secure designation. This creates another powerful lobby to continue the extremely permissive programs for attracting IMGs.

There is no question that individual IMGs have established themselves as key providers in selected underserved rural areas and in so doing have provided critical services to needy populations (White, 1993; Verghese, 1994). However, IMGs have been less likely than U.S. medical graduates (USMGs) to end up in nonmetropolitan areas, and most settle in large cities. For certain areas of the United States, including rural counties with high infant mortality and low physician-to-population ratios, IMGs do represent a disproportionate percentage of the rural physicians (Mick and Sutnick, 1996; Mick and Lee, 1997). But it is important to note that restricting the future entry of IMGs into this country will have no impact on the current cohort of practicing rural physicians.

The problem with using IMGs to address geographic maldistribution is that it significantly exacerbates the impending physician oversupply in the United States and deprives other countries of talented clinicians (GAO, 1997a). The Council on Graduate Medical Education (COGME) recommended that the size of the physician residency pool be reduced from 140% of the number of the U.S. medical graduates in 1993 to 110%. As part of this process, COGME has also recommended the elimination of Medicare DME and IME payments for new exchange visitor residents.

If there were no other changes, a decrease in the entry number of foreign IMGs would affect rural areas, but the impact would be very slow and modest. In addition, other mechanisms exist to increase the flow of USMGs to underserved rural areas. COGME has recommended that a portion of the savings realized from the elimination of Medicare GME support be diverted to incentives to make residency programs more effective at training physicians likely to practice in underserved areas and also be used to bolster the NHSC and Community Health Center (CHC) programs.

The Influence of Managed Care

Managed care is a major emerging influence on the delivery of rural health care, as discussed in Chapter 10, Rural Managed Care. Although managed care has become dominant in many urban areas of the United States, its impact in rural areas is just beginning to be felt. The more rural the area, the less the penetration of managed care. But this is changing rapidly, and over 90% of all rural counties were in the service area of at least one health maintenance organization (HMO) by the end of 1995. Managed care is not a creature of the private sector only; nationally, about one tenth of rural Medicaid recipients are enrolled in Medicaid HMOs and prepaid plans, and the number is increasing rapidly.

Managed care is a two-edged sword, with regard to both geographic maldistribution and rural medical underservice. Managed care networks have the potential to provide organizational vehicles for hiring and deploying physicians in areas that could not support independent physicians on their own. By emphasizing primary care services and raising the status and the salary of primary care providers, managed care systems favor the type of generalists who are more likely to practice in rural areas. And by creating economies of scale—and providing on-call coverage, continuing medical education, and locum tenens service—they can markedly improve the conditions of employment for isolated physicians and the economic viability of marginal groups.

The potentially negative impacts of managed care systems on rural health derive from two factors: the loss of local control of health care systems and the reluctance of private managed care systems to provide care to the uninsured. Most managed care systems are sponsored by large metropolitan organizations, and these entities may have little understanding of or empathy for isolated rural areas. In the past, many rural health care systems—particularly those that received federal assistance—have been sponsored by nonprofit community groups. As physicians are absorbed into health care systems managed from distant urban locations, physician loyalties may shift from the towns where they work to the organizations that pay their salaries.

Managed health care systems also exist in a brutally competitive marketplace and are unlikely to provide much uncompensated care for those who cannot afford to pay. The presence of physicians hired through vertically integrated systems may mean that the community has health professionals, but they may be of little use to the working poor who have neither Medicaid nor conventional health insurance. Again, the remoteness—physical and cultural—of the managed system from the distant rural scene may make it much more difficult for the rural provider to offer subsidized or sliding-scale services to the needy in the community.

The managed care industry is in rapid flux, and it is difficult to predict the extent to which managed care will ultimately dominate rural areas as it has dominated some urban ones. The extent to which Medicare and Medicaid make managed care more or less attractive in rural areas will have an immense impact on its extension into these areas. Whatever decision is made, it is critical that there be some sensitivity to the impact on rural areas. Most rural places are too small to have more than one or two clinics offering care. The plurality and choices that exist in urban areas are often simply unavailable in rural areas, and individual rural areas are at risk for losing what little autonomy and local control they currently enjoy.

Chronic Shortage Areas

One of the reasons that shortage areas persist in rural America is that some parts of the country present problems more severe and recalcitrant than the norm. Four major factors make rural areas of the United States difficult to staff with physicians: (1) a sparse population, (2) a lack of conventional physical and cultural amenities, (3) extreme and persistent poverty, and (4) a population consisting primarily of ethnic or racial minorities.

Often these factors exist simultaneously: African Americans in the rural South, Hispanics in the Southwest, and American Indians in the Plains often live in communities that are poor, suffer weather extremes, and have few sources of employment. Life in these places is hard, and it is difficult to attract and retain professionals of any kind, including physicians and other health professionals.

The sources of persistent rural poverty are numerous and are bound up in the history of this country, racial and ethnic polarities, and the economic disadvantages of remote isolated places. Health care is just one of the basic human services that are needed to allow these places to advance, along with improved education and economic development. Until these places join the economic mainstream, it is highly unlikely that they will ever attract an adequate retinue of health professionals without the direct intervention of programs such as the NHSC, the CHC, or the Indian Health Service that support the direct provision of services. And it should be recognized that long-term practice in these areas by physicians, no matter how altruistic, is a rare event.

As the Physician Payment Review Commission (PPRC) pointed out in its 1994 *Annual Report to Congress*, rural poverty may be a better marker of effective physician shortage than the HPSA designation (PPRC, 1994). Even the development of universal health insurance, in and of itself, might not translate into the migration of sufficient physicians to some areas perceived as unattractive. In these cases, government will continue to be the provider of the last resort under almost every possible scenario, an entirely proper role given the importance of health care as a basic human need.

POTENTIAL SOLUTIONS TO THE PERSISTENT PROBLEM OF RURAL GEOGRAPHIC MALDISTRIBUTION

The vast expansion in the number and size of medical schools in the 1960s and 1970s was to a large extent a direct response to the perception of widespread physician shortages. During the 1970s it became apparent that the shortages were more due to specialty and geographic maldistribution. Expansion of medical student class sizes contributed directly to the growing oversupply of physicians but did not, in and of itself, do very much to remedy geographic shortages.

The most far-reaching federal intervention was support for the creation of generalist specialties: family medicine, general internal medicine, and general pediatrics. Through grants to medical schools and teaching hospitals, the government catalyzed the creation of a growing cadre of generalist physicians. Although initial progress was halting, the emergence of managed care—and the resultant demand for generalists to work in these systems—has translated into a major change in the preference of medical students for primary care careers. This shift would not have been possible without the sustained commitment and creative leadership of those who crafted the federal programs and the very creative partnerships among federal, state, and private entities.

One of the most powerful ways to remedy problems of rural geographic maldistribution is to change the medical education system so that it selects, trains, and deploys more health care workers who choose to practice in rural areas. Four basic conceptual models underlie many of the physician recruitment and retention programs designed as a way to address rural physician shortages: affinity, economic incentive, practice characteristics, and indenture (Crandall, Dwyer, and Duncan, 1990). The power of educational interventions derives basically from the "affinity" model, the notion that physicians choose rural practice because it is their preferred choice. To the extent that we train health professionals who prefer rural practice over other alternatives, it may be possible to improve physician distribution without the need to create special delivery systems or invoke some element of coercion in location choice.

Much of the federal support incorporated within the Title VII programs—the major federal vehicle for generalist training—is based on the premise that this is an achievable goal. (Title VII programs are discussed in more detail in Chapter 5, Federal Programs and Rural Health) Talley has discussed the four basic "truths" about rural health: (1) students with rural origins are more likely to train in primary care and return to rural areas, (2) residents trained in rural areas are more likely to choose to practice in rural areas, (3) family medicine is the key discipline of rural health care, and (4) residents practice close to where they train (Talley, 1990). To the extent that these relationships are accurate—and evidence supports associations between these characteristics and the decision to practice in rural areas—modifications of the training milieu to incorporate these factors make sense.

The advantage of this approach is that instead of requiring the establishment of federal or state delivery systems that may be controversial, complex, and expensive, it takes optimum advantage of free-market solutions to the problem of geographic physician maldistribution; graduating residents gravitate to underserved areas to fill their personal desires. In taking advantage of the affinity model, recruitment is streamlined, and long-term retention enhanced (Pathman, Konrad, and Agnew, 1994). Even in cases in which graduates do not elect to serve in places of shortage, programs that encourage generalist careers address other problems within the health care system and provide opportunities for advanced professional training for rural students and minorities who might otherwise not pursue the health professions.

Although this type of intervention does not lend itself to controlled experiments, there is ample evidence that the affinity model works. The enormous difference in the extent to which medical schools send physicians into rural practice is powerful indirect proof of Talley's postulates. Publicly owned medical schools in rural states—particularly those that see their mission as training future family physicians—have very high proportions of their graduating classes ultimately practicing in rural areas. By contrast, research-intensive private schools in metropolitan areas with no commitment to family medicine have virtually no rural graduates (Rosenblatt et al., 1992).

The range of educational interventions is limited only by the creativity of those designing the courses, but a few themes have been repeated with success in a variety of settings. The key seems to be the creation of a pipeline that reaches out to rural communities to encourage the selection and success of rural students, gives these students opportunities throughout medical school and residency to work in rural settings, and supports them in practice after they settle in rural areas. This, coupled with a medical school and residency training environment that values generalism, community-responsive practice, and rural life, is a recipe for improving the flow of medical practitioners to underserved rural areas. Federal and state investments in these areas have been very effective, a fact reflected in the popularity and ubiquity of these programs.

CHANGES IN REIMBURSEMENT STRATEGIES OF MEDICARE AND MEDICAID

The Balanced Budget Act (BBA) of 1997 contains a set of provisions that will affect those who train and employ health care providers, the organizations that insure patients, and the people and institutions that provide medical care. The provisions are so multifaceted and complex that it is impossible to predict exactly how they will affect the location patterns of practitioners or the access barriers experienced by the rural and urban underserved (Mueller, 1997). It is clear, however, that these modifications will affect both the Medicare and Medicaid programs and how they interact with the educational and provider institutions that train and deploy the health professionals discussed in this report.

The creation of the bonus payments as part of the Omnibus Budget Reconciliation Act of 1987 and implemented in 1989 increased even more the importance of ensuring that designation of shortage areas is valid and objective. Because the HPSA designation has an immediate and substantial effect on the flow of funds to areas designated, it becomes an even more attractive status sought after by organizations or governmental entities delivering health services. One possible reason that the number of HPSAs has not declined is that as the penalty for designation loss has increased, organizations have become more adept at making the case for retaining or attaining this coveted status.

Another important incentive is designation as a rural health clinic (RHC). Such designation allows entities to receive cost-based reimbursement through Medicare and Medicaid, which can amount to a substantial increase in revenues for clinics so designated. However, the BBA made two changes in RHC reimbursement that seem likely to decrease the importance of this incentive. For the first time, there is now a cap on cost-based reimbursement to facility-owned RHCs (if owned by a hospital with >50 beds) as there has always been on independent RHCs. Also, cost-based reimbursement of RHCs by Medicaid is to be phased out by 2004.

Although educational interventions have the proven ability to improve the flow of health professionals to underserved rural areas, they cannot overcome all the barriers that exist that prevent physicians from settling in these places. A powerful additional mechanism is the use of targeted incentives, an adaptation of the economic incentive model in Crandall's taxonomy. Central to this approach is the belief that physicians and others act as rational economic beings. If some form of economic inducement enhances the reimbursement for rural services, then physicians are more likely to locate in these areas. This approach has been used with some success in Britain, Canada, and Australia, where a variety of bonuses increase reimbursement for selected rural practitioners.

The major example of this approach in the American setting is the locational effects of the Medicare reimbursement system. Effective January 1997, Medicare greatly reduced the number of payment localities by consolidation of areas including rural and urban areas in a number of states. The net effect is to reduce urban/rural payment differentials that led to relatively lower payments for rural providers, thus serving as a disincentive for rural practice.

A significant economic incentive was the establishment in 1989 of Medicare bonus payments to physicians providing care in urban and rural HPSAs (PPRC, 1994). Beginning in 1989 as a 5% bonus payment—also known as Medical Incentive Payments (MIPs)—the amount was raised to 10% in 1991, the level at which it remains. It is clear that the bonus payments are an important inducement for at least some physicians who locate in HPSAs and have become an increasingly popular tool to help establish and sustain practices in underserved areas.

The presence of this 10% supplement to the usual fee scale seems to have had a stabilizing influence in certain rural areas, though it is difficult to tease out the independent effect. Part of the problem may be the difficulty in targeting the MIPs to those areas and individuals with the greatest need. It is also possible a larger monetary incentive will be needed to counter the gravitational pull of our larger cities.

Changes in Existing Direct Federal and State Programs

When educational interventions and economic incentives fail to remedy geographic maldistribution, the major recourse is the creation of programs that provide direct services to underserved areas. There are numerous examples of such programs, the largest of which are the community health centers and the NHSC; these programs are discussed in depth elsewhere in this volume. There is no question that these two remain the preeminent safety net programs for rural America. Studies by the Rural Health Research Centers in Chapel Hill, North Carolina, and Seattle, Washington, demonstrate that about one in four of new primary care physicians entering an HPSA in the late 1980s was placed there under NHSC auspices (Konrad, 1994) and that one in five physicians practicing independently in many of the smallest rural communities was initially brought to those areas through service in the NHSC (Cullen et al., 1997). CHCs provided care to 3.9 million rural people in 1996.

The optimal size of the CHC and NHSC programs in rural areas is difficult to determine. Even the most precise methodological tool will never produce an estimate that will satisfy everyone's need. Shortages are, by definition, relative, and what constitutes adequate service is highly dependent on subjective criteria. From a pragmatic standpoint, the NHSC, CHCs, and related direct-service programs exist to plug the largest cracks in a system that is highly porous. Providing health insurance for an individual will always be a much more precise intervention than establishing a clinic for an underserved population or sending a physician to practice in a place of need. But in the absence of universal health insurance, there is really no other recourse.

Given the realities of the present system, future efforts should concentrate on improving the fit between need and services, enhanced coordination—and reduced duplication—of services provided, better identification of students to ultimately serve in the NHSC, and improved effectiveness and efficiency of governmental-sponsored health care services, including those of rural health clinics (GAO, 1996b). The wide variety of programs available—and the natural variability in the way they are organized and administered—leads to enormous complexity in the provision of services. It is certainly worth the effort to simplify programs and their administration and to ensure that governmental resources follow human need, not the administrative prowess of officials who excel at the bureaucratic skills that can obtain these services for their communities.

New Technologies—The Potential Impact of Telemedicine

Telemedicine is an emerging technology with enormous potential for mitigating the impact of the geographic maldistribution of health professionals. Telemedicine—by transcending spatial and temporal barriers—eliminates some of the isolation felt by patients and providers in remote and/or underserved rural areas. By bringing together patients, primary care physicians, and specialists through telecommunications, it is possible to solve complex clinical problems, increase professional collaboration and training, support continuing medical education, and foster network development. The development of new information management technologies is closely tied to telemedicine and will improve sharing of paperless records, clinical research, and medical education. There is no question that telemedicine has a legitimate, important, and growing role in rural medicine (Balas et al., 1997).

But the path to the future is neither clear nor simple. As pointed out in the Second Invitational Consensus Conference on Telemedicine and the National Information Infrastructure (Bashshur, Puskin and Silva, 1995), multiple and significant obstacles exist that make the current efforts uncoordinated, expensive, inaccessible, and, at times, even illegal. Although a full discussion of the issues surrounding telemedicine are well beyond the scope of this chapter, there are certain issues that should be addressed in order to ensure that this promising innovation can be effectively and appropriately used.

The current state of telemedicine could be characterized as creative but relatively unstructured, with a wide variety of public and private sector experiments proceeding simultaneously. Some applications—such as reading electrocardiograms or fetal monitoring strips at a distance—have become commonplace. Others—such as dermatology consults or teleradiology—are being performed in many different places but without standard protocols for transmission, interaction, evaluation, or charging. And others—such as doing an appendectomy at a distance—remain in the realm of science fiction, if just barely. If roving spacecraft can perform atomic spectroscopy on rocks on Mars, there are no conceptual barriers to devising complex interventions at a medical facility 100 miles removed from the base station.

The next stage in the process of telemedicine is to codify, standardize, and evaluate the experimental and practical applications that exist. The major issues have been raised in the report cited and by the Government Accounting Office (GAO, 1997b). From the standpoint of geographic maldistribution, several topics rise to the fore. First, some resolution of the professional licensure regulations is needed so that physicians in metropolitan areas can make their expertise available to remote rural areas, even if state lines are crossed. Second, clear protocols for a unified technological infrastructure are needed, both to reduce costs and to allow rural providers to have the option of communicating with multiple providers of these distant services without being captives of any single information provider. And finally, third-party payers need to resolve reasonable standards for reimbursing those who provide medical services at a distance.

SUMMARY AND CONCLUSION

Geographic maldistribution of health providers is one of the most deep-seated characteristics of the American health care system. Even though the 1990s were marked by rapid expansion in the absolute and relative number of practicing physicians, significant rural shortages have persisted. Many rural communities still struggle to attract an adequate number of health professionals to provide high-quality care to local people. As vertically integrated health care systems providing managed care to defined populations rapidly become the norm for the majority of the American population, it is not clear what will happen to rural populations. To the extent that these systems of care penetrate into isolated rural areas, it is possible that they will provide vehicles through which to make health care more available to historically underserved areas. On the other hand, if managed care systems restrict themselves to areas with ample health insurance and large aggregations of population, it is entirely possible that disadvantaged rural communities will be left further behind.

The situation is further complicated by the wide variety of federal, state, and private programs that have been developed to address—either directly or indirectly—problems associated with rural health professional shortages. Starting with the establishment of community and migrant health centers and the NHSC over 25 years ago, the federal government has invested billions of dollars to remedy some of the effects of geographic maldistribution. These programs have been supplemented by major changes in the education of physicians, with an overdue attention to the production of primary care providers. Although major forces have improved the supply of health professionals in some rural areas, there is no question that the safety net will be critical in rural America until the nation more directly tackles the persistent problem of health insurance. Even then, rural areas will have structural barriers that will require special programs to assist in the training, deployment, and support of health professionals.

REFERENCES

Balas EA, Jaffrey F, Kuperman GJ, et al. 1997. Electronic communication with patients: evaluation of distance medicine technology. JAMA 278: 152–158.

Bashshur RL, Puskin D, Silva J. 1995. Telemedicine and the national information infrastructure. Telemedicine Journal 1: 321–375.

Bureau of Health Professions. 1992. Rural Health Professions Facts. Supply and Distribution of Health Professions in Rural America. Rockville, MD: Health Resources and Services Administration.

Bureau of Health Professions. 1997. Area Resource File March. Rockville, MD: Health Resources and Services Administration, U.S. DHHS.

Bureau of Health Professions. 1998. Area resource file. March. Rockville, MD: Health Resources and Services Administration, U.S. DHHS.

Bureau of Primary Health Care. 1997. Unpublished table provided by BPHC, September, 1997. Rockville, MD: Health Resources and Services Administration, U.S. DHHS.

Center for the Evaluative Clinical Sciences, Dartmouth Medical School. 1996. The Dartmouth Atlas of Health Care. Chicago, Ill: American Hospital Publishing.

Council on Graduate Medical Education. 1992. Third Report: Improving Access to Health Care Through Physician Workforce Reform: Directions for the 21st Century. Washington, DC: Government Printing Office.

Council on Graduate Medical Education. 1995. Fifth Report: Women and Medicine. Washington, DC: Government Printing Office.

Council on Graduate Medical Education. 1997. Ninth Report: Graduate Medical Education Consortia: Changing the Governance of Graduate Medical Education to Achieve Physician Workforce Objectives. Washington, DC: Government Printing Office.

Crandall LA, Dwyer JW, Duncan RP. 1990. Recruitment and retention of rural physicians: issues for the 1990s. Journal of Rural Health 6: 19–38.

Cullen TJ, Hart LG, Whitcomb ME, Lishner DM, Rosenblatt RA. 1997. The National Health Service Corps: rural physician service and retention. Journal of the American Board of Family Practice 10: 272–279.

Doescher M, Ellsbury K, Hart LG. 1998. The distribution of rural female physicians in the United States. WWAMI Rural Health Research Center Working Paper no. 44. Seattle, WA: WWAMI Rural Health Research Center, University of Washington.

Federal Register. 1998. Designations of Medically Underserved Population and Health Professional Shortage Areas; Proposed Rule. Federal Register 63: 46538–46555.

General Accounting Office. 1995. Health Care Shortage Areas: Designations not a Useful Tool for Directing Resources to the Underserved. Washington, DC: General Accounting Office GAO/HEHS-95-200.

General Accounting Office. 1996a. Foreign Physicians: Exchange Visitor Program Becoming Major Route to Practicing in US Underserved Areas. Washington, DC: General Accounting Office GAO/HEHS-97–26.

General Accounting Office. 1996b. Rural Health Clinics: Rising Program Expenditures Not Focused on Improving Care in Isolated Areas. Washington, DC: General Accounting Office GAO/HEHS-97–24.

General Accounting Office. 1997a. Private Health Insurance: Continued Erosion of Coverage Linked to Cost Pressures. Washington, DC: General Accounting Office GAO/HEHS-97–122.

General Accounting Office. 1997b. Telemedicine: Federal Strategy Is Needed to Guide Investments. Washington, DC: General Accounting Office GAO/NSIAD/HEHS-97–67.

Konrad TR. 1994. The Rural HPSA Physician Retention Study: Final Report for Grant No. RO HS 06544–0 from Agency for Health Care Policy and Research. Cecil G. Sheps Center for Health Services Research, University of North Carolina, Chapel Hill.

Konrad TR. 1997. Shortages of physicians and other health professionals in rural areas. Background paper produced for COGME. Chapel Hill, NC: Cecil G. Sheps Center for Health Services Research, University of North Carolina at Chapel Hill: Unpublished.

Mick SS, Sutnick AI. 1996. International medical graduates in rural America: the 1987 distribution of physicians who entered the US medical system between 1969 and 1982. Journal of Rural Health 12: 423–431.

Mick SS, Lee SYD. 1997. The safety-net role of international medical graduates. Health Affairs 16: 141–150.

Mueller K. 1997. Rural Implications of the Balanced Budget Act of 1997. RUPRI Health Panel, Rural Policy Research Institute, University of Missouri.

Nesbitt T, Connell F, Hart LG, Rosenblatt RA. 1990. Access to obstetric care in rural areas: effect on birth outcomes. American Journal of Public Health July: 814–823.

Norris TE, Acosta DA. 1997. A fellowship in rural family medicine: program development and outcomes. Family Medicine 29: 414–420.

Pathman DE, Konrad TR, Agnew CR. 1994. Studying the retention of rural physicians. J Rural Health 10: 183–192.

Physician Payment Review Commission. 1994. Annual Report to Congress: 1994. Washington, DC: Government Printing Office.

Rosenblatt RA, Whitcomb ME, Cullen TJ, Lishner DM, Hart LG. 1992. Which medical schools produce rural physicians? JAMA 268: 1559–1565.

Talley RC. 1990. Graduate medical education and rural health care. Academic Medicine 65: 522–525.

Verghese A. 1994. My Own Country: A Doctor's Story. New York, NY: Vintage Books.

White O. 1993. This could end the rural doctor shortage. Medical Economics Dec. 13: 42–44, 47–49.

4

Nonphysician Professionals and Rural America

LEONARD D. BAER AND LAURA M. SMITH

Nonphysician professionals—nurse practitioners (NPs), physician assistants (PAs), certified nurse midwives (CNMs), and certified registered nurse anesthetists (CRNAs)—are an important component of health care resources in rural communities. These professionals have found a place in the health care delivery structure of rural and urban communities because they are able to provide a substantial proportion of the primary care needs of a general population within the resource constraints of many rural communities (Denham and Pickard, 1979; Spitzer et al., 1974; U.S. Congress, Office of Technology Assessment, 1986). Physician assistants, nurse practitioners, and certified nurse midwives have been promoted as especially suited to work in smaller rural communities because they require a lower level of capital support than physicians and often prefer the greater autonomy afforded by rural practice (Cooper, Henderson, and Dietrich, 1998). The numbers of these professionals practicing in the United States have grown rapidly since their general acceptance in practice during the 1980s and future growth in these professions is expected to accelerate as the result of a rapid expansion of training programs (Cooper, Laud, and Dietrich, 1998) (Table 4.1). The distribution of NPs, PAs, CRNAs, and CNMs slightly favors nonmetropolitan counties in the United States with 24.7 NPs per 100,000 population across nonmetropolitan counties compared with 20.1 in metropolitan counties (Table 4.2). Physician assistants are evenly distributed geographically, with CRNAs favoring nonmetropolitan counties 10.8 compared with 9.7 per 100,000. Nurse midwives are more represented in the population of nonmetropolitan counties, 2.47 per 100,000 compared with 1.9 per 100,000, but there are far fewer of these professionals in practice.

The Rural Health Clinics Program of Medicare and Medicaid, which allows for cost-based reimbursement to clinics located in underserved rural areas, requires these clinics to employ at least a half-time nurse practitioner, physician assistant, or certified nurse practitioner. This program, initiated in 1977 by an act of Congress, has grown rapidly and is one factor that has affected the number of these health professionals practicing in rural communities. In November 1997, there were approximately 5,200 NPs, PAs, or CNMs practicing in the 3,484 certified clinics operating at that time.

NURSE PRACTITIONERS

The formal nurse practitioner (NP) role was created in the 1960s with support from the medical community to extend service capacity to communities with physician shortages (National Advisory Council on Nurse Education and Practice, 1997). NPs are registered nurses (RNs) with advanced education and clinical training in a specialty area including primary care.

Originally, NPs received their training primarily through post-RN certificate programs, but today most NP training is at the master's or post-master's level (Na-

Table 4.1 Recent and Projected Numbers of U.S. NPs, PAs, CRNAs, and CNMs, 1990–2015

	1990	*1995*	*2005*	*2015*
Nurse Practitioners	27,000	52,000	106,500	151,000
Physician Assistants	19,000	27,500	53,200	78,500
Nurse Anesthetists	21,000	22,300	14,100	11,600
Nurse Midwives	3,100	5,100	8,900	12,400

Source: Derived from figure in Cooper RA, Laud P, Dietrich CL. 1998. Current and projected workforce of nonphysician clinicians. JAMA 280(9):788–794.

tional Advisory Council on Nurse Education and Practice, 1997). Length of NP training varies by prior experience and full- or part-time status of students, ranging from 9 months to 2 years, but usually averages about 18 months (Physician Payment Review Commission, 1994).

Nurse practitioner associations and organizations have made some progress in collecting data about the numbers of practicing NPs, but the absence of a consistent definition of NPs makes reliable and accurate data difficult to collect and report. Estimates of the total number of NPs vary due to definitional inconsistencies among federal and state agencies. Often NPs practice under different titles or serve in roles other than those with the title of NP. Estimates derived from the National Sample Survey of Registered Nurses (U.S. Department of Health and Human Services, 1996) indicated a total of 63,191 active NPs in March 1996 (Table 4.2). Of these, 55,730 were employed in nursing. Even fewer—32,844—had the position title of NP. Only 23,946 NPs had both the position title of NP and state recognition as advanced practice nurses (U.S. Department of Health and Human Services, 1996).

Lin and colleagues (1997) reported that approximately 15% of all NPs practice in nonmetropolitan counties. According to weighted estimates based on the National Sample Survey of Registered Nurses, the percentage is higher: 20.6% of all NPs practice in nonmetropolitan counties; 67.6% practice in metropolitan counties; and 11.8% are not employed in nursing (U.S. Department of Health and Human Services, 1996). Intercounty variation in population per NP shows where there is less supply (Plate 4.1).

As of 1997, the American Association of Colleges of Nursing (1998) reported that of 339 institutions offering master's degrees in nursing, 295 offer master's degree programs for NPs. This represents a substantial increase from the 119 NP training programs reported in the United States in 1992 by the National Organization of Nurse Practitioner Faculty (Henderson and Fox-Grage, 1997). The Physician Payment Review Commission (1994) estimated that 80% of NP training programs offer master's degrees, a percentage that may be on the rise as the profession continues to grow. The annual number of NP graduates has sharply increased in recent years. A recent report from the National Conference of State Legislatures (Henderson and Fox-Grage, 1997) found a 130% increase in the annual number of NP graduates between 1993 and 1995, with 3,105 graduates in the latter year. By the 1996–97 academic year, the number of newly awarded master's degrees for NPs increased even further to 5,907 (American Association of Colleges of Nursing, 1998).

The number of NPs practicing in rural areas has been linked to targeted training programs (Fowkes, 1993). Interdisciplinary, collaborative training efforts could facilitate the practices of NPs in rural areas. In some cases, an elective or required course for NPs may be taught by a PA or CNM, or team-taught by several health professionals. Distance education can also be an important component of training in underserved areas, through use of electronic bulletin boards, the Internet, two-way interactive television, videotapes, laptop computers, textbooks, or other resources. Cost, however, remains a major impediment to distance education in many underserved areas (Lewin-VHI, Inc., 1995). Community-based and distance education programs have particular advantage in reaching out to rural and underserved areas where health professions supply and training re-

Table 4.2 Distribution of NPs, PAs, CRNAs, and CNMs in U. S. Metropolitan and NonMetropolitan Counties, 1996

	Nonmetro	*Professionals/100,000 Nonmetro Population*	*Metro*	*Professionals/100,000 Metro Population*
Nurse Practitioners	13,011	24.72	42,719	20.08
Physician Assistants[a]	6,268	11.91	24,816	11.66
Nurse Anesthetists	5,687	10.80	20,656	9.71
Nurse Midwives	1,301	2.47	4,036	1.90

Sources: American Academy of Physician Assistants, 1998; U.S. Department of Health and Human Services, 1996; U.S. Census Bureau, 1998.

[a]Includes clinically practicing PAs only, as of year's end 1997.

sources may be more limited. For example, the Robert Wood Johnson Foundation is funding eight projects in 41 institutions throughout the country. These are multi-university partnerships for training projects for community-based training of NPs, PAs, and CNMs. The partnerships are aimed at increasing recruitment and retention of nonphysicians, and most focus on rural areas (Partnerships for Training, 1998). Numerous other programs also seek to increase the supply of nurse practitioners in rural and underserved areas through community-based and distance education.

The growth of managed care may contribute somewhat to the increase in demand for NP graduates because of their lower salaries relative to physicians (McGrath, 1990; Yurkowski, 1997). Public and legal acceptance, as well as interprofessional cooperation, may further contribute to the increase in NP graduates.

NPs practice in a variety of health care settings such as ambulatory care, nursing homes, and hospitals. Weighted estimates from the Sixth National Sample Survey of Registered Nurses (U.S. Department of Health and Human Services, 1996) indicate 23.8% of all NPs practice in ambulatory care, 23.0% in hospitals, and 18.7% in public health, with 11.8% not practicing. Approximately two thirds (66.9%) of all nationally certified or state-recognized NPs in ambulatory settings have "primary responsibility for a specific group of patients" (Washington Consulting Group, 1994). Among NPs in general, the majority focus on primary care but there are also growing specialties in areas such as psychiatric and neonatal care (National Advisory Council on Nurse Education and Practice, 1997). Pan and colleagues (1997) found that 37.4% of all primary care NPs have more than one practice location. As is true of the nursing profession in general, the overwhelming majority of NPs (95.0%) are female (National Sample Survey of Registered Nurses, 1996).

States have different educational and licensure requirements, along with variations in practice autonomy and prescription authority for nurse practitioners (Washington Consulting Group, 1994; Rothouse, 1998; Gilliam, 1994). In a recent study, Sekscenski and colleagues (1994) found that states with more favorable practice environments for NPs tend to have greater numbers of NPs per 100,000 population. The Sekscenski study produced similar findings for CNMs and PAs, showing that legal constraints do impact interstate distribution. Favorable practice environments were determined based on legal status (e.g., supervision, practice independence, scope of practice), reimbursement, and authority to prescribe medicine. It is not known whether state laws and policies differentially influence where rural or urban providers choose to locate.

Various policies may limit practice in rural and nonrural areas because of concerns about reimbursement. Some state laws and policies prevent direct payment to nurse practitioners and other advanced practice nurses, allowing direct payment only to the supervising physicians (Safriet, 1994). Some states require private insurers to pay NPs directly for their services, but often such payment is optional (Sandvold, 1994). Under the national reconciliation spending bill, Medicare Part B now reimburses nurse practitioners directly at a rate that is 85% of physician payments (Pearson, 1998). The estimated mean salary for nurse practitioners in 1996 was $44,533 (U.S. Department of Health and Human Services, 1996).

NPs have statutory authority to prescribe medicine in all states except Georgia. Yet there is substantial variation from state to state in the degree of physician supervision and the ability of NPs to prescribe controlled substances (Pearson, 1998). The most tolerant laws are in the very rural states, including West Virginia, Wyoming, Montana, and North Dakota as well as several predominantly urban states such as New Jersey, Connecticut, and the District of Columbia (Pearson, 1998). Safriet (1994, 1992) notes that state laws and policies often vary in their applicability within states based on geographic and clinical setting. For example, an NP in a remote, rural area may have less stringent supervision requirements than in places having an abundance of physicians (Safriet, 1992).

Legal and geographic concerns are consistent with the uncertain status of NPs as substitutes or complements for physicians. Many NPs strive for a more independent role from physicians (Cawley, 1996). Substitutability of NPs varies from state to state, depending not only on state laws and policies but on educational training, health care behavior, and interprofessional competition or cooperation.

CERTIFIED REGISTERED NURSE ANESTHETISTS

Certified Registered Nurse Anesthetists (CRNAs) are advanced-practice nurses with specialized training in the administration of anesthesia. CRNAs present an interesting case in which the professional and social status of health professions may outweigh financial concerns. On the one hand, CRNAs are less expensive than physician anesthesiologists (MDAs), a fact that could increase utilization of CRNAs. On the other hand, federal and third-party payment structures that favor MDs can make cost a less important factor for hospitals making decisions about whether to hire an MD or CRNA. There is a trend among many hospitals in favor of MDAs over CRNAs (Cromwell, 1996).

Estimates derived from the National Sample Survey of Registered Nurses (U.S. Department of Health and Human Services, 1996) indicate that there were 30,386 nurse anesthetists in the country in 1996 (Table 4.2). Of these, 26,342 are employed in nursing. A total of 21,485 professionals have the position title of nurse anesthetist, of whom 21,240 have national certification. Only 12,121 CRNAs are recognized by a state board of nursing (U.S. Department of Health and Human Services, 1996).

An estimated 18.7% of all nurse anesthetists practiced in nonmetropolitan counties in 1996; 67.9% practiced in metropolitan counties; and 13.3% were not then employed in nursing. Among nurse anesthetists employed in nursing, the overwhelming majority practiced in hospital settings (84.4%), but there were also nurse anesthetists working in ambulatory care (10.8%) and other settings (U.S. Department of Health and Human Services, 1996).

Of 95 CRNA training programs in the US in 1995, two thirds were in nursing schools. Accreditation goals for 1998 may have led many schools to drop certificate programs in favor of master's programs (Hawkins and Thibodeau, 1996). As of 1996, an estimated 69.8% of nurse anesthetists were female, and 30.2% male (U.S. Department of Health and Human Services, 1996). The estimated mean salary for nurse anesthetists in 1996 was $74,845 (U.S. Department of Health and Human Services, 1996).

CERTIFIED NURSE MIDWIVES

Certified Nurse Midwives (CNMs) are registered nurses who have graduated from accredited programs specializing in prenatal, perinatal, newborn, and gynecological care and have passed a certification exam administered by the American College of Nurse-Midwives (ACNM). CNMs typically provide care for all stages of pregnancy and birth, lower genital tract infections, and contraception/family planning to their patients (Kraus, 1997). In addition, patients seek care for gynecology, nutritional counseling, primary care, and mental wellness (Kraus, 1997). In 1997, The proportion of CNMs who reported that well-woman gynecology and primary care visits make up part of their monthly practice was 5% higher than in 1993 (Kraus, 1997). Core to the philosophy of certified nurse-midwifery is the idea that pregnancy and birth are normal processes in human development. As part of that core philosophy, CNMs advocate nonintervention in uncomplicated pregnancy and birth, and the empowerment of women as participants in their own care (ACNM, 1997b).

The percentage of CNM-attended births was 5.6% of all births in 1995, which is estimated to have risen slightly from the 1975 level (ACNM, 1997a). However, evidence exists that in certain settings CNMs are responsible for a larger percentage of deliveries and other care in rural areas. For example, a 1990 study found that CNMs attended more than 12% of births in rural Arizona counties compared to 4% of births for the state as a whole (Gordon, 1990).

Nurse midwifery in the United States has its roots in the service of rural areas. Mary Breckenridge, a pioneer in nurse midwifery, showed in the late 1920s the effectiveness of the professional nurse midwife in reducing maternal and infant mortality in rural areas of the United States—specifically remote regions of Kentucky—with the establishment of the Frontier Nursing Service, which employed British nurse midwives and sent American nurses to England for training (Rooks, 1986). In the United States, professional nurse midwifery training was not found until the early 1930s, when the Maternity Center Association of New York City, in response to high infant and maternal mortality rates reported by the Children's Bureau, opened the first U.S. nurse midwifery school for the education of public health nurses. A goal of the Maternity Center school was to provide states with the highest infant and maternal mortality rates, and high numbers of untrained or "granny" midwives, with nurse midwives who would establish public health programs to train and supervise the 45,000 lay midwives who provided most of the obstetric care in the United States at that time (Hogan, 1975). It was not until 1971, when the ACNM formally established certification measures, that Certified Nurse Midwifery was recognized as a profession (Office of Inspector General [OIG], 1992). Because professional midwifery has only recently been accredited in the United States, the profession has had to define itself in an environment where lay midwifery, which was for the most part isolated from nursing and medical science, has been more commonly known (Rooks, 1986). General acceptance of certified nurse midwifery has been slow but accelerated as the profession gained visibility as a result of the feminist movement of the 1970s and 1980s (Ricketts, 1990). The perceptions of the medical community and of the general public as a whole in regard to the lay or "granny" midwife may constitute a barrier to the acceptance and growth of this profession (Rooks, 1986; Department of Health and Human Services, 1993; OIG, 1992).

The National Sample Survey of Registered Nurses (U.S. Department of Health and Human Services, 1996) shows that an estimated 61.8% of nurse midwives practice in metropolitan counties and 19.9% in nonmetropolitan counties, with 18.3% not practicing. In slightly different terms, approximately one in four employed nurse midwives practices in nonmetropolitan counties. The majority of CNMs work in hospitals and physician-owned practices, with about 10% working for HMOs and only approximately 10% to 12% in private CNM practices (ACNMb, 1997; OIG, 1992). The shift away from independent practice by nurse midwives may be attributed to various causes, such as burdensome malpractice insurance costs or lack of admitting privileges (OIG, 1992).

Estimates derived from the National Sample Survey of Registered Nurses (U.S. Department of Health and Human Services, 1996) indicate a total of 6,534 nurse midwives, including 5,745 with national certification (Table 4.2). Similarly, as of 1996, the ACNM reported more than 6,400 members, 5,200 of whom were in clinical practice. An additional 400 nurse midwives are certified each year. With few if any exceptions, all nurse midwives are female (U.S. Department of Health and Human Services, 1996). The estimated mean salary for nurse midwives in 1996 was $55,309 (U.S. Department of Health and Human Services, 1996).

Several studies have shown that CNMs can supply childbirth services to low-risk women at a quality equivalent to their physician counterparts (MacDorman and Singh, 1998; Knedle-Murray et al., 1993). A recent study published in the *Journal of Epidemiology and Community Health*, looking at national data for births in 1991, found that after controlling for risk factors, CNM-attended births have a 19% lower incidence of infant mortality, and a 31% lower rate of low-birthweight infants than physician (MDs and DOs)-attended births (MacDorman and Singh, 1998). In a study comparing the styles of care among CNMs, obstetrician-gynecologists, and family physicians, Rosenblatt (1997) found that certified nurse midwives make fewer interventions (e.g., fetal monitoring, epidural anesthesia) and have a lower cesarean section rate than both physician specialties. Such reductions in operations and resultant prolonged hospital stays translate into lower costs and minimize patient exposure to associated risks (Rosenblatt, 1997).

According to the ACNM, approximately 68% of CNMs have master's degrees and 4% have doctoral degrees (ACNM, 1997). Between 1994 and 1997, the number of accredited CNM programs increased from 35 to 50 (Henderson and Chovan, 1994; ACNM 1997a). These numbers include two distance learning programs, which are particularly useful to individuals in rural areas who otherwise would have to travel great distances to get to class: The Frontier School of Midwifery and Family Nursing Community-based Nurse-midwifery Education Program (CNEP) and The State University of New York at Stony Brook (SUNY-SB) Pathways to Midwifery Program. Both programs utilize audio and video tapes, texts, and internet resources. The SUNY-SB program in particular uses computer-mediated discussions between faculty and students (Treistman et al., 1996). Such programs allow students access to education in remote settings, although cost may be a barrier in some locations.

A 1991 survey of 1,879 clinically active CNMs found that 80% of the CNMs served patients who met five or more of the criteria used to define vulnerable populations—for example, patients with a greater risk of poorer-than-average birth outcomes. The ACNM considers patients vulnerable if they meet one or more of the following characteristics: under 16 years of age, fewer than 8 years of education, race/ethnicity other than white, migrant/immigrant, poor, living in an underserved area, and uninsured (Scupholme et al., 1992). The same survey reported that 56% of CNM patients lived in areas designated as underserved. Scupholme and colleagues (1992) suggest that increasing the CNM workforce could increase availability of care to vulnerable women and children.

Despite their potential for reducing physician shortages, CNMs remain a largely untapped source of care for underserved areas, though changes in regulatory legislation are broadening opportunities for practice by CNMs (Reed, 1997). CNMs are eligible for reimbursement under Medicare and Medicaid programs in all practice settings (OIG, 1992), though the percentage of physician fee schedule for Medicaid reimbursement varies among states (Reed, 1997). Private insurance reimbursement is mandatory in only 29 states (Reed, 1997). As of 1997, as many as 47 states granted varying degrees of prescriptive authority to CNMs (Fig. 4.1) (Reed, 1997). However, in 16 states there are limits to the degree of autonomy CNMs have in prescribing drugs and medications. In some cases, CNM prescriptive authority is distinguished in legislation as a delegated medical act and the law allows them to prescribe only under a selected set of conditions that are considered "exceptions." In some states CNMs are granted only limited authority under physician control and seven states do not allow CNMs to prescribe controlled substances (Reed, 1997) (Fig. 4.1).

Legal constraints are inconsistent among states because of variations in regulatory authority and function (Henderson and Chovan, 1994). For example, some CNMs are regulated by the state Board of Nursing (BON) alone but others are regulated jointly by the BON and Board of Medicine (BOM) or solely by the BOM or

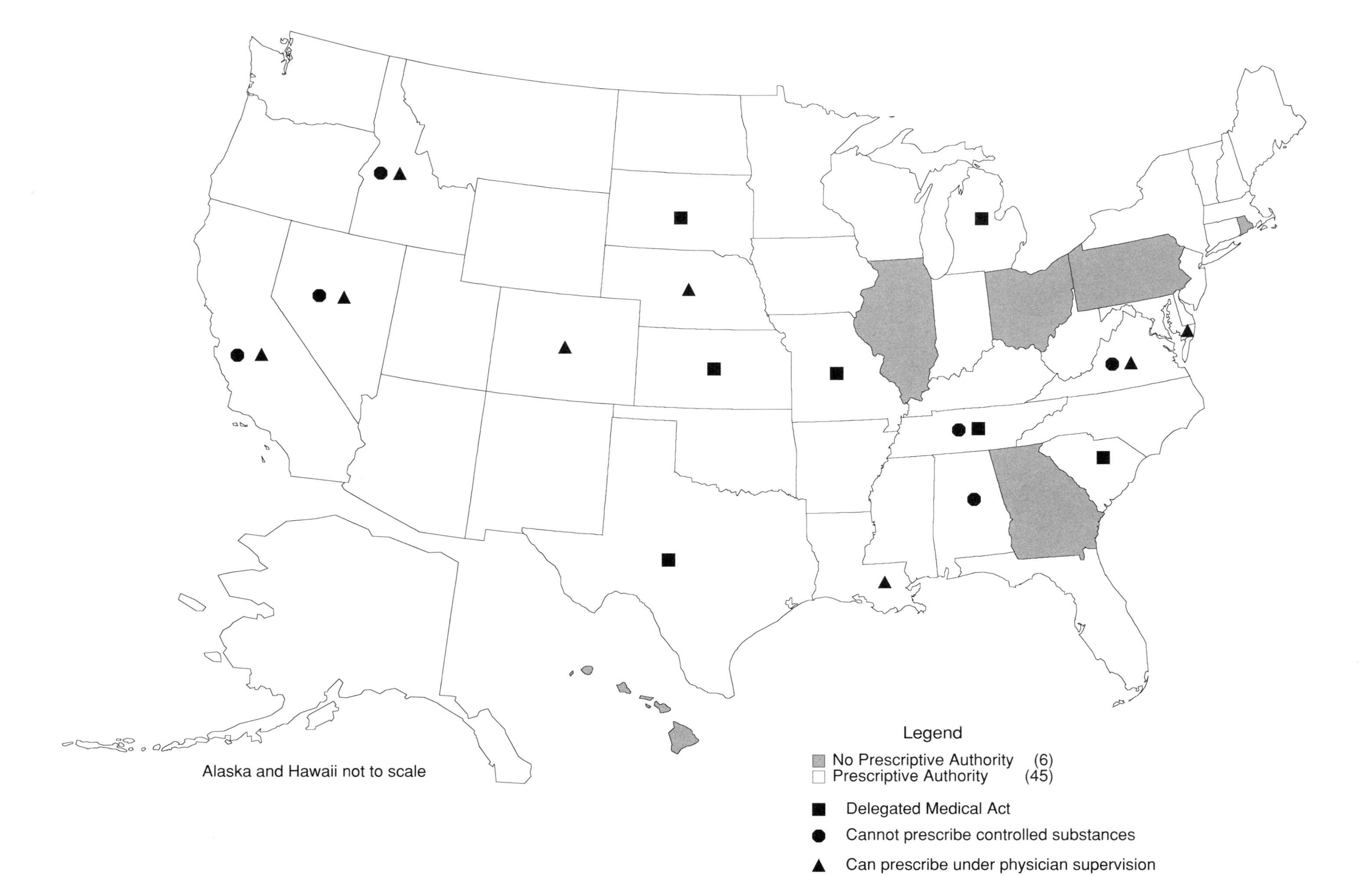

Figure 4.1. Prescriptive authority of certified nurse midwives, 1997. Source: Reed A. 1997. Journal of Nurse-Midwifery 42(5): 421–426. Produced by North Carolina Rural Health Research and Policy Analysis Center, Cecil G. Sheps Center for Health Services Research, University of North Carolina at Chapel Hill.

the Department of Public Health/Board of Health. Only Utah and New York regulate CNMs through midwifery boards (Reed, 1997). Regulatory authority can affect the distribution of services and professionals; a 1994 study indicated that state laws and policies do influence the geographic distribution of CNMs (Sekscenski et al., 1994).

Measures have been implemented on federal and state levels to increase the utilization of CNMs in rural areas. As with other nonphysician professionals, there are funds available for education through the National Health Services Corps (NHSC) in exchange for working in underserved areas (NHSC, undated). State contingency programs similar to the NHSC also provide scholarships and loan repayment in exchange for working in underserved areas (Association of American Medical Colleges, 1995). North Carolina has included CNMs in its Rural Obstetrical Care Incentive Program, which supplies a malpractice insurance subsidy to obstetrical care professionals. Under this program, participating CNMs receive up to $3,000 to help cover malpractice insurance costs in return for working with the local health department in implementing maternity care coverage plan for that community (Taylor, 1993). CNMs have the capacity not only to complement, but also to supplement physicians for supply of gynecological and obstetrical care, particularly for low-risk pregnancies. It has been recognized that provider collaboration can improve quality of care (Keleher, 1998) and that it is becoming part of the restructured health care system (Bureau of Health Professions, 1997).

PHYSICIAN ASSISTANTS

Whereas NPs, CNMs, and CRNAs are advanced-practice nurses, physician assistants (PAs) developed as an extension of the MD profession. The PA profession began in the 1960s with the goal of improving access to health care for the underserved (Cawley, 1996). The contribution of PAs to primary health care was a central concern in the profession's establishment, given the dwindling numbers of general practitioners and perceptions of a national physician shortage at that time.

As of year's end 1997, there were 31,083 clinically active PAs (American Academy of Physician Assistants, 1998). Figures compiled in 1996 indicated 34,748 individuals were trained as PAs (though perhaps not employed or practicing), compared with 25,211 in 1991 (American Academy of Physician Assistants, 1997). Similarly, the number of PA programs reporting new graduates increased from 53 in 1991 to 71 in 1996. During the same period, the number of new PA graduates nearly doubled to 2,532 per year (American Academy of Physician Assistants, 1997).

There has also been a steady increase in salaries. The American Academy of Physician Assistants (1997) reported that the mean salary in 1991 for its members in nongovernmental clinical practice was $45,188; by 1996, the actual mean salary was $64,584, unadjusted for inflation. Any growth in the PA profession might have only a limited influence on primary care in rural areas, if PA trends away from rural practice continue beyond the 1990s. Nearly 60% of all PAs whose first practice site was rural reported their most recent practice site in an urban area. (Larson et al., 1998). With rural defined as nonmetropolitan, Larson and colleagues (1998) found that 9.1% of general practice PAs with four to seven years experience have practiced entirely in nonmetropolitan areas. By comparison, 21.1% of general practice PAs with 12 or more years' experience have practiced entirely in nonmetropolitan areas. As of year's end 1997, 79.8% (24,816) of all clinically practicing PAs were practicing in metropolitan areas, and 20.2% (6,269) were practicing in nonmetropolitan areas (American Academy of Physician Assistants, 1998) (Plate 4.2). Any tendency away from rural practice could potentially mirror physician practice patterns, such as greater specialization and economic opportunities in metropolitan areas.

Physician assistant training usually takes 2 years. A survey of clinically practicing PAs who belong to the American Academy of Physician Assistants (1997) found that 69.8% have training at the bachelor's level, 18.1% at the master's level or higher, and 12.1% have an associate's degree or certificate. The survey also showed that approximately half (50.6%) of all clinically practicing PAs are male (1997). However, recent graduates from PA programs are more likely to be female: 64.5% of all PAs with less than 4 years' experience are female, as are 65.2% of all PAs with 4 to 7 years' experience (Larson et al., 1998).

The proportion of PAs employed by hospitals has grown substantially from one in seven in 1974 to nearly one in three in 1996 (Sekscenski, 1994; American Academy of Physician Assistants, 1997). The percentage practicing in hospitals has remained relatively stable throughout the 1990s, with substantial variation in employment from one region of the country to another. For example, approximately 46% of PAs in the Northeast practice in hospital settings, compared with approximately 16% in the West (American Academy of Physician Assistants, 1997). Policy makers may find that such regional differences warrant a closer look to understand why there is variation in the practice patterns of PAs.

The percentage of all PAs in primary care declined from 57% in 1980 to 46% in 1993 (Advisory Group on

Physician Assistants and the Workforce, 1994). As of year's end 1997 in metropolitan areas, 43.9% (10,892 of 24,816) of clinically active PAs practice in primary care (general practice, family practice, internal medicine, or general pediatrics). In nonmetropolitan counties, the comparable figure is 70.5% (4,421) (American Academy of Physician Assistants, 1998). Such a contrast among counties may be the result of a number of factors, such as limited opportunity for specialized practice beyond primary care in rural areas; the specialization of precepting or supervising physicians; or greater opportunities for primary practice in rural areas.

Muus and colleagues (1996) found that rural PAs have greater independence from physicians than their urban counterparts. In support of this conclusion, the authors found that rural PAs were more likely than urban PAs to be located in a separate facility from the supervising physician. Furthermore, rural PAs spend less time than urban PAs talking with the supervising physician (Muus et al., 1996).

PAs serve primarily within a medical context that recognizes the physician as the referent provider (Cawley, 1996). As such, PAs are often restricted by law to act in complementary or supplementary roles (Pan et al., 1997). Every state licenses PAs except Mississippi (Rothouse, 1998). State restrictions often focus on prescriptive authority or scope of practice (Cawley, 1996).

State laws and policies do affect where PAs practice (Sekscenski et al.,1994). Because PAs are in a dependent relationship with physicians, the geographic distribution of physicians can have a substantial influence on the geographic distribution of PAs in rural areas. Insurance regulations that specify the degree of physician supervision also influence where and whether PAs find opportunities to practice in rural areas.

REFERENCES

Advisory Group on Physician Assistants and the Workforce. 1994. Physician assistants in the health workforce/1994. Submitted to: Council on Graduate Medical Education (COGME). U.S. Department of Health and Human Services, Public Health Service, Health Resources and Services Administration, Bureau of Health Professions, Division of Medicine, Special Projects and Data Branch.

American Academy of Physician Assistants. 1997. Physician assistants: Statistics and trends, 1991–96. Alexandria, VA: American Academy of Physician Assistants.

American Academy of Physician Assistants. 1998. Unpublished table, 1998. Estimated number and percent distribution of clinically practicing physician assistants at year-end 1997 by state.

American Association of Colleges of Nursing. 1998. 1997–1998 enrollment and graduations in baccalaureate and graduate programs in nursing. Publication no. 97–98–1. Washington, DC: American Association of Colleges of Nursing.

American College of Nurse-Midwives. 1997a. Basic facts about certified nurse-midwives. Fact Sheet (M&PR 97—10/28). ACNM.

American College of Nurse-Midwives. 1997b. The core competencies for basic midwifery practice: Adopted by the American College of Nurse-Midwives May 1997. Journal of Nurse-Midwifery 42(5): 373–376.

Association of American Medical Colleges, Division of Student Affairs and Education Services. 1995. State and Other Loan Repayment/ Forgiveness and Scholarship Programs, 2nd ed. Washington, DC: AAMC.

Bureau of Health Professions. 1997. National Advisory Council on Nurse Education and Practice Report to the Secretary of Health and Human Services: Federal Support for the Preparation of the Nurse Practitioner Workforce through Title VIII.

Cawley JF. 1996. The evolution of new health professions: a history of physician assistants. In: Osterweis M, McLaughlin CJ, Manasse HR Jr, Hopper CL, eds. The US Health Workforce: Power, Politics, and Policy. Washington, DC: Association of Academic Health Centers: 189–207.

Cooper RA, Henderson T, Dietrich CL. 1998. Roles of nonphysician clinicians as autonomous providers of patient care. JAMA 280(9): 795–802.

Cooper RA, Laud P, Dietrich CL. 1998. Current and projected workforce of nonphysician clinicians. JAMA 280(9): 788–794.

Cromwell J. 1996. Health professions substitution: a case study of anesthesia. In: Osterweis M, McLaughlin CJ, Manasse HR Jr, Hopper CL, eds. The US Health Workforce: Power, Politics, and Policy. Washington, DC: Association of Academic Health Centers: 219–228.

Denham JWm Pickard CG. 1979. Clinical Roles in Rural Health Centers. The Rural Health Center Development Series. Cambridge, MA: Ballinger.

Department of Health and Human Services. 1993. 9th Report to Congress: Health Personnel in the United States. DHHS Publication No. P-OD-94–1.

Fowkes V. 1993. Meeting the needs of the underserved: the roles of physician assistants and nurse practitioners. In: Clawson DK and Osterweis M, eds. The Roles of Physician Assistants and Nurse Practitioners in Primary Care. Washington, DC: Association of Academic Health Centers: 69–83.

Gilliam JW. 1994. A contemporary analysis of medicolegal concerns for physician assistants and nurse practitioners. Legal Medicine: 133–180.

Gordon RJ. 1990. The effects of malpractice insurance on certified nurse-midwives: the case of rural Arizona. Journal of Nurse-Midwifery 35(2): 99–106.

Hafferty FW, Goldberg HI. 1986. Educational strategies for targeted retention of nonphysician health providers. Health Serv Res 21(1): 107–25.

Hawkins JW, Thibodeau JA. 1996. The Advanced Practitioner: Current Practice Issues, 3rd ed. New York: Tiresias Press.

Henderson T, Chovan T. 1994. Removing Practice Barriers of Nonphysician Providers: Efforts by States to Improve Access to Primary Care. Intergovernmental Health Policy Project. George Washington University.

Henderson TM, Fox-Grage W. 1997. Training nurse practitioners and physician assistants: how important is state financing? Washington, DC: National Conference of State Legislatures, November 1997.

Hogan A. 1975. A Tribute to the Pioneers. Journal of Nurse Midwifery 10(2): 6–11.

Keleher KC. 1998. Collaborative Practice: characteristics, barriers, benefits, and implications for midwifery. Journal of Nurse-Midwifery 43(1): 8–11.

Knedle-Murray ME, Oakley DJ, Wheeler JRC, Petersen BA. 1993. Production process substitution in maternity care: issues of cost, quality, and outcomes by nurse-midwives and physician providers. Medical Care Review 50(1): 91–112.

Kraus N. 1997. Practice profile of members of the American College of Nurse-Midwives. Journal of Nurse-Midwifery 42(4): 355–363.

Larson EH, Hart GL, Goodwin MK, Geller J, Andrilla C. 1998. Dimensions of retention: a national study of the locational histories of physician assistants. WWAMI Rural Health Research Center Working Paper No. 47. Seattle, WA: WWAMI Rural Health Research Center, University of Washington.

Lewin-VHI, Inc. 1995. Expanding the capacity of advanced practice nursing education: Final report. Submitted to US Department of Health and Human Services, Public Health Service, Division of Acquisition Management, ASC/OM.

Lin G, Burns PA, Nochajski TH. 1997. The geographic distribution of nurse practitioners in the United States. Applied Geographic Studies 1(4): 287–301.

MacDorman MF, Singh GK. 1998. Midwifery care, social and medical risk factors, and birth outcomes in the USA. Journal of Epidemiology and Community Health 52(5): 310–317.

McGrath S. 1990. The cost-effectiveness of nurse practitioners. Nurse Pract 15(7): 40–42.

Muus KJ, Geller, JM, Ludtke RL, Pan S, Kassab C, Lusloff AE, Hart GL. 1996. Implications for recruitment: comparing urban and rural primary care PAs. JAAPA 9: 49–60.

National Advisory Council on Nurse Education and Practice, Report to the Secretary of Health and Human Services. 1997. Federal support for the preparation of the nurse practitioner workforce through Title VIII. Washington, DC: Health Resources and Services Administration.

National Health Service Corps, Bureau of Primary Health Care, Health Resources and Services Administration, Public Health Service, U.S. Department of Health and Human Services. Report to the Congress for Years 1990–1994. Undated.

Office of Inspector General, Department of Health and Human Services. 1992. A survey of certified nurse-midwives.

Pan S, Geller JM, Gullicks JN, Muus KJ, Larson AC. 1997. A comparative analysis of primary care nurse practitioners and physician assistants. Nurse Pract 2(1): 14–15.

Partnerships for Training. 1998. Update and project summary. Association of Academic Health Centers.

Pearson LJ. 1998. Annual update of how each state stands on legislative issues affecting advanced nursing practice. Nurse Practitioner 23(1): 14–66.

Physician Payment Review Commission (PPRC). 1994. Annual report to Congress. Washington, DC: U.S. Government Printing Office.

Reed A. 1997. Trends in state laws and regulations affecting nurse-midwives: 1995–1997. Journal of Nurse-Midwifery 42(5): 421–426.

Ricketts TC. 1990. Education of Physician Assistants, Nurse Midwives, and Nurse Practitioners for Rural Practice. Journal of Rural Health 6(4): 537–543.

Rooks J, Haas JE. 1986. Nurse-Midwifery in America. American College of Nurse-Midwives Foundation, Inc, Washington, DC, 1986, pp. 17–20.

Rosenblatt RA, Dobie SA, Hart GL, Schneeweiss R, Gould G, Raine TR, Benedetti TJ, Pirani MJ, Perrin EB. 1997. Inerspecialty differences in the obstetric care of low-risk women. American Journal of Public Health 87(3): 344–351.

Rothouse M. 1998. Scope of Practice/Prescriptive Privileges. Health Policy Tracking Service.

Safriet BJ. 1994. Impediments to progress in health care workforce policy: license and practice laws. Inquiry 31(3): 310–17.

Safriet BJ. 1992. Health care dollars and regulatory sense: the role of advanced practice nursing. Yale Journal on Regulation 9: 417–488.

Sandvold I. 1994. Analysis of selected barriers to expansion of clinical practice by nurse practitioners and certified nurse-midwives. In: US Department of Health and Human Services, Public Health Service, Health Resources and Services Administration. Health Personnel in the United States: Ninth report to Congress: 1993. DHHS Pub. No. P-OD-94–1. Washington, DC: DHHS, 21–26.

Scupholme A, DeJoseph J, Strobino DM, Paine LL. 1992. Nurse-midwifery care to vulnerable populations, phase 1: Demographic characteristics of the national CNM sample. Journal of Nurse-Midwifery 37(5): 341–348.

Sekscenski ES, Sansom S, Bazell C, Salmon ME, Mullan F. 1994. State practice environments and the supply of physician assistants, nurse practitioners, and certified nurse-midwives. New England Journal of Medicine 331(19): 1266–1271.

Sekscenski ES. 1994. Physician assistants. In: US Department of Health and Human Services, Public Health Service, Health Resources and Services Administration. Health Personnel in the United States: Ninth report to Congress: 1993. DHHS Pub. No. P-OD-94–1. Washington, DC: DHHS, 59–62.

Spitzer WO, Sackett, DL, Sibley JC, Roberts RS, Gent M, Kergin DJ, Hackett BC, Olynich A. 1974. The Burlington randomized trial of nurse practitioners. N Engl J Med 290: 251–256.

Stone SE, Brown MP, Westcott JP. 1996. Nurse-midwifery service in a rural setting. Journal of Nurse-Midwifery 41(5): 377–382.

Taylor DH, Ricketts TC. 1993. Helping nurse-midwives provide obstetrical care in rural North Carolina. American Journal of Public Health. 83(6): 904–905.

Treistman J, Watson D, Fullerton J. 1996. Computer-mediated distributed learning design in midwifery education. Journal of Nurse-Midwifery 41(5): 389–392.

US Census Bureau. URL: *http://www.census.gov/population/estimates/nation/popclockest.txt*

U.S. Congress, Office of Technology Assessment. 1986. Nurse practitioners, physician assistants, and certified nurse-midwives: a policy analysis—Health Technology Case Study #37, NTIS-PB87–177 465/AS. Springfield, VA: National Technical Information Service.

U.S. Department of Health and Human Services, Division of Nursing, Nursing Data and Analysis. 1996. Sixth national sample survey of registered nurses 1996. PB97–503320.

Washington Consulting Group. 1994. Survey of certified nurse practitioners and clinical nurse specialists: December 1992. NTIS-PB94–158169. Prepared for Division of Nursing, Bureau of Health Professions, Health Resources and Services Administration. Springfield, VA: National Technical Information Service.

Yurkowski W. 1997. The use of nonphysician providers in managed care settings. JAMA 13: 1095.

5

Federal Programs and Rural Health

THOMAS C. RICKETTS III

The federal government has long been involved in the support of programs and projects that target rural populations and places. Although there is no comprehensive national rural policy (Bonnen, 1992) for the main sectors of economic development, agriculture, energy, communications, and transportation, there has been a concerted effort to coordinate policy and combine and coordinate programs in health policy. The establishment of the Office of Rural Health Policy (ORHP) in 1987 signaled a desire on the part of Congress and the Administration to bring together the various elements of federal rural health policy to eliminate duplication of effort and to apply policies consistently. This chapter describes the federal programs and projects that focus on rural health. Programs that are part of more comprehensive legislation such as Medicare and Medicaid will be touched on but the specific aspects of those programs that affect rural populations are covered in other chapters.

The U.S. Department of Agriculture (USDA) was, for the latter part of the nineteenth and early part of the twentieth century, the primary sponsor of federal programs for rural populations. Although there were no specific rural health care delivery initiatives prior to the New Deal, the USDA did promote health-related activities through its extension and education activities. The first specific rural health policy initiative was the voluntary prepaid health plans established by the Farm Security Administration (FSA) in the USDA, which, at its peak, enrolled over 600,000 people in 1,100 rural counties. Another program of the FSA set up cooperative structures of physicians, clinics, and hospitals and provided care to low-income farmers across the United States and Puerto Rico. That program declined in the 1940s as the farm economy strengthened, making fewer farmers eligible for support. The program was abandoned when the FSA became the Farm Home Administration.

The Hill-Burton Act, formally known as the Hospital Survey and Construction Act of 1946 (P.L. 79–725 amended in 1964, P.L. 88–443) was the next major initiative to support rural health care delivery. Over 30 years, the program provided $3.7 billion federal dollars for the construction or modernization of health facilities and stimulated an additional $9.1 billion in matching state and local funds. One goal of the program was to equalize the ratio of hospital beds–to-population between urban and rural areas. Of the more than 10,700 projects funded under the program, 75% were in communities of fewer than 50,000 people and 43% in communities with fewer than 10,000 people. Over half of the funds spent under the program went to communities of fewer than 25,000 people. The Hill-Burton program did increase the number of hospital beds in rural areas to the point where, in 1986, the number of beds per 1,000 population was 4.0 for nonmetropolitan compared to 4.1 for metropolitan counties.

In the 1970s, a number of programs were initiated either by Congress or by the Administration to address the special needs of underserved populations, including the Health Underserved Rural Areas (HURA) and Rural Health Initiative (RHI). The HURA program was meant to demonstrate innovative approaches to the delivery of health services and the RHI was an attempt to bring together the rapidly fragmented health programs that were beginning to expand and overlap, including the new Community Health Centers (CHC), Migrant

Health Centers (MHC), the National Health Service Corps (NHSC), and funds targeted for capital expansion through the USDA and the Department of Housing and Urban Development (HUD). These approaches to coordination lacked specific congressional authorization and were abandoned by the 1980s.

Programs that were initiated in the 1970s and that proved of lasting importance in rural health care delivery and policy fall into three major categories: (1) policy development and support of rural health infrastructure center through the ORHP, (2) reimbursement of rural providers through Medicare and Medicaid or direct services provision and support, including the Community and Migrant Health Services (C/MHS) and Indian Health Service authorizations, and (3) support for health professions training and placement that grew out of the Health Professions Educational Assistance Acts, including the NHSC, Title VII and VIII training support, and the Area Health Education Centers (AHEC).

POLICY DEVELOPMENT

The Federal Office of Rural Health Policy

As a part of the Health Resources and Services Administration (HRSA) in the Department of Health and Human Services (DHHS), the ORHP has a central responsibility for rural health policy advocacy and information development. The ORHP works both within government at federal, state, and local levels, and with the private sector—with associations, foundations, providers, and community leaders—to seek solutions to rural health care problems. ORHP activities are funded directly through congressional appropriations and they are charged with administering or providing input to a broad range of programs.

The Office of Rural Health Policy supports research and policy analysis and policy coordination in health care delivery. The ORHP has funded rural health research centers since the initiation of the office in 1988 with three research and two policy analytic centers being funded under cooperative agreements for the period 1996–1999.

ORHP also manages a telemedicine program, funding innovative telemedicine demonstrations in rural health care facilities. The program is designed to expand network development and improve access to health care services through the use of telecommunications technology or through systematic evaluations of the costs and benefits of telemedicine as applied in rural communities. In fiscal 1998, the ORHP allocated $5.8 million in grants to 18 organizations and institutions across the United States.

The Rural Outreach and Networks Grants Program

The Rural Health Outreach grant initiative, administered by ORHP, was authorized by the 1991 Appropriations Bill for DHHS (P.L. 101–517). The program provides grants to nonprofit, public, or private health care facilities located in rural areas. The program goals include:

- Facilitate the provision of services to rural underserved populations
- Enhance the capacity or expand service areas to increase access to rural health services
- Promote integration and coordination of services in or among rural communities
- Enhance linkages, integration and cooperation among the various entities eligible to receive grants.

The program is designed to support projects demonstrating new and innovative models of outreach and health services delivery in rural areas that lack basic services.

The program has dispersed more than $170 million to over than 300 rural communities for health care delivery. These have been demonstration projects for how to deliver services in an innovative manner to rural people in need. In 1996, the program was expanded by Congress to include grants for developing formal, integrated health care networks in rural areas. More than 70% of all projects funded by ORHP have continued after the completion of federal support.

The Network Development Grants have a different focus from the Outreach Grants, which support service delivery. Authorized by Section 330A, Title III of the Public Health Service Act as amended by the Health Centers Consolidation Act of 1996 (Public Law 104–299), Rural Health Network Development Grants were designed to develop organizational capacity in the rural health sector through formal collaborative partnerships involving shared resources and possible risk-sharing. Funds are used to develop formalized, integrated networks of providers that in combination may offer a range of primary care and acute care services. For example, a rural hospital in one community used the funds to create a vertically integrated network that includes local physicians, and a community-incorporated clinic. Grant funds have also been used to acquire staff, contract with technical experts, and purchase other resources needed to build the network. Grants under this program may be made to support either a one-year planning phase or a three-year implementation process. In October 1997, awards were made to health providers in 144 communities, 34 of whom are creating formal networks and 110 of whom are new and continuing Outreach grantees. In fiscal year 1998, $14.1 million was allocated by the Congress to the Rural Health Outreach Program and $5.7 million to Rural Health Network Grant projects at various locations (Plate 5.1).

The ORHP also administers a State Office of Rural Health Grant Program, which began in 1991. That program has resulted in the creation or expansion of 50 state offices. The state offices have organized a coordinating organization, the National Organization of State Offices of Rural Health (NOSORH), which meets annually and has developed an information network to compare programs. By administering the State Office program, ORHP helps coordinate federal and state strategies to improve rural health. The State Office Program received an allocation of $3.0 million in each of fiscal years 1996 through 1998. The individual state grants require a three-to-one match from state funds, which helps leverage support from the states.

REIMBURSEMENT AND DIRECT SERVICES

Medicare and Medicaid

The Medicare and Medicaid programs pay for health care delivery in rural communities, reimbursing hospitals, physicians, nursing homes, and other professionals and institutions that provide health care. The Medicare program pays hospitals through its Part A system, which is supported by the Medicare Trust Fund into which most working Americans pay a designated tax. Hospitals are paid from this fund through a prospective payment system (PPS) based on specific diagnoses and adjustments for the number and types of patients. Physician services are paid through the Part B system, which is supported by a separate funding system and which pays on a fee schedule that is adjusted according to local payment levels. Of the total 38,115,000 Medicare beneficiaries in the United States in 1997, over 9.7 million (25.7%) resided in nonmetropolitan counties. Medicare paid $35 billion in reimbursements for rural beneficiaries in 1995 (22% of the total). The passage of the Medicaid and Medicare legislation in 1965 created a system of payments for health care services that, from its inception, treated rural and urban areas differently. The differences in payment levels for hospital and physician services were originally based on costs, and the system implemented regulations that would adjust for cost differentials. The assumption was that rural places had lower costs and thus received lower payments. This approach of geographic price discrimination resulted in larger and larger discrepancies between urban and rural payment rates. Eventually, Congress addressed these differences with a series of adjustments and special classifications within the hospital payment system, Part A, and attempted to adjust physician payments through a relative value scale in Part B. Special rural systems of hospital payments were implemented in stages creating Rural Referral Centers (RRC), Sole Community Hospitals (SCH), Essential Access Community Hospitals (EACH), and Rural Primary Care Hospitals (RPCH), which provided enhanced reimbursement to rural hospitals meeting certain criteria (Table 5.1). As part of the Balanced Budget Act of 1997 (BBA), several more changes were made to these focused rural initiatives, including the creation of Critical Access Hospitals (CAH) as part of the Medicare Rural Hospital Flexibility Program. These hospital-related programs are described more fully in Chapter 9, Hospitals in Rural America.

The Medicaid program is a state-federal partnership with varying program components and eligibility criteria among states. In 1995, there were 35,311,000 total Medicaid beneficiaries. Because states report aggregate totals, there is no reliable estimate of the numbers of Medicaid beneficiaries or expenditures in nonmetropolitan counties in the United States.

Medicaid is a combined state and federal program that pays for health care for certain low-income populations. The program is administered by each of the states, with the federal government contributing 50% to 79% of the total costs, depending on the relative per capita income of the states. In 1995, the Medicaid Program paid $121.14 billion for all services for 36.3 million persons. The largest number of recipients were low income children (47.3%), followed by low-income adults (21%), low-income aged (11.4%), and low-income disabled

Table 5.1 Hospitals and Units/Status Under the Prospective Payment System (PPS), 1997

Total hospitals	6,345
Hospitals under PPS	5,233
Hospitals receiving special consideration	800
Rural referral centers	129
Sole community hospitals	671

Sources: Health Care Financing Administration, Bureau of Data Management and Strategy: data from the Division of Health Care Information Services; Bureau of Policy Development: Division of Hospital Payment Policy; and the Health Standards and Quality Bureau: data from the Division of Systems Management and Data Analysis.

(16.1%). However, the payments for the low-income aged and disabled were 71% of the total Medicaid state and federal budget. Because nonmetropolitan areas are, overall, poorer than metropolitan areas, a higher proportion of the nonmetro population is enrolled in Medicaid, 15.9% compared to 12.5% in 1996 (U.S. Census, Current Population Survey, March 1997). The Medicaid program in rural areas is treated in greater detail in Chapter 7, State Laws and Programs that Affect Rural Health Delivery, and Chapter 8, Medicaid Managed Care in Rural Areas.

The Health Care Financing Administration (HCFA) operated the Rural Hospitals Transitions grants programs, which provided funds to rural hospitals through fiscal year 1996, when funding was withdrawn. The program was designed to assist rural hospitals cope with changes in markets and the federal reimbursement system. Under the program, hospitals were granted up to $50,000 per year for up to 3 years. Over the course of 7 years of funding, 1,921 hospitals were identified as eligible to receive funds, and over 900 had been or were being funded through January 1996.

Alternative Hospital Configurations under Medicare

The growing complexity of health care delivery and the increasing dependence on technology have made the operation of small hospitals increasingly difficult. This is due to the intensity of capital investment necessary to operate a modern hospital that meets ever more stringent regulatory requirements and provides the range of services demanded by both patients and practitioners. This reality gave rise to the development of alternative configurations for hospitals, a subject treated more completely in Chapter 9, Hospitals in Rural America. The dependence of rural hospitals on Medicare revenues means that any restructuring of small hospitals would require accommodation in Medicare regulations to allow for payment to institutions that did not meet all the normal requirements of that program. The Omnibus Budget Reconciliation Act (OBRA) of 1989 established the Essential Access Community Hospital–Rural Primary Care Hospital (EACH-RPCH) program and directed the Heath Care Financing Administration (HCFA) to approve up to seven demonstration states to implement this new, limited-service hospital experiment. Under that program, seven states received grants to develop rural health networks consisting of Rural Primary Care Hospitals (RPCHs) and EACHs. RPCHs are limited-service rural hospitals that provide outpatient and short-term inpatient hospital care on a urgent or emergency basis, then release patients or transfer them to an EACH or other full-service hospital. To be designated as RPCHs, hospitals had to meet certain criteria, including requirements that they not have more than six inpatient beds for acute (hospital-level) care and maintain an average inpatient length of stay of no more than 72 hours.

Montana created a separate, limited-service hospital program called the Medical Assistance Facility (MAF) program, which has been in operation since 1988. The program operated under demonstration authority granted HCFA by the same OBRA 1989 Act that allows these limited-service hospitals (MAFs) to be reimbursed for providing treatment to Medicare beneficiaries even though they do not meet all requirements applicable to hospitals.

Congress, as part of the 1997 BBA, created the Medicare Rural Hospital Flexibility Program. This legislation recognized the alternative hospital as an appropriate way to ensure that inpatient services would remain in smaller rural communities through the creation of Critical Access Hospitals (CAH). The EACH/RPCH and MAF hospitals automatically qualify for approval under this program. The CAH program requires each state to develop a Rural Plan, outlining the need for Critical Access Hospitals and the conditions for their approval. The program, through September 1998, has created the stimulus to expand the alternative model hospital concept to many more than the original EACH/RPCH and MAF states. Up to 25 states had shown interest in the program and 20 will have submitted Rural Health Plans and moved toward qualifying hospitals for cost-based reimbursement.

Rural Health Clinics

Public Law 95–210 created the Rural Health Clinic Program, which provides exceptions to normal reimbursement rules for clinics and primary care delivery units that make use of nurse practitioners, physician assistants, and nurse midwives and are located in areas designated as underserved by the Bureau of Primary Health Care or the governor of the state in which it is located. The program was created to increase the number of primary care practitioners in rural, underserved communities by allowing for payment under Medicare and Medicaid for the services of these professionals.

The Rural Health Clinic Program started slowly with only 285 clinics designated in 1980, and grew to 581 by 1990. After 1990, the pace of designation increased, with over 1,300 clinics being designated between 1990 and 1993. By 1997 there were 3,538 clinics certified (Table 5.2).

Table 5.2 Number of Rural Health Clinics and Medicare Payments, 1993–1997

Year	*Number of Rural Health Clinics*	*Medicare Payments (in millions)*
1993	1,322	$56
1994	1,969	76
1995	2,642	125
1996	3.209	182
1997	3,538	220

Source: HCFA, Office of Designations, 1998.

Under rules current as of 1997, clinics could be either "provider-based," usually part of an institutions such as a hospital or skilled nursing facility, or "freestanding"—an independent clinic or practice of medicine. The freestanding clinics had caps placed on their payment levels and the Balanced Budget Act of 1997 extended those caps to provider-based clinics. Originally, provider-based clinics were paid on a cost-based formula without a cap. The characteristics of counties with Rural Health Clinics, those designated as Health Professional Shortage Areas (HPSA), and all nonmetropolitan counties are summarized in Table 5.3. The locations of Rural Health Clinics in 1997 are mapped in Plate 5.2 and the founding dates for the clinics described in Figure 5.1.

Swing-Beds

The Medicare and Medicaid programs also permit the use of "swing-beds," which allow rural hospitals to use their beds interchangeably for acute and long-term care. Hospitals are restricted in the number of beds they may use in this program: a maximum of 15 beds may be so designated. In 1997 there were 1,383 hospitals participating in the swing-bed program, almost one half of all eligible rural hospitals (MEDPAC, 1998). The availability of swing-beds is important to the new Critical Access Hospital (CAH) program. Critical access hospitals with swing-bed agreements are allowed to have up to 25 inpatient beds and to furnish both acute (hospital-level) and SNF-level care, provided that no more than 15 of those beds are used at any one time for acute care.

CONSOLIDATED RURAL HEALTH PROGRAMS

HRSA's Consolidated Health Centers Program—funded at $826 million in fiscal year 1998—is composed of four initiatives: Community Health Centers, Migrant Health Centers, the Health Care for the Homeless Program, and the Health Care for Residents of Public Housing Program. These programs are administered by the Bureau of Primary Health Care (BPHC) and guarantee the delivery of basic health care services, including prenatal care, immunizations, physical exams, and other preventive health care, to families who lack access to health care, migrant and seasonal farm workers and their families, and children and adults who are homeless or are at risk for homelessness.

The Bureau of Primary Health Care estimates that over 43 million persons are medically underserved and it is this population that is targeted by the Centers. There are over 630 centers operating approximately 1,600 sites; 60% of the grantees are located in rural areas providing direct services to approximately 4 million persons. The Migrant Health Center program involves 120 community-based and statewide organizations that either deliver services or coordinate services for migrant and seasonal farm workers. Health services are provided in the cultural context of the approximately 1.5 million migratory and 2.5 million seasonal workers. Table 5.4 describes the characteristics of the center programs as of 1995.

Table 5.3 Characteristics of Rural Health Clinic Counties

	Counties with Active RHCs (median)	*Rural whole- or part-county HPSAs, (N=1484) (median)*	*All Nonmetro Counties (median)*
Physicians/10,000 population	3.1	3.0	3.3
General hospitals	1	1	1
Medicare payment per beneficiary, 1991	$2,847	$2,771	$2,740
Per capita income, 1993	$15,605	$15,050	$15,581
Percent 65 years of age or older	15.3%	15.1%	15.5%
Population/sq mi, 1990	35.5	24.4	27.1
Percent in Frontier (<6 persons per sq mi)	8.2%	19%	17%

Source: Bureau of Health Professions. Area Resource File. Rockville, MD; Health Resources and Services Administration, March 1998. HCFA. Office of Designations, 1998.

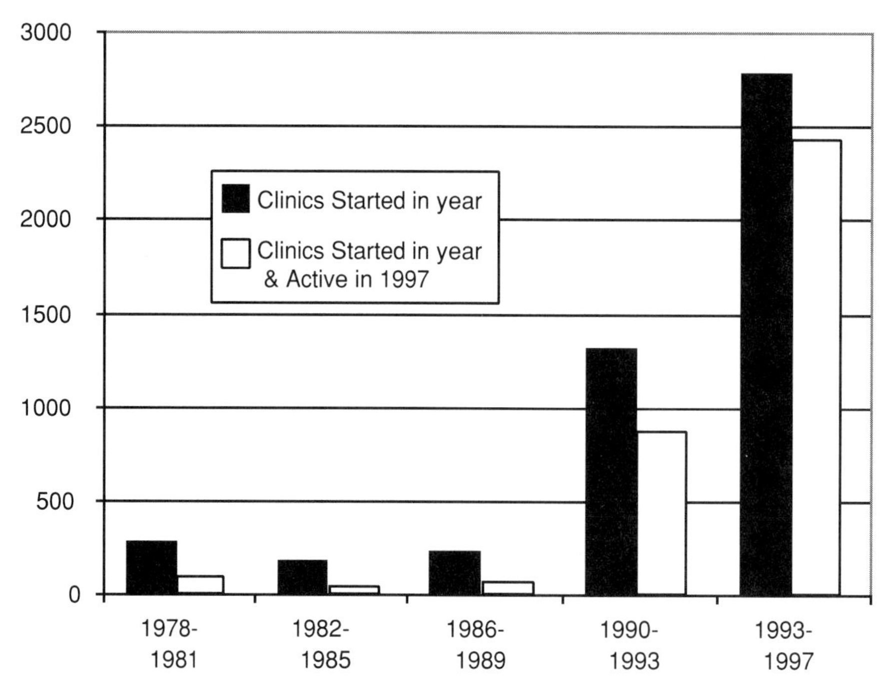

Figure 5.1. Founding dates of rural health clinics, 1978 to 1997. Source: Cheh and Thompson, 1997.

HEALTH PROFESSIONS TRAINING

National Health Service Corps

The NHSC was created in 1970 to directly address the problem of the maldistribution of physicians and other health professionals. The Corps places health professionals into communities and facilities identified as having a critical health professional shortage. The Corps provides scholarships or loans for students who then pay for all or part of that support with service in Health Professional Shortage Areas (HPSAs). Many of the HPSAs also include a Community or Migrant Health Center (C/MHC) site and, in 1996, roughly half of the 2,331 physicians, nurse practitioners, physician assistants, nurse midwives, dentists, and mental health professionals serving in the Corps were working in a CHC to fulfill their obligation.

The field strength of the NHSC scholarship program peaked in 1981. Between 1978 and 1981, just under 6,700 scholarships were awarded. Predictions that a physician surplus by 1990 would cause a natural diffusion of the surplus physicians to shortage areas persuaded Congress to scale back the program. Only 653 scholarships were awarded between 1981 and 1988. Even with the very rapid growth of the overall physician supply, the diffusion of practitioners to rural and underserved areas did not materialize. Recognizing that quick solutions for critical shortages were necessary, Congress authorized the NHSC Loan Repayment Program in 1987. This enabled the recruitment of providers who had completed their training and could begin work in urban and rural shortage areas immediately.

The NHSC Revitalization Act of 1990 expanded the scholarship and loan repayment programs, providing the NHSC with additional personnel resources to help meet the needs of underserved communities. More than 21,000 health professionals have served in the Corps since its inception in 1970. Of these, over 13,500 received NHSC scholarship or loan repayment support. Field strength at present is close to 1,900 professionals as of 1997 (Plate 5.3); the annual rate of assignment for physicians and nurse practitioners and physician assistants is displayed in Figures 5.2 and 5.3. The types of professionals placed include:

- allopathic and osteopathic physicians with specialties in family medicine, general internal medicine, general pediatrics, psychiatry, and obstetrics-gynecology
- nurse practitioners, physician assistants, certified nurse midwives
- dental professionals, including dentists, dental hygienists
- mental health professionals, including clinical psychologists, clinical social workers, psychiatric nurse specialists, and marriage and family therapists.

Table 5.4 BPHC Centers, 1995 Statistics

	Urban		*Rural*		
	Number	*Percent*	*Number*	*Percent*	*Total*
Grantees organizations	333	46%	389	54%	722
Grant awards	405	44%	508	56%	913
People served	4,313,000	53%	3,806,000	47%	8,119,000
Service delivery sites	1,032	47%	1,172	53%	2,204
Health center grant funds (millions)	$412.0 5	4%	$344.5	46%	$756.5
Other funds (millions)	$912.4	54%	$841.1	48%	$1,753.5
Total funds (millions)	$1,324.4	53%	$1,185.6	47%	$2,510.0

Source: Bureau of Primary Health Care. Unpublished data, 1998.

The Corps now provides competitive scholarships to U.S. citizens who attend an accredited U.S. school of allopathic or osteopathic medicine, nurse midwifery or nurse practitioner program or physician assistant program that awards either master's or bachelor's degrees. Students are paid a monthly stipend; tuition, fees, books, and supplies are covered for up to 4 years in exchange for a 2-year commitment to serve in a Health Professional Shortage Area (HPSA). The NHSC placed nearly 2,000 health professionals in underserved rural and urban areas in 1997. On average, nearly 50% of all NHSC placements have been retained in underserved areas over the past 4 years. NHSC members provided care to over 3 million patients, and made nearly 7 million patient visits to residents of underserved urban and rural areas in just the past year.

Title VII and Title VIII Health Professions Support

The Health Professions Educational Assistance Act of 1976 created Title VII of the Public Health Service Act, which initially provided grants to medical schools to encourage them to increase the number of primary care physicians they trained. Since then, the range of programs funded under Title VII has expanded to include policy development through the Council on Graduate Medical Education (COGME); interdisciplinary, community-based linkage programs including AHECs and rural interdisciplinary grants; health professions training for diversity; primary care medicine; dentistry; public health workforce development; and student assistance scholarships, loans, and programs. These 40 separate

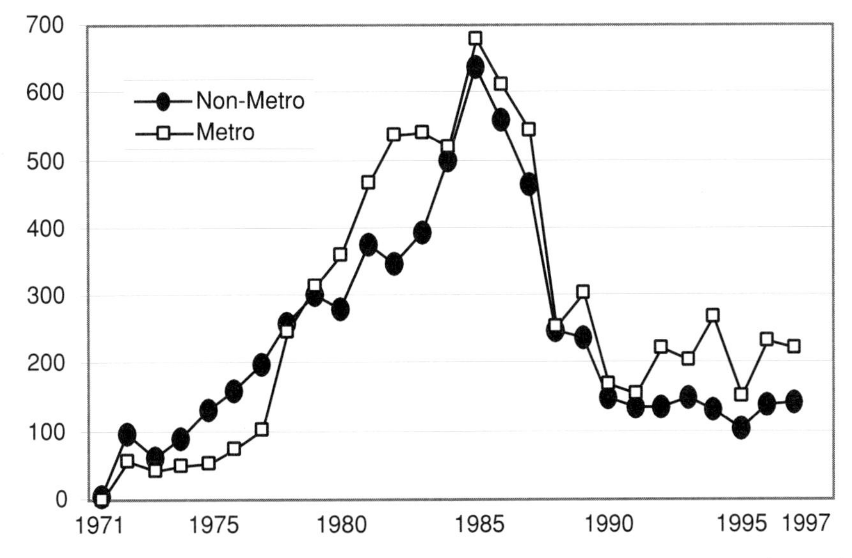

Figure 5.2. National Health Service Corps assignments for physicians by year, metropolitan and nonmetropolitan counties, 1971 to 1997. Source: Bureau of Primary Health Care, unpublished data, 1998.

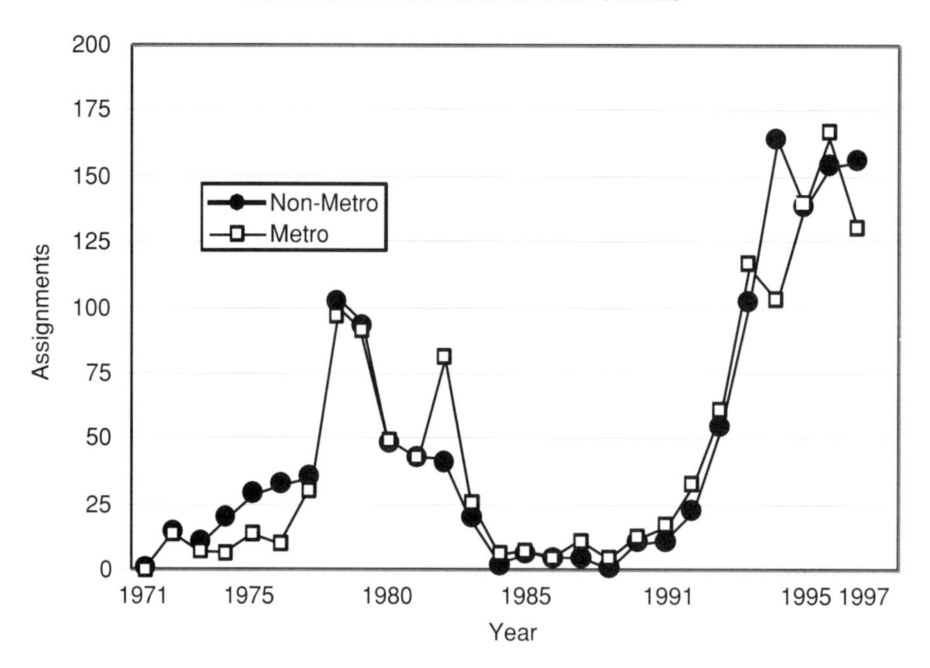

Figure 5.3. National Health Service Corps assignments for physicians assistants and nurse practitioners by year, metropolitan and nonmetropolitan counties, 1971 to 1997. Source: Bureau of Primary Health Care, unpublished data, 1998.

programs are administered through the Bureau of Health Professions.

Many of the programmatic efforts funded through Title VII are not specifically targeted to rural areas; however, they are an important part of the federal effort to improve the equitable distribution of health care resources across rural and urban communities. The AHEC program, described below, directly benefits many rural communities through extension of the resources of academic health centers. The effectiveness of most of the Title VII programs is measured by their impact on underserved areas, HPSAs and MUAs, and, because the majority of those areas are rural, there is strong emphasis on rural issues in Title VII administration and oversight.

Nursing Workforce Development is supported by Title VIII of the Public Health Service Act. Title VIII has funded more than 60% of all current nurse practitioner programs and 83% of the existing nurse-midwifery programs over the past 20 years in the United States. Title VIII has provided funding for the development and/or expansion of nearly 20% of all nurse-anesthetist educational programs, and supported over 75% of nurse-anesthetist graduates in the past year. Nurse anesthetists provide 65% of the 26 million anesthetics administered each year and are the sole providers of anesthesia in 85% of rural hospitals. Last year, 34% of nurse-anesthetists practiced in communities with populations of less than 50,000.

Area Health Education Centers

During the development of health professions training programs, it became apparent to Congress that there needed to be support for the practicing physician as well as a mechanism to regionalize training of health professionals away from the medical schools and academic health centers. The Area Health Education Centers (AHEC) Program was initiated in 1972 after passage of the Comprehensive Health Manpower Training Act of 1971 (P.L. 92–157). The program began with an explicit focus on improving geographic access to health services through the decentralization of health professional education. AHEC support from the federal government initially was intended to create a set of demonstration programs that would eventually establish themselves in their host states and regions.

During the period 1992–1997, the Congress expanded AHEC funding from $17.3 million to $27.2 million and the number of active awardees rose from 20 to 36. Many of these states use substantial state appropriations to support outreach activities, which include rural placements and externships, support for distance learning, the transportation of preceptors to distant sites, and the capital expenses for the building of regional centers. Congress appropriated $32.4 million to the AHEC and Health Education Training Centers programs in 1998.

AHEC programs have coordinated and supported the

training of nearly 1.5 million health professions students and primary care residents in underserved areas with an explicit focus on rural areas in most state programs. AHEC provided community-based clinical training to nearly 10,000 medical school students, or 13% of the nation's total medical school enrollment, in 1996. In the same year, 32 AHEC programs assisted in providing community-based training experiences at 1,400 rural and urban areas nationwide for 2,900 primary care residents, 600 physician assistant students, 1,100 nurse practitioner students, and 8,800 other health professions students. Over 16% of all 1996 National Health Service Corps (NHSC) personnel utilized AHEC supported training.

RURAL INTERDISCIPLINARY TRAINING PROGRAM

The Congress created in the 1988 Health Professions Reauthorization Act a program to support the training and education of health professionals for practice in rural communities. Administered by the Bureau of Health Professions, the program provides grants intended to encourage and prepare a range of health professionals, especially those working in teams, to enter into and/or remain in practice in rural America where health care professionals are currently in short supply. Not more than 10% of the individuals receiving training with these grants can be trained as doctors of allopathic or osteopathic medicine. Grant funds are available to fund interdisciplinary training projects designed to (1) use new and innovative methods to train health care practitioners to provide services in rural areas, (2) demonstrate and evaluate innovative interdisciplinary methods and models designed to provide access to cost-effective comprehensive health care, (3) deliver health care services to individuals residing in rural areas, (4) enhance the amount of relevant research conducted concerning health care issues in rural areas, and (5) increase the recruitment and retention of health care practitioners in rural areas and make rural practice a more attractive career choice. Grants can be made to public health units and nonprofit organizations as well as colleges and universities. All projects must have formal working agreements with rural delivery organizations and rural communities for placement and community-based training. In 1994, 54% of the graduates from the interdisciplinary training programs were employed in rural or frontier areas 3 years after their training. In fiscal year 1997, there were 20 rural interdisciplinary grant awards and four contracts totaling $4.1 million. The fiscal year 1998 appropriation remained at $4.2 million in total program costs.

REFERENCES

Bonnen JT. 1992. Why is there no coherent U.S. rural policy? Policy Studies Journal 20(2): 190–201.

Cheh V, Thompson R. 1997. Rural Health Clinics: Improved Access at a Cost. Princeton, NJ: Mathematica Policy Research.

MEDPAC. 1998. Health Care Spending and the Medicare Program: A Data Book. Washington, DC: Medicare Payment Advisory Commission.

6

The Medicare Program in Rural Areas

CURT D. MUELLER, JULIE A. SCHOENMAN, AND ELIZABETH DOROSH

Medicare provides health insurance coverage for over 38 million Americans. Program payments in 1995 were $184 billion, over 20% of personal health care expenditures (United States Department of Health and Human Services [USDHHS], 1997). Medicare is an important part of the nation's health care financing system, but it is especially important for rural America because a higher proportion of the rural population is elderly. Estimates obtained by the Walsh Center for Rural Health Analysis from the U.S. Bureau of the Census indicate that in 1997, about 14% of the population in nonmetropolitan counties was over age 65, versus 11% in metropolitan counties. Although Medicare has brought health insurance security to the rural elderly and other beneficiaries, some observers believe that payment disparities and inequities persist between urban and rural communities. Overall, the Medicare program pays less per rural than per urban beneficiary, and pays less for the same service provided in rural than in urban places. The importance of these disparities is magnified because rural providers depend more on the Medicare program than on other payers.

The Health Care Financing Administration (HCFA), an agency within the Executive Branch of the federal government, is charged with administering the Medicare program. In this capacity, HCFA produces an annual program review and other publications that describe the Medicare program in detail.* Program oversight on the congressional side is provided by the Medical Payment Advisory Commission (MedPAC), which was formed by the Balanced Budget Act of 1997 by combining the Physician Payment Review Commission (PPRC) and the Prospective Payment Assessment Commission (ProPAC). MedPAC will continue to provide significant sources of information and background data on the Medicare program, as did its predecessors.†

Although publications and data releases by HCFA, MedPAC, PPRC, ProPAC, and others have been very useful and informative, they have not routinely provided much detail on the Medicare program from the rural perspective. This chapter is intended to help fill this gap.

*In particular, see the *Medicare and Medicaid Statistical Supplement*, published annually as a supplement to HCFA's Health Care Financing Review (e.g., USDHHS, 1997). The supplement contains textual descriptions of the program, as well as numerous charts and tables. Another invaluable reference on the Medicare program is the *Overview of Entitlement Programs,* or "Green Book," periodically updated by the Committee on Ways and Means.

†Publications by MedPAC, PPRC, and ProPAC are extremely valuable as guides to current program policies and expected policy changes (e.g., MedPAC, 1998a,b; ProPAC, 1997; PPRC, 1997). A new commission, the National Bipartisan Commission on the future of Medicare, is expected to release its report in March 1999. Aspects of the program from the beneficiary perspective are presented in the form of survey estimates from the Medicare Current Beneficiary Survey (MCBS) (Laschober, 1997). Finally, a number of texts are useful in placing the program in an historical context (e.g., Moon, 1996, and Davis et al., 1990).

It provides an overview of how the Medicare program affects rural areas. Administrative data from HCFA on program payments and use of services are examined. These data are provided because HCFA program data of this type are not readily available for rural areas. Estimates of beneficiary access and satisfaction, generated from the Medicare Current Beneficiary Survey (MCBS) are also reported. Finally, data on payment rates under Medicare risk plans are presented. It is important to note that data presented in this chapter are a selected overview of the program from the rural perspective. Related topics and issues are addressed in Chapter 10, Rural Managed Care, and Chapter 2, Access to Health Care.

PROGRAM STATISTICS

Data on enrollments and program expenditures for 1995 and 1990 were provided by HCFA's Office of Research and Demonstrations. Separate estimates were provided for "rural" and "urban" counties based on definitions that are routinely employed by HCFA. For Tables 6.1 through 6.3 and Figures 6.1 through 6.4, urban counties are defined as counties included in standard metropolitan statistical areas (SMSAs) or metropolitan state economic areas (SEAs, in New England), as defined by the Office of Management and Budget using data from the 1980 census. The 1980s definition of urban-rural is used to allow for stable comparisons because the number of counties in each category varies from year to year. "Rural" counties include those not contained in SMSAs or SEAs.

Program Payments and Numbers of Beneficiaries

In 1995, total Medicare payments, including payments for the aged and disabled, were $35.23 billion and $123.75 billion in rural and urban counties, respectively. Payments per person using services were $4,477 for rural and $5,487 for urban beneficiaries.

Most Medicare beneficiaries generated relatively small payments to providers. In rural areas, about 43% of Medicare enrollees with a reimbursement generated payments of less than $500 during 1995 (Fig. 6.1). The total of these expenditures for all low-payment enrollees accounted for about 2% of total program payments (Fig. 6.2). Forty-four percent (44%) of rural beneficiaries generated payments ranging from $500 to $10,000 per person, accounting for about 28% of total program payments; 38% of program expenditures were incurred by only 4% of rural beneficiaries, who generated average payments in excess of $25,000 per person.

The relationship between numbers of service recipients and payments in rural areas differs from the pattern for urban beneficiaries. Larger relative numbers of persons in urban areas generated larger per person payments. In urban areas, only 37% of beneficiaries generated payments of $500 or less in 1995 (compared to 43% in rural areas); 27% of beneficiaries used services with per capita payments in the $500 to $2,000 range in urban areas, versus 23% in rural areas (Fig. 6.1). In urban areas, 6% of beneficiaries generated payments of $25,000 or more, versus 4% in rural areas (Fig. 6.2). This larger percent (which represents a considerably larger absolute number of beneficiaries than in rural ar-

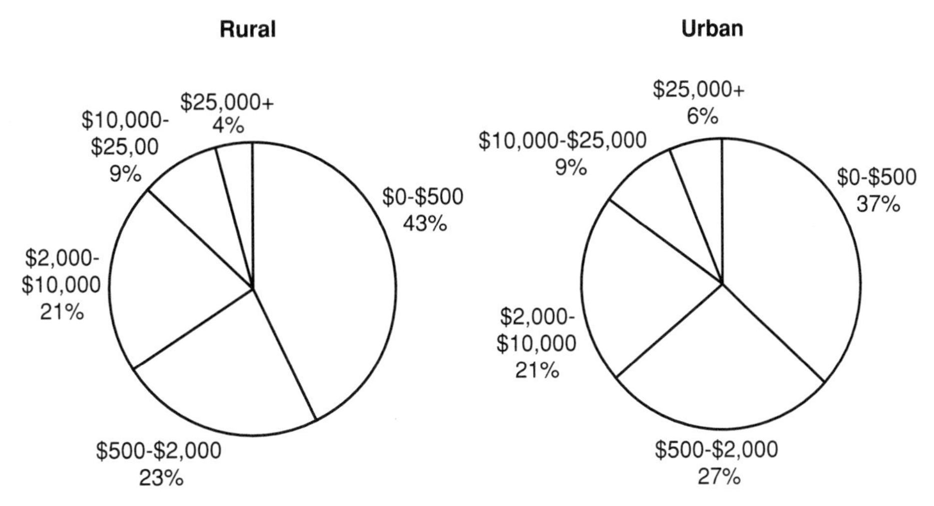

Figure 6.1. Percent distribution of program beneficiaries served, by medical expenditures per beneficiary, rural and urban areas, 1995.

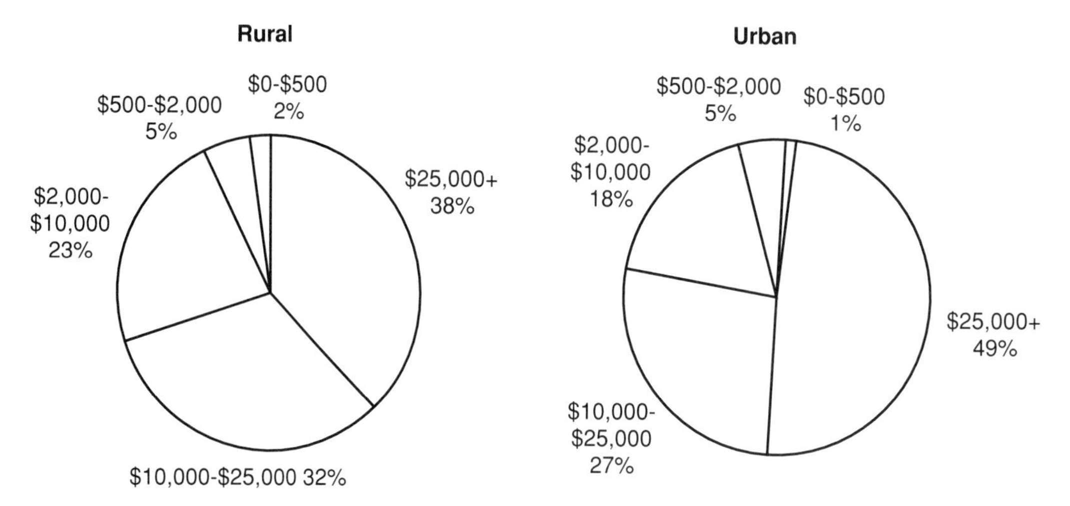

Figure 6.2. Percent distribution of Medicare program payments by medical expenditures per beneficiary, rural and urban areas, 1995.

eas) accounted for 49% of total payments, versus only 39% in rural areas.

Observed relationships between numbers of beneficiaries and levels of spending are consistent with what is known about barriers of access to care and the nature of care consumed in urban versus rural settings. The relative supplies of many medical resources, including the numbers of physicians, hospitals, hospital beds, and tertiary care systems are larger in urban areas, which may reduce nonmonetary barriers such as travel time. Furthermore, payment rates tend to be greater in urban areas to compensate providers for geographic differences in the costs of practice as defined and measured by HCFA.

Program Payments by Type of Service

The Medicare program separates payments for hospital services and physician or professional services into two linked but distinct systems. Payments to hospitals come from Part A, and professional services from Part B. Part A dollars come from the Medicare Trust Fund, which is supported by payroll deductions. Part B dollars are from a "premium" paid by the enrollee and through general federal tax revenues. (See USDHHS, 1997, for more information on the benefit structure of the program.)

Almost half of total Medicare payments—49% in urban areas and 50% in rural areas—were for inpatient hospital services (Table 6.1). Residents of rural and urban areas spent comparable relative amounts on Part B physician services (25% of total payments by rural residents, and 27% of total payments by urban residents). Rural and urban residents also spent comparable relative amounts on skilled nursing services (4% and 5% in rural and urban areas, respectively). Home health agency services accounted for a greater share of dollars in rural areas (12% versus 9% in urban areas), as did outpatient department services (11% and 9% in rural and urban areas, respectively).

A comparison of the distributions of payments by type of service indicates that the shares of payments for inpatient care and physician services have decreased from 1990 to 1995, whereas payment shares for outpatient care and skilled and home care have increased (Table 6.1). The share of payments for outpatient services to residents of rural areas increased from 9% of payments to 11% of payments in 1995. Meanwhile, the combined share of payments for hospital inpatient and physician services declined 13% in rural areas (from 85% in 1990 to 74% in 1995) and 10% in urban areas (from 86% to 77%).

The most dramatic changes in program payments between 1990 and 1995 were for home health and skilled nursing services. From 1990 to 1995, home health payments (under Parts A and B, combined) increased from $1.0 billion to $4.1 billion in rural areas, and from $2.9 to $11.2 billion in urban areas; skilled nursing facility payments increased from $0.4 to $1.5 billion in rural areas, and from $1.6 to $6.3 billion in urban areas. Payment shares for skilled nursing and home health services also increased dramatically during the 5-year period (Table 6.1). The payment share for home health services tripled in rural areas. In 1990, 4% of payment dollars were for home health services; by 1995, 12% of payments were for these services. In urban areas, the home health payment share increased 75% from 4% to 7% of program payments. In a similar fashion, payment shares for skilled nursing services doubled in rural areas and more than doubled in urban areas during the 5-year period.

Table 6.1 Percent Distributions of Medicare Program Payments, by Type of Service, Urban and Rural Areas, 1990 and 1995

	Urban		*Rural*	
Type of Service	*1990*	*1995*	*1990*	*1995*
Inpatient	56%	50%	56%	49%
Skilled Nursing Care	2%	5%	2%	4%
Home Health Agency	4%	7%	4%	12%
Physician	30%	27%	29%	25%
Outpatient	9%	9%	9%	11%

Although changes in the level of program payments reflect program growth in rural areas, the changes do not reveal trends in factors that underlie program growth. Expenditure growth reflects changes in the numbers of beneficiaries who receive each type of service, changes in service intensity (e.g., type of physician visit or hospital stay), and increases in payments that account for general health care inflation.

The average hospital inpatient payment on behalf of rural beneficiaries who used inpatient services was $9,242 in 1995 (Table 6.2). This amount reflects care received by rural residents in rural and urban areas, just as payments for urban residents includes payment for services received in rural areas. Over 1.8 million rural residents received inpatient services during the year. About 7.6 million beneficiaries used physician services, and payments on their behalf averaged $1,151. Payments on behalf of urban residents were 31% greater for inpatient services and 30% greater for physician services, on average. These differences do not reflect differences in the numbers of users (they are on a per user basis), but reflect differences both in service intensity and urban-rural differences in payment levels. Urban payments per recipient are higher than rural payments for all services except home health.

Under the Balanced Budget Act of 1997, most home health benefits will be covered under Part B of the Medicare program. In 1995, however, Parts A and B of the Medicare program covered home health services. Most home health benefits were provided under Part A. Part A covered most visits following an inpatient hospital stay, and Part B provided benefits when home health service use was not preceded by a hospital stay. Rural payments per recipient for in-home services covered under Part A were $4,416, versus $4,399 in urban areas in 1995. The proportion of service recipients who lived in rural places was higher for this category than for any other service category. Payments for home health care under Part B—generally equipment and supplies—were $5,659 in rural areas in 1995, 21% greater than in urban areas ($4,675). Clearly, home health services are very important in rural areas. Home health care services substitute for services that have traditionally been provided during longer, more expensive hospital stays. For rural residents, hospitalization sometimes means stays that are a considerable distance from family and community. These stays impose burdens on family members by virtue of their distance from home. In rural areas, availability of home health services can permit patients to return home more quickly, reducing travel and time burdens on supportive family members and friends.

The largest rates of growth in payments per rural recipient have been for long-term care services (Fig. 6.3). Between 1990 and 1995, payments per recipient for skilled nursing facility use have increased by 21% and payments for home health services under Part A have increased by 26%. Similar rates of increase were experienced in urban areas.

Table 6.2 Program Payments per Recipient and Number of Recipients, by Type of Service, Rural and Urban Areas, 1995

	Rural		*Urban*	
Service	*Payment*	*Recipients*	*Payment*	*Recipients*
Any Service	$4,477	7,368,500	$5,437	22,334,640
Inpatient	$9,242	1,867,800	$12,104	5,090,100
Physician	$1,151	7,574,800	$1,498	21,903,920
Outpatient	$659	5,309,520	$825	14,118,240
Skilled Nursing Facility	$4,757	314,780	$6,863	918,180
Home Health				
Part A	$4,416	412,940	$4,399	2,514,340
Part B	$5,659	6,800	$4,675	34,520

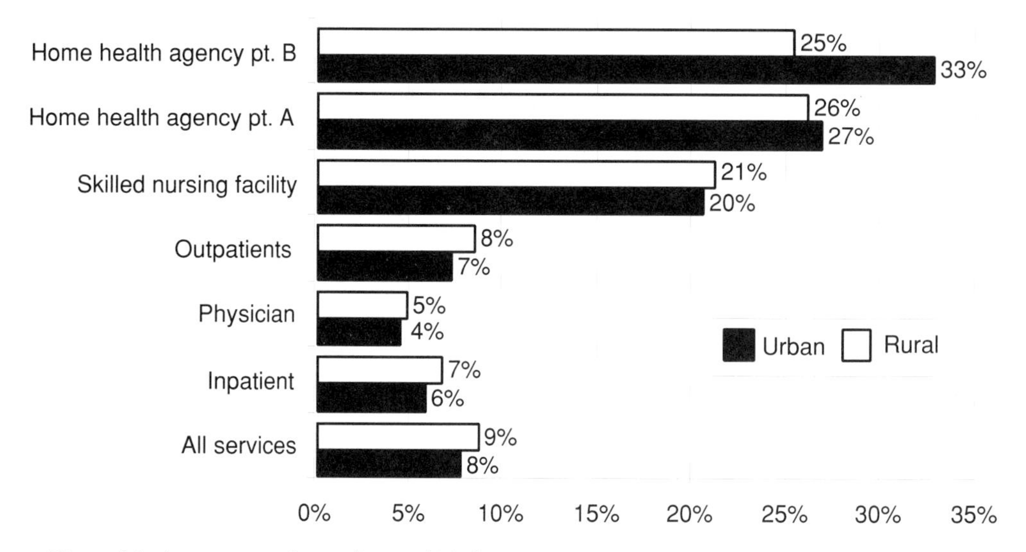

Figure 6.3. Average annual growth rate of Medicare program payments per recipient, 1990 to 1995, by type of service, rural and urban areas.

Urban-rural differences in the rates of change in the number of service recipients are more dramatic than differences in the growth rates of payment per recipient. Overall, the number of program service recipients in rural areas increased by 1% per year between 1990 and 1995. By contrast, average annual growth in the number of service recipients in urban areas was greater by a factor of three. Numbers of rural recipients of inpatient services and Part B home health services, however, fell between 1990 and 1995 as corresponding numbers in urban areas increased (Fig. 6.4).

BENEFICIARY ISSUES

Administrative program data are useful in indicating the size of the Medicare program and differences in expenditure levels and trends, overall and by service type, between rural and rural areas. These data, however, are not routinely used to study issues of beneficiary access and satisfaction with the program. Instead, beneficiary issues have been addressed with data from HCFA's ongoing Medicare Current Beneficiary Survey (MCBS) and with administrative claims data that are used to study

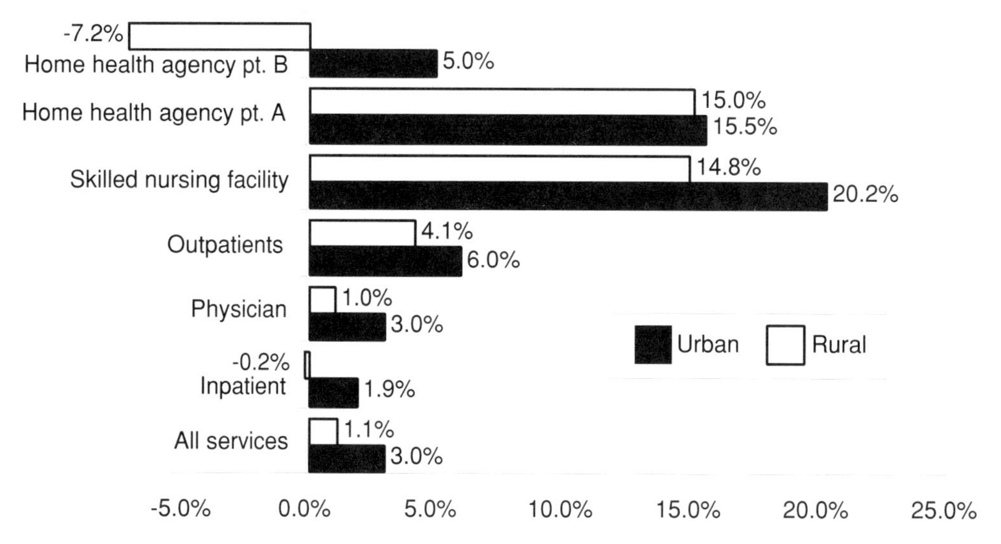

Figure 6.4. Average annual rate of growth in beneficiaries receiving Medicare benefits, 1990 to 1995, by type of service, rural and urban areas.

use of specific services by beneficiaries (e.g., Physician Pay-ment Review Commission [PPRC], 1996, 1992). Although these analyses sometimes present estimates for metropolitan and rural areas, little information is presented on how access and satisfaction vary within different types of rural and urban areas. In the remainder of this section, estimates on access and beneficiary satisfaction are presented for different types of rural and urban areas, based on data from the MCBS.

Data

The MCBS is an ongoing panel survey of Medicare beneficiaries. Sampled respondents are followed up over time and questioned each year. In addition, the sample is refreshed each year to adjust for changing demographic characteristics of the elderly population. The sample's composition is designed to be representative of various Medicare populations, such as all program beneficiaries and aged, non-institutionalized beneficiaries. The survey covers a variety of health care topics related to the use of and access to medical care, health status and chronic conditions, and information on the beneficiary's household and assets. It is also possible to link the survey data with the sampled respondent's Medicare claims. These can be used to study the types of services received, expenditures on medical care, and how these relate to personal and family characteristics described by survey responses.

In order to obtain estimates for persons residing in different types of rural areas, data on MCBS survey respondents were linked with the U.S. Department of Agriculture's (USDA) "urban influence" system of classifying counties (Ricketts and Johnson-Webb, 1997). This system classifies U.S. counties into one of nine categories, depending on the county's population and whether it is part of, or adjacent to, a county that has a sufficient population to be deemed metropolitan. Examination of the linked MCBS data revealed that some of the nonmetropolitan county group categories contained too few respondents to represent certain types of rural areas sufficiently, so several of the categories were combined to avoid the lack of precision that accompanies small samples.* Additional investigation revealed little variation across the newly defined nonmetropolitan areas. Therefore, estimates below are presented for the following four county-level urban-rural categories. Categories 1 and 2 are for metropolitan counties (and are defined as categories 1 and 2 under the urban influence coding system). Categories 3 and 4 are for nonmetropolitan counties.

Metropolitan:

1. Counties with a resident population of at least 1 million persons.
2. Counties with a resident population of fewer than 1 million persons.

Non-metropolitan:

3. Counties adjacent to a metropolitan county.
4. Counties not adjacent to a metropolitan county.

In the analysis that follows, category 3 is the aggregate of counties under the urban influence system that are adjacent to metropolitan areas (urban influence categories 3 through 6); category 4 is counties that the urban influence system categorizes that are non-adjacent to metropolitan areas (categories 7 through 9).

In the remainder of this section, estimates from the linked MCBS are presented. First, estimates for several dimensions of access are presented: the percentages of the elderly beneficiary population who use selected types of care, including physician office visits, outpatient department and clinic services, and hospital inpatient services. Second, estimates of the percentage of elderly beneficiaries who claim to have had influenza and pneumonia vaccinations are reported as indicators of access to preventive services. Third, survey findings on how beneficiaries rate their health status are presented. Finally, estimates of the percentage of beneficiaries who are satisfied with various aspects of the health care system are discussed. For each set of estimates, results are presented for residents of the four metropolitan/nonmetropolitan county groups. Statistical tests on differences were performed, as noted, using t-tests of differences in population proportions; for purposes of this discussion, an alpha level of 0.01 is used to determine statistical significance.*

Traditional Access Measures

Access to care is a concept traditionally used by health care policy makers and researchers to refer to the availability and accessibility of medical care.† A number of factors can influence access to care, including geographic location, the supply of health care workers and facilities, family income and insurance status, cultural beliefs, and other sociodemographic characteristics of the population. The Medicare program eliminates some barriers to access based on ability to pay by virtue of its insurance features. At the same time, out-of-pocket expenses can be

*This problem is addressed in Stearns, Slifkin, and Walke (1997).

*An alpha-level of 0.05 is not used because standard errors have not been adjusted for complete survey design effects.

†A discussion of the appropriateness of access as a measure is discussed in detail in Chapter 2, Access to Health Care for Rural Patients.

Table 6.3 Percentage of Elderly Medicare Beneficiaries with an Ambulatory Physician Contact, by Type of Contact, Urban and Rural Areas, 1994

	Modified Urban Influence Code Categories				
	Metro		*Nonmetro*		
Type of Contact	*1*	*2*	*3*	*4*	*All*
Office	71.5%	80.5%	80.4%	78.4%	76.2%
Hospital Outpatient	45.7%	52.4%	59.4%	63.6%	51.6%
Office, Outpatient or Emergency Room	75.0 %	83.6%	86.0%	85.8%	80.4%

Source: Project HOPE Walsh Center for Rural Health Analysis, MCBS data linked with Modified categories of the Urban Influence Codes.

substantial for the rural elderly (Laschober, 1997). Given that the rural population has a higher proportion of older persons and that Medicare is a vital component of rural health care revenue, Medicare beneficiaries constitute a significant segment of the demand for medical care in rural health areas. Beneficiary contact with physicians is examined to measure how well program beneficiaries are accessing health care in rural areas.

Eighty percent (80%) of elderly Medicare beneficiaries had a physician contact through an office visit, visit to a hospital outpatient department, or an emergency room in 1994 (Table 6.3). The percent of beneficiaries with at least one physician contact varies from 75% in metropolitan counties with one million or more residents (residents of counties in urban influence category 1) to 86% of residents of counties adjacent to metropolitan areas. This difference is statistically significant at the 0.01 level. Beneficiaries in nonmetropolitan counties appear to enjoy access to office and hospital outpatient visits that is similar or better than in metropolitan counties. Seventy-eight percent (78%) had office contacts in the non-adjacent counties; 72% of beneficiaries in the most populated metropolitan counties had an office contact ($p < 0.01$). Sixty-four percent (64%) in the most rural counties, and 46% in the most urban counties, had outpatient visits (difference significant, $p < 0.01$).

The average Medicare beneficiary had 5.1 office visits and the average beneficiary with at least one office visit had 6.7 visits (Table 6.4). The number of physician contacts does not exhibit much variation across geographic areas.

Another access measure is the percent of the population with a hospital inpatient stay. A greater percentage of elderly beneficiaries in the most rural counties had an inpatient stay than in the most urban counties. Over 18% of the elderly in the most nonmetropolitan counties were hospitalized, versus about 16% in metropolitan counties (Table 6.5), but these differences are not statistically significant at the 0.01 level. The greatest rates of hospitalization appear to be in counties that are not adjacent to a metropolitan county (counties in categories 5 and 6).

Table 6.4 Mean Number of Physician Office Visits per Medicare Beneficiary, Urban and Rural Areas, 1994

	Modified Urban Influence Code Categories				
	Metro		*Nonmetro*		
Mean Number of Office Visits by	*1*	*2*	*3*	*4*	*All*
All beneficiaries	5.2	5.3	4.7	4.8	5.1
Beneficiaries with at least 1 office visit	7.3	6.5	5.8	6.2	6.7

Source: Project HOPE Walsh Center for Rural Health Analysis, MCBS data linked to Modified urban influence code categories.

Table 6.5 Percentage of Elderly Medicare Beneficiaries with an Inpatient Hospital Stay, Urban and Rural Areas, 1994 (percent)

	Modified Urban Influence Code Categories				
	Metro		*Nonmetro*		
	1	*2*	*3*	*4*	*All*
Percent with Inpatient Stay	16.4	15.5	15.3	18.5	16.1

Source: Project HOPE Walsh Center for Rural Health Analysis, MCBS data linked to Modified urban influence code categories.

Estimates of the percentage of elderly beneficiaries receiving influenza and pneumonia vaccines show that overall, 59.0% of beneficiaries reported receiving an influenza vaccine in winter 1993, and 24.1% reported having received the pneumonia vaccine (Table 6.6). Nonmetropolitan counties not adjacent to metropolitan areas had the lowest percentage of beneficiaries receiving the influenza vaccine—55%. Vaccinations in the most populated urban areas also were below average; 58% of beneficiaries reported having received the influenza vaccine. The pattern for receipt of the pneumonia vaccine is similar. Although urban-rural differences may be indicated by these estimates, differences appear to be small. Furthermore, there appears to be as much variation within metropolitan and nonmetropolitan areas as across the metropolitan and nonmetropolitan areas. Estimates of traditional access measures presented above do not reveal large urban-rural differentials, with the possible exception of inpatient admissions. Data indicate that admissions may more frequently occur among beneficiaries who reside in counties that are nonadjacent to metropolitan counties. One explanation for this pattern of utilization is that the rural population is a sicker population. In rural areas, nonprice barriers of access, such as longer travel times, cause people to postpone visiting the physician. The rural population might delay visits to the physician, which leads to the need for a different kind and more intensive care later on. Although ambulatory care visit rates are comparable to rates in urban areas (see above), nonmonetary price barriers that may not exist in urban areas may have been overcome in rural areas because of greater needs of rural residents. Alternatively, access to hospital care may be facilitated in many nonmetropolitan areas through the availability of small, rural hospitals.

Evidence in support of a less healthy rural population from the MCBS is mixed. On the one hand, health status of rural beneficiaries may be poorer than in metropolitan areas (Table 6.7). The fraction of beneficiaries in excellent health in each of the nonmetropolitan county groups (ranging from 15% to about 17%) is less than the fraction for metropolitan counties (ranging from 18% to 19.3% of elderly beneficiaries). In a similar fashion, the percent of persons in fair or poor health in each of the nonmetropolitan areas (25% to about 27%) exceeds the metropolitan rates (22% and 23%). The percent of beneficiaries in fair/poor health in nonadjacent counties, 27%, exceeds the percent in the most metropolitan coun-

Table 6.6 Percentage of Elderly Medicare Beneficiaries Receiving an Influenza Vaccination the Previous Winter and Percentage Ever Vaccinated for Pneumonia, Urban and Rural Areas, 1994

	Modified Urban Influence Code Categories				
	Metro		*Nonmetro*		
	1	*2*	*3*	*4*	*All*
Percent receiving influenza shot	57.5	61.5	60.3	55.4	59.0
Percent receiving pneumonia shot	22.3	25.3	27.6	24.9	24.3

Source: Project HOPE Walsh Center for Rural Health Analysis. Calculations of MCBS data linked with Modified urban influence codecategories.

Table 6.7 Health Status of Elderly Medicare Beneficiaries, Urban and Rural Areas, 1994 (percent)

	Modified Urban Influence Code Categories				
	Metro		*Nonmetro*		
	1	*2*	*3*	*4*	*All*
Excellent	19.3	18.0	15.0	16.6	18.0
Very Good/Good	58.7	59.5	59.8	56.7	59.0
Fair/Poor	22.0	22.5	25.2	26.7	23.1

Source: Project HOPE Walsh Center for Rural Health Analysis. Calculations of MCBS data linked with Modified urban influence code categories.

ties, 22% (p<0.01). However, urban versus rural differences are not very large.

Beneficiary Satisfaction

Data from the MCBS reveal that program beneficiaries—both in rural and in urban areas—are satisfied with the Medicare program. Ninety-six percent (96%) of beneficiaries indicate satisfaction with the overall quality of medical care, and little variation in the level of satisfaction over quality exists within and across residents in metropolitan and nonmetropolitan counties. Contrary to expectations, the rural elderly are not less satisfied with the availability of care on nights and weekends. Although somewhat fewer elderly beneficiaries in the most remote counties are satisfied with the ease of commuting to receive medical care than residents of metropolitan areas (91.9% in remote counties, versus 94.3% in the largest metropolitan counties), the difference is small and not statistically significant. Although these findings suggest that rural and urban residents do not significantly differ in their levels of satisfaction, it is important to note that satisfaction is relative to expectations, and that rural and urban residents may have different expectations concerning their needs and provider behavior.

PROGRAM PAYMENTS TO MANAGED CARE PLANS

Medicare beneficiaries have been permitted to enroll in qualified Health Maintenance Organizations (HMOs) since 1982 (PPRC, 1997). Of the HMOs choosing to enroll Medicare beneficiaries, the vast majority have what are known as "risk contracts" with the Medicare program. Under this arrangement, the HMO agrees to provide all Medicare-covered services to enrolled beneficiaries in exchange for a fixed monthly capitation payment from Medicare. Because health plans with these types of contracts accept all insurance risk for enrolled beneficiaries, they are commonly referred to as "risk plans." The discussion below describes the methods used to compute the monthly capitation payments for Medicare risk plans, and presents results of simulations describing the expected impact of recent legislative changes to the payment method while highlighting rural-urban differences.

The AAPCC Method

Prior to the Balanced Budget Act (BBA) of 1997, the monthly capitation payment received by Medicare risk plans was based on the adjusted average per capita cost (AAPCC). The AAPCC rates for each county—or state, in the case of the End-Stage Renal Disease (ESRD) program—were set annually by HCFA, using historical expenditure data to project what Medicare would expect to pay during the next year if the beneficiary remained in the traditional Medicare fee-for-service (FFS) system. Each county's base payment was actually set at 95% of its AAPCC. This county base payment was then translated into a capitation payment for a given Medicare risk plan enrollee by applying a series of individual risk adjustments to account for factors such as the enrollee's age, gender, institutional status, and so forth.

From a rural perspective, the AAPCC payment method resulted in two key problems. First, the payment rates in rural areas were, on average, lower than rates in urban areas, reflecting the historically lower Medicare expenditures in rural areas compared to urban areas. Second, payment rates in many rural areas tended to fluctuate dramatically from year to year because of the small number of Medicare beneficiaries residing in many rural counties and the fact that a change in expenditures for even a few beneficiaries could dramatically affect the mean expenditures for the county. The relatively lower payment rates and higher rate volatility in rural areas contributed to plans' reluctance to enter these areas (Casey, 1997; Serrato, Brown, and Bergeron, 1995), and this relative unavailability of managed care plans in rural areas is reflected in their low Medicare HMO enrollment rates (see Chapter 10, Rural Managed Care).

The limited availability of managed care options for rural beneficiaries is of concern largely because Medicare HMOs have typically offered their enrollees benefits that extend beyond the standard Medicare benefit package (e.g., outpatient prescription drug coverage, routine

Plate 1.1. Percent Rural Population by County, 1990

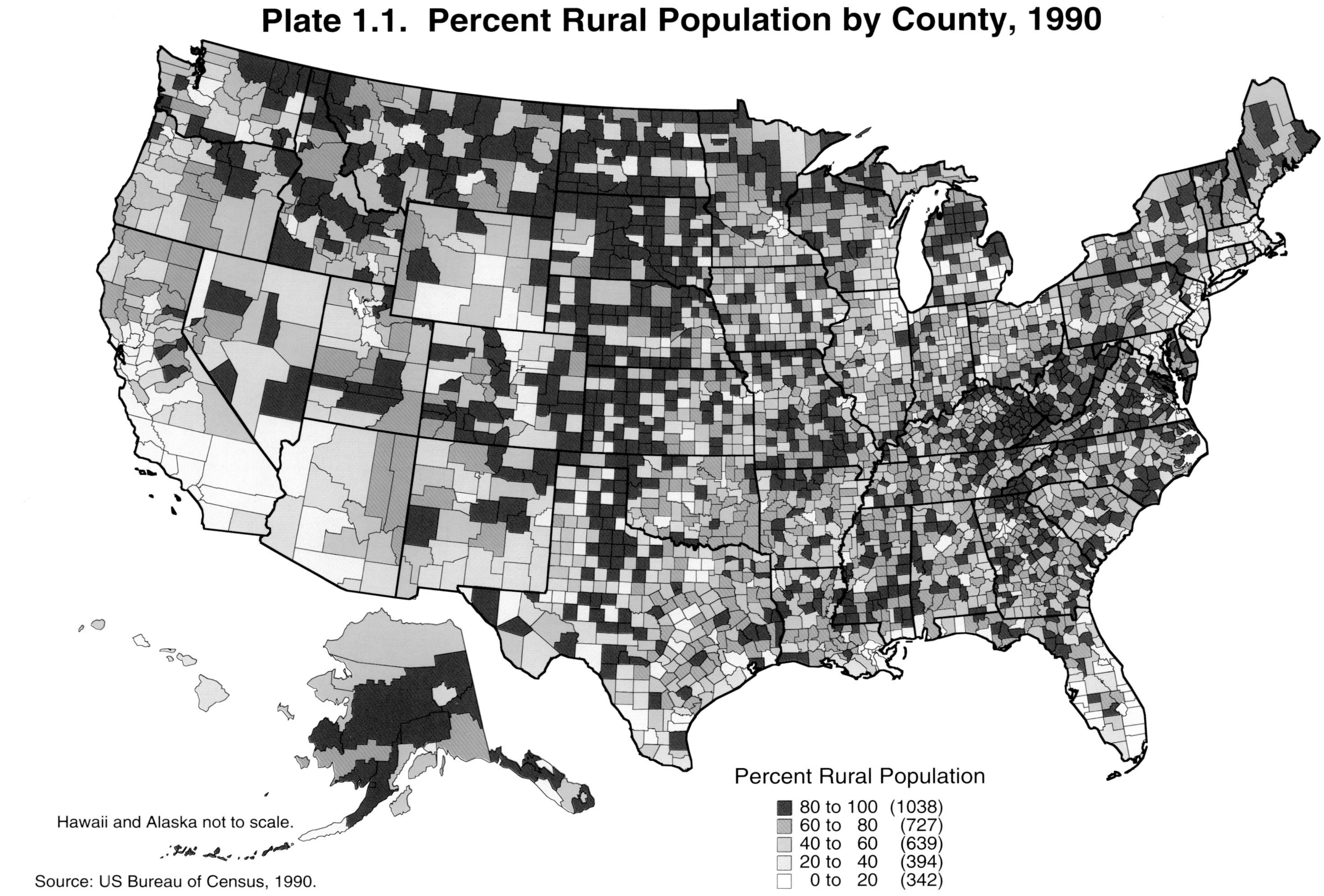

Source: US Bureau of Census, 1990.

Produced by: North Carolina Rural Health Research and Policy Analysis Center, Cecil G. Sheps Center for Health Services Research, University of North Carolina at Chapel Hill, with support from the Federal Office of Rural Health Policy, HRSA, US DHHS.

Plate 1.2. Nonmetropolitan Counties, 1998

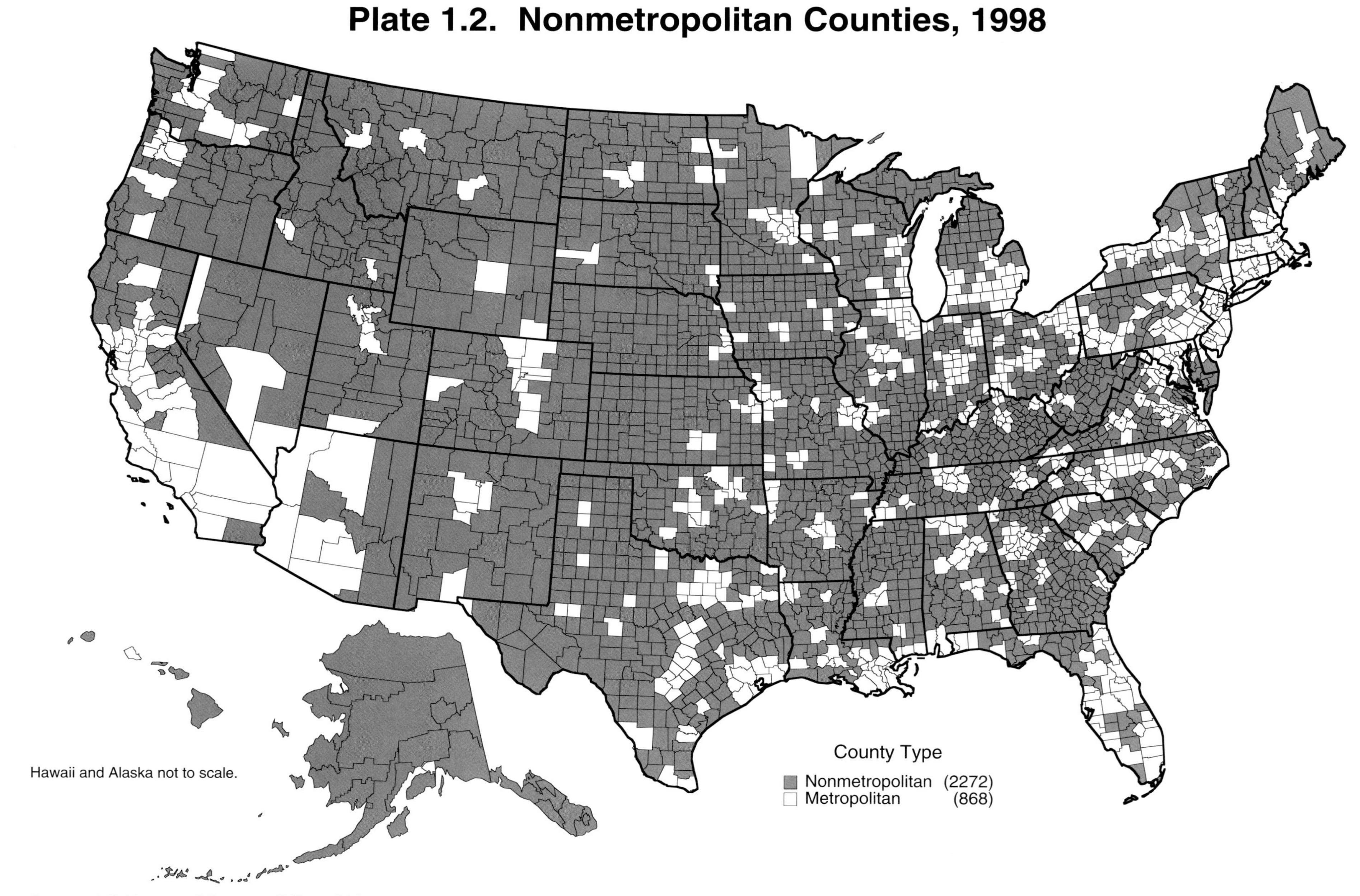

Source: US Bureau of Census; Office of Management and Budget, 1998.

Produced by: North Carolina Rural Health Research and Policy Analysis Center,
Cecil G. Sheps Center for Health Services Research, University of North Carolina at Chapel Hill.

Plate 1.3. Urban Influence Codes, 1997

Metropolitan and Nonmetropolitan Counties

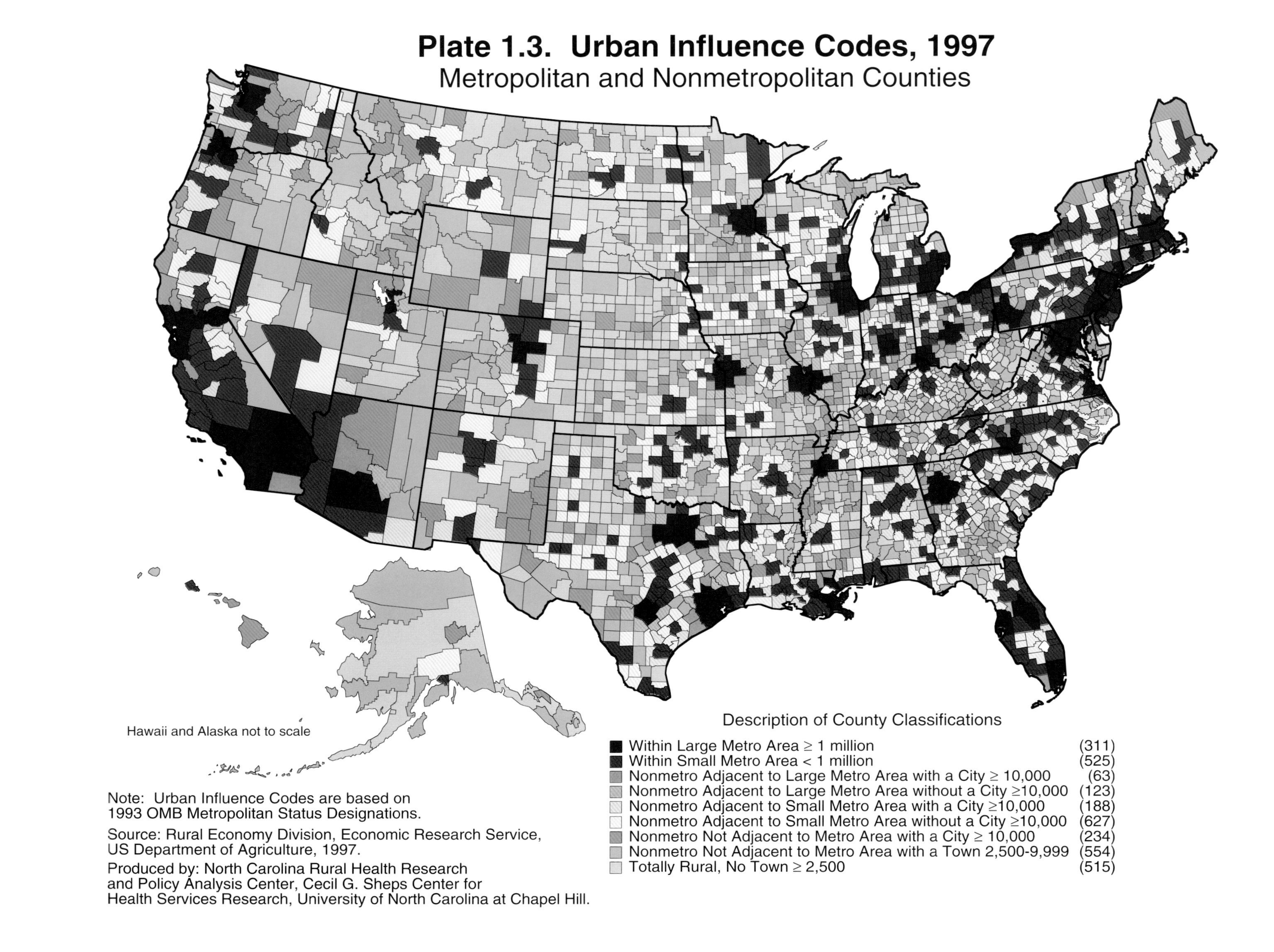

Note: Urban Influence Codes are based on 1993 OMB Metropolitan Status Designations.

Source: Rural Economy Division, Economic Research Service, US Department of Agriculture, 1997.

Produced by: North Carolina Rural Health Research and Policy Analysis Center, Cecil G. Sheps Center for Health Services Research, University of North Carolina at Chapel Hill.

Plate 1.4. Rural-Urban Continuum Codes, 1994

Metropolitan and Nonmetropolitan Counties

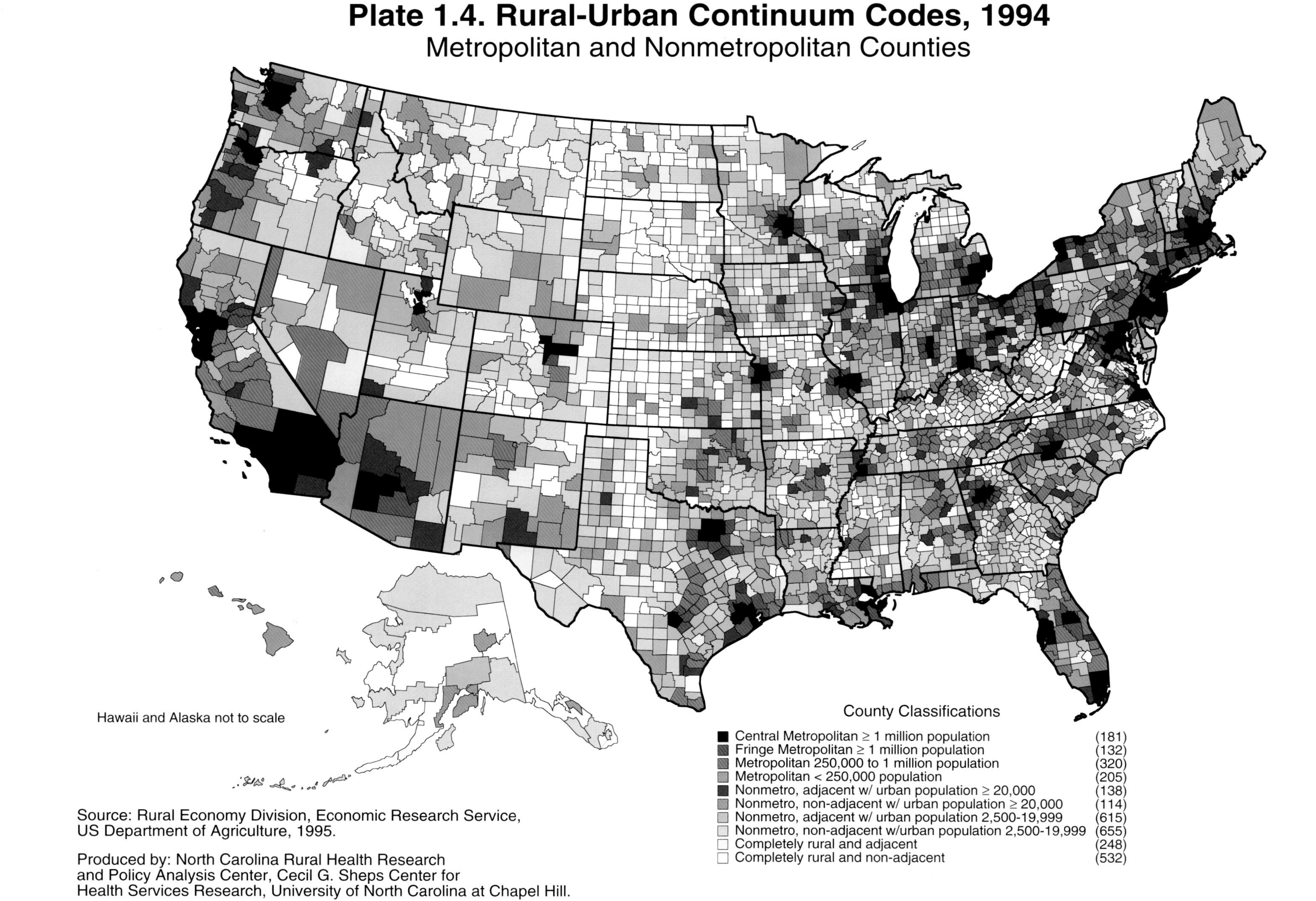

Source: Rural Economy Division, Economic Research Service, US Department of Agriculture, 1995.

Produced by: North Carolina Rural Health Research and Policy Analysis Center, Cecil G. Sheps Center for Health Services Research, University of North Carolina at Chapel Hill.

Plate 1.5. Mortality Rates, All Causes, 1990-1994

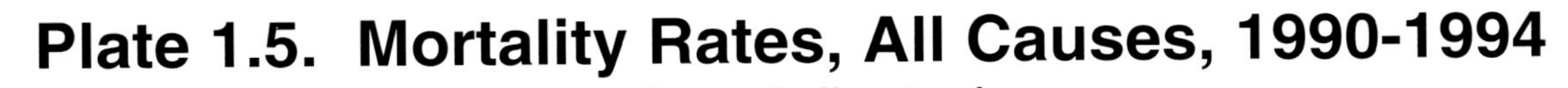

Age-Adjusted

Nonmetropolitan Counties

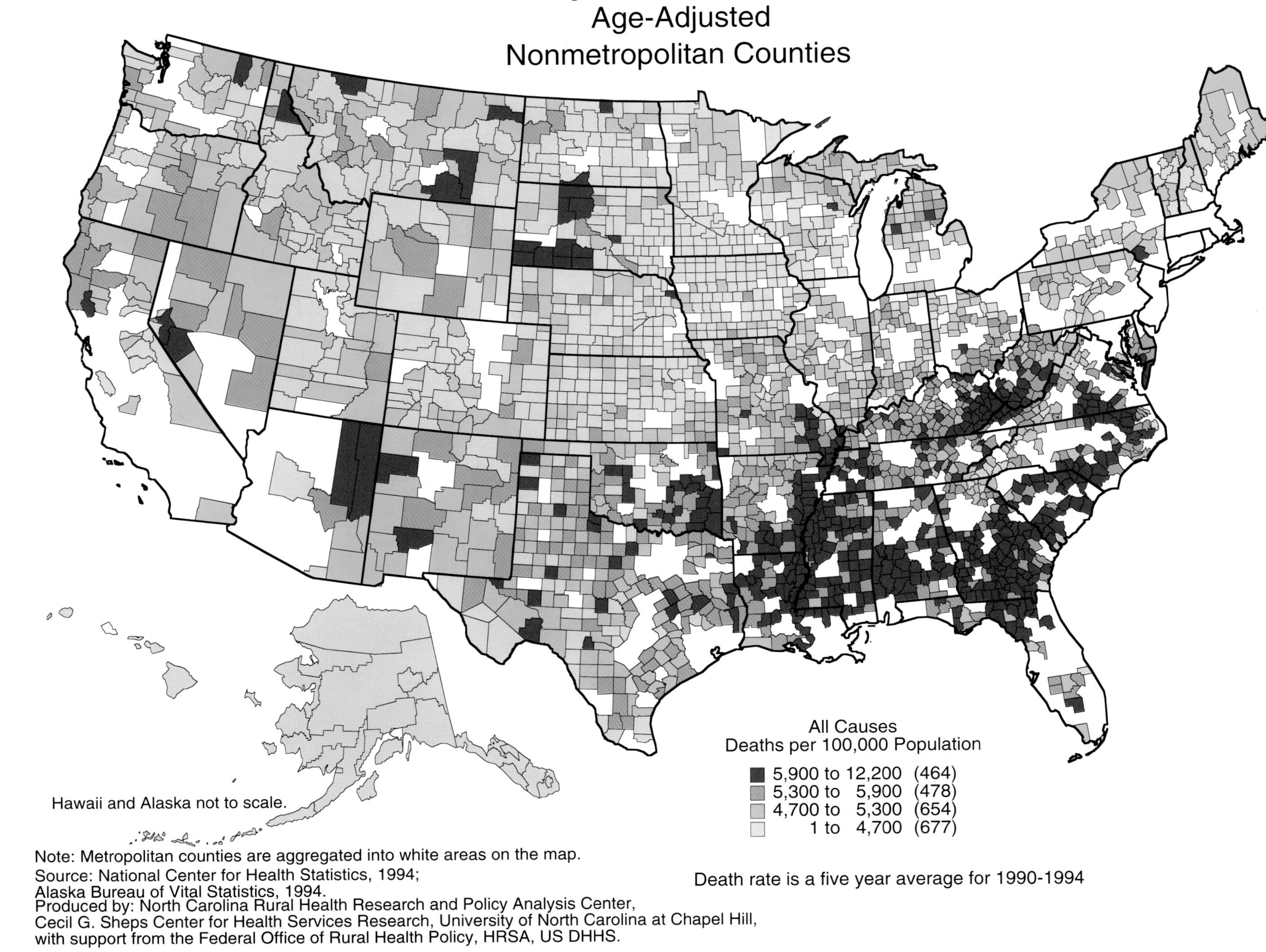

Note: Metropolitan counties are aggregated into white areas on the map.

Source: National Center for Health Statistics, 1994;
Alaska Bureau of Vital Statistics, 1994.

Produced by: North Carolina Rural Health Research and Policy Analysis Center,
Cecil G. Sheps Center for Health Services Research, University of North Carolina at Chapel Hill,
with support from the Federal Office of Rural Health Policy, HRSA, US DHHS.

Plate 3.1. Primary Care Health Professional Shortage Areas (HPSAs), 1997

Nonmetropolitan Counties

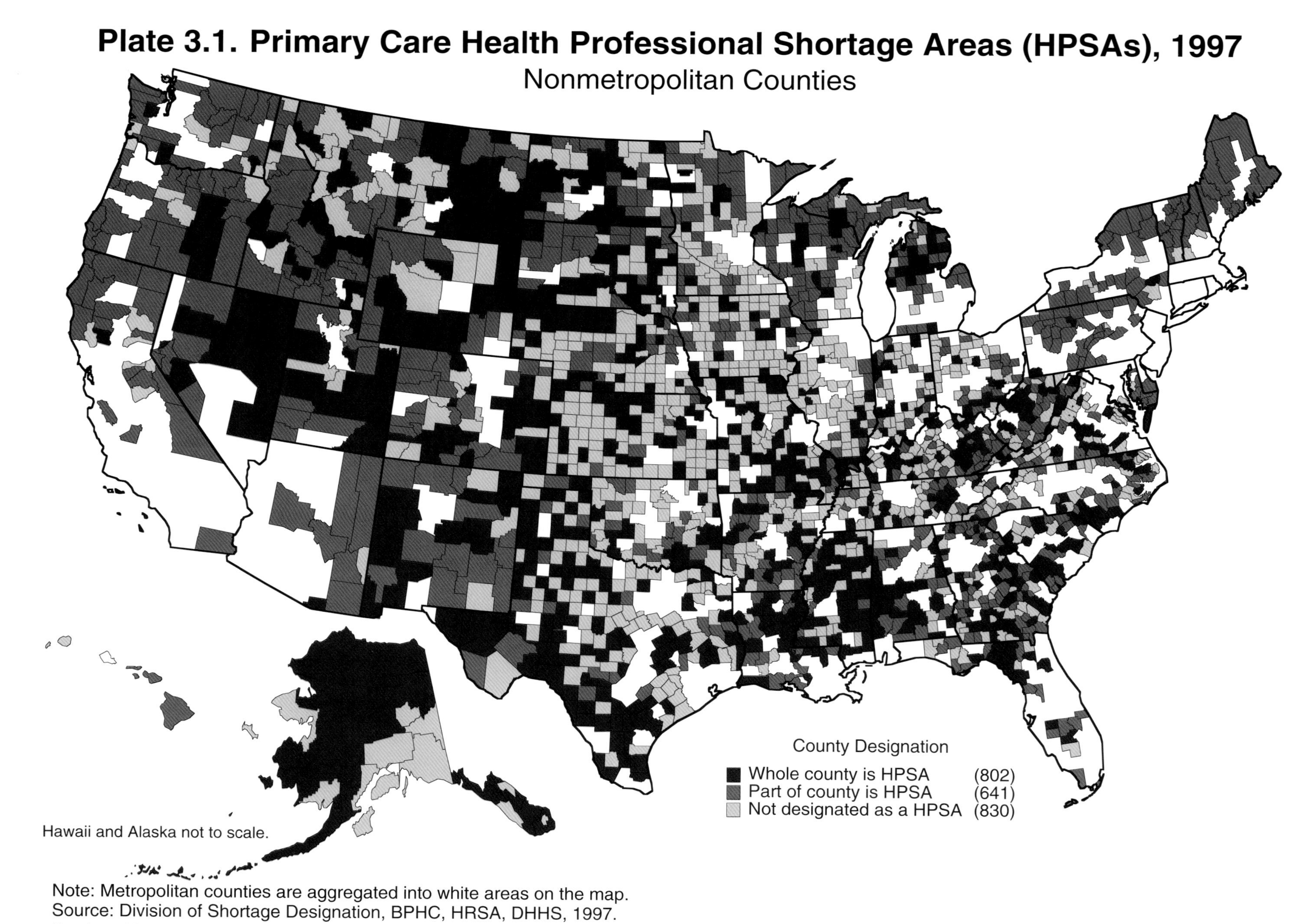

Note: Metropolitan counties are aggregated into white areas on the map.

Source: Division of Shortage Designation, BPHC, HRSA, DHHS, 1997.

Produced by: North Carolina Rural Health Research and Policy Analysis Center, Cecil G. Sheps Center for Health Services Research, University of North Carolina at Chapel Hill, with support from the Federal Office of Rural Health Policy, HRSA, US DHHS.

Plate 4.1. Population Per Nurse Practitioner, 1994

Nonmetropolitan Counties

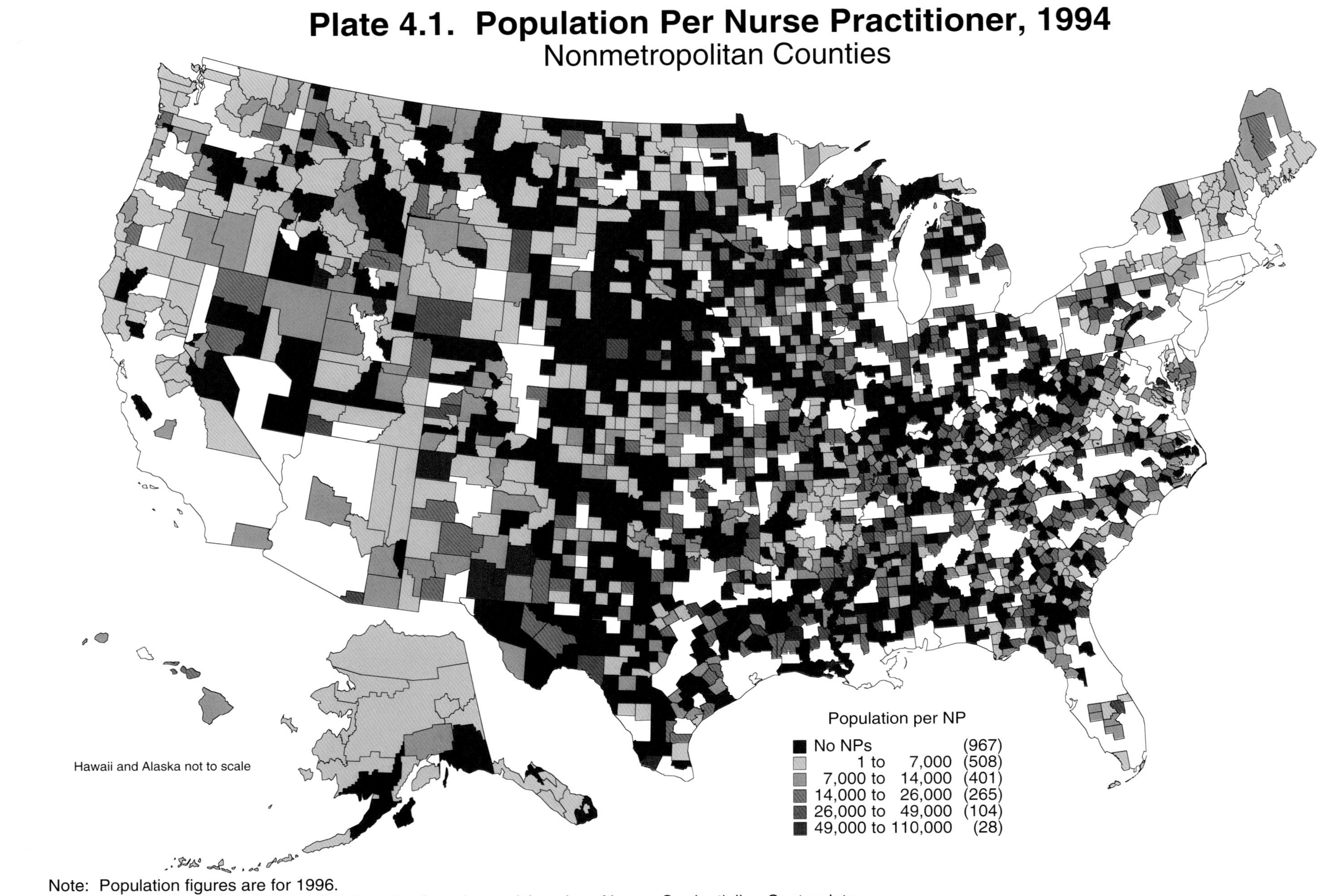

Note: Population figures are for 1996.
Source: Lin et.al., 1996, based on state boards of nursing and American Nurses Credentialing Center data; Area Resource File, OHPAR, HRSA, BHPr, PHS, US DHHS, February, 1997.
Produced By: North Carolina Rural Health Research and Policy Analysis Center, Cecil G. Sheps Center for Health Services Research, University of North Carolina at Chapel Hill.

Plate 4.2. Nonmetropolitan Population per Primary Care Physician Assistant, 1997

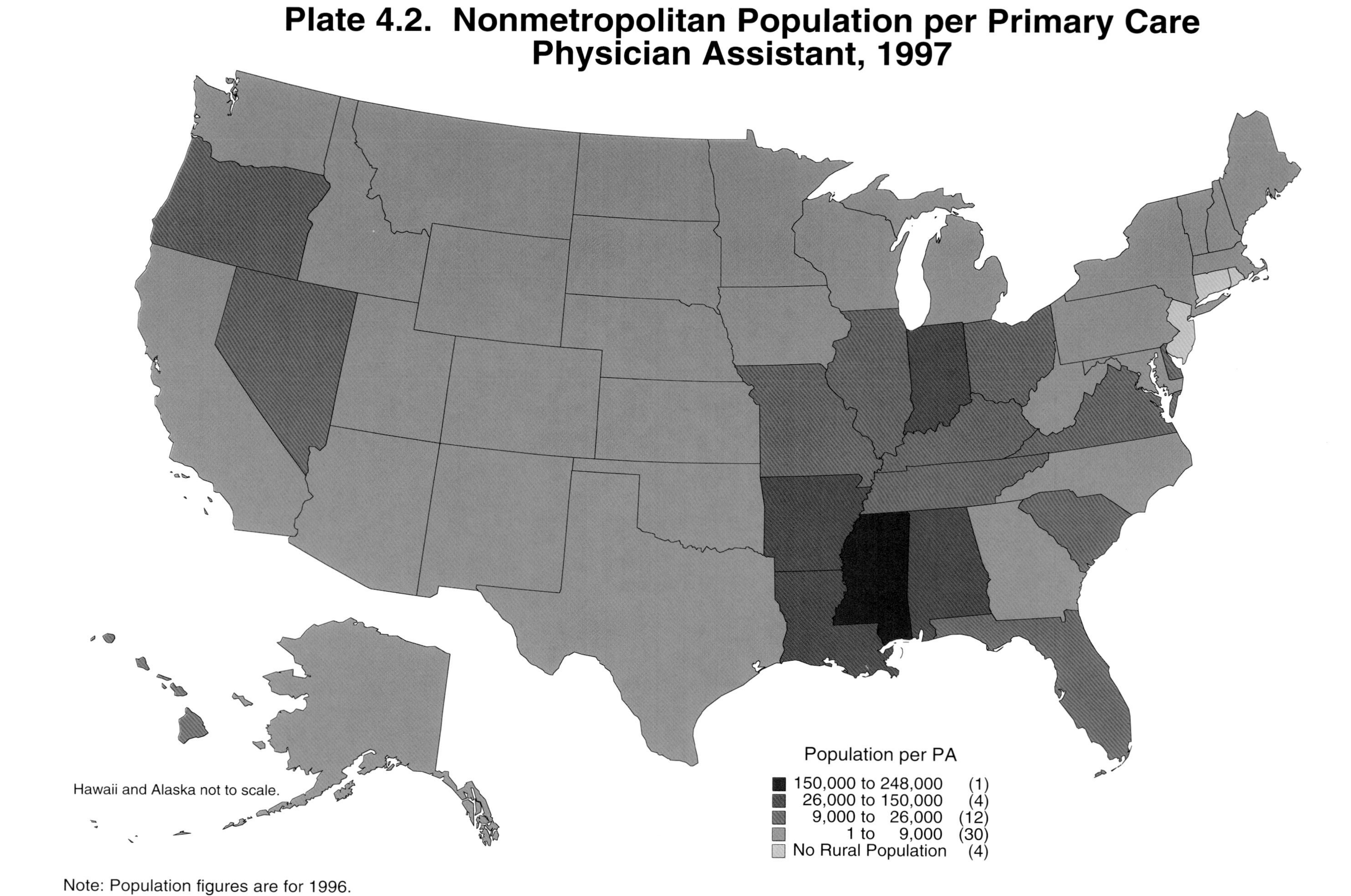

Note: Population figures are for 1996.

Source: American Academy of Physician Assistants, 1998; Area Resource File, OHPAR, BHPr, HRSA, PHS, US DHHS, February, 1997. Produced by: North Carolina Rural Health Research and Policy Analysis Center, Cecil G. Sheps Center for Health Services Research, University of North Carolina at Chapel Hill, with support from the Federal Office of Rural Health Policy, HRSA, US DHHS.

Plate 5.1. Rural Health Outreach and Network Development Award Communities, 1997

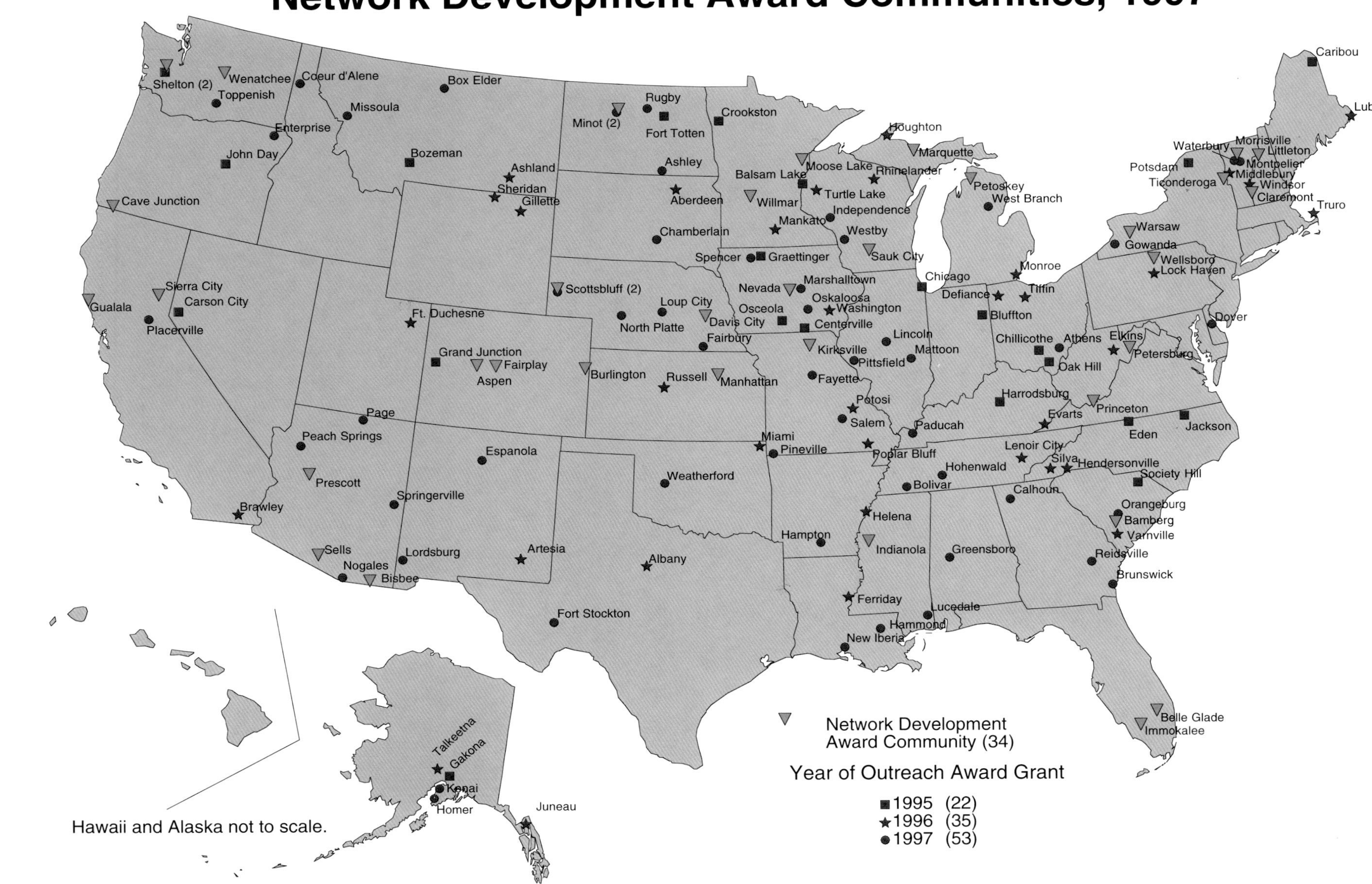

Source: US Office of Rural Health Policy, HRSA, PHS, US DHHS, 1997.

Produced by: North Carolina Rural Health Research and Policy Analysis Center, Cecil G. Sheps Center for Health Services Research, University of North Carolina at Chapel Hill.

Plate 5.2. Certified Rural Health Clinics, 1997

Independent and Provider-Based

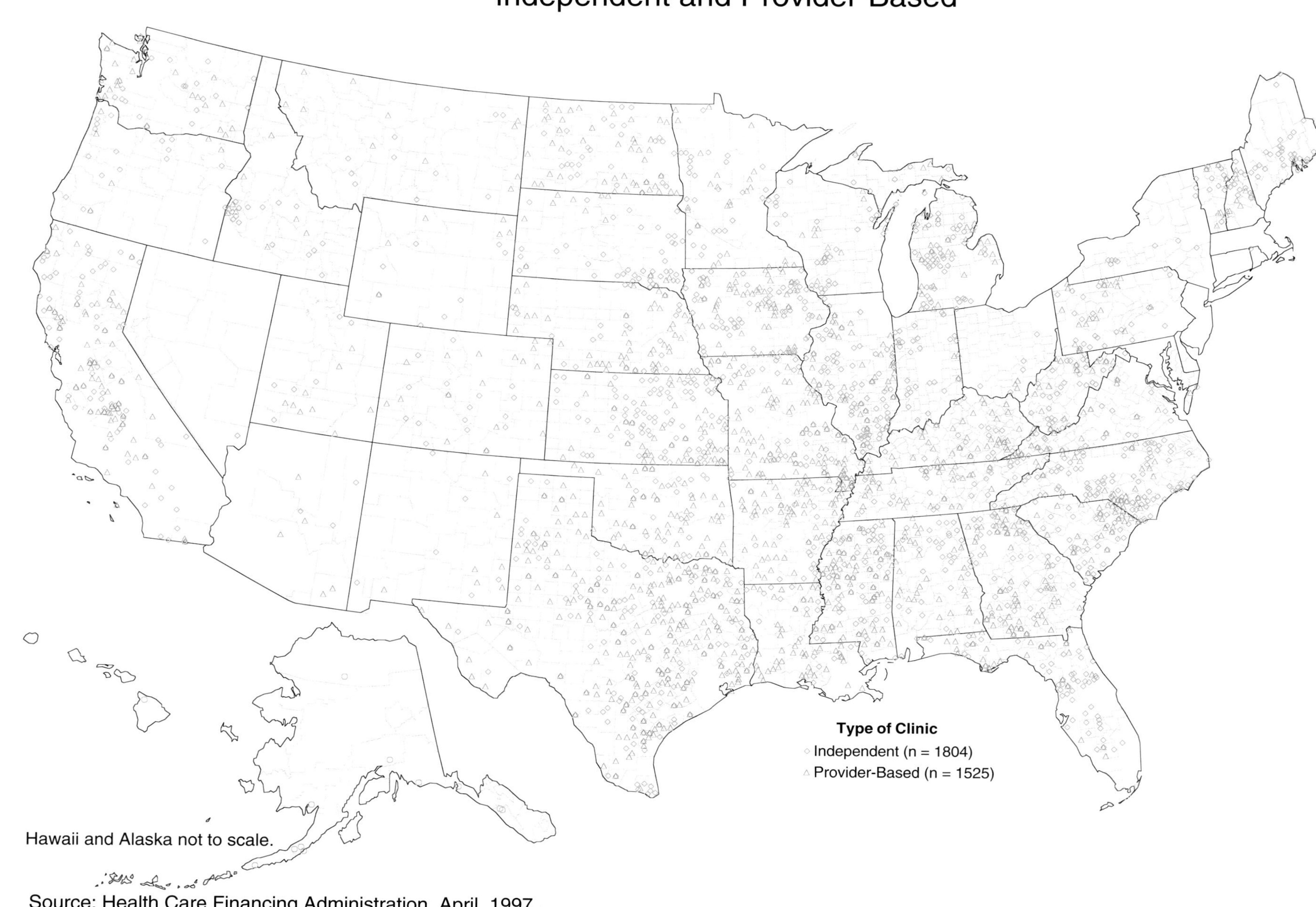

Source: Health Care Financing Administration, April, 1997.

Produced by: North Carolina Rural Health Research and Policy Analysis Center, Cecil G. Sheps Center for Health Services Research, University of North Carolina at Chapel Hill, with support from the Federal Office of Rural Health Policy, HRSA, US DHHS.

Plate 5.3. Location of All National Health Service Corps Placements, 1971-1998*

By Type of Health Professional Placed

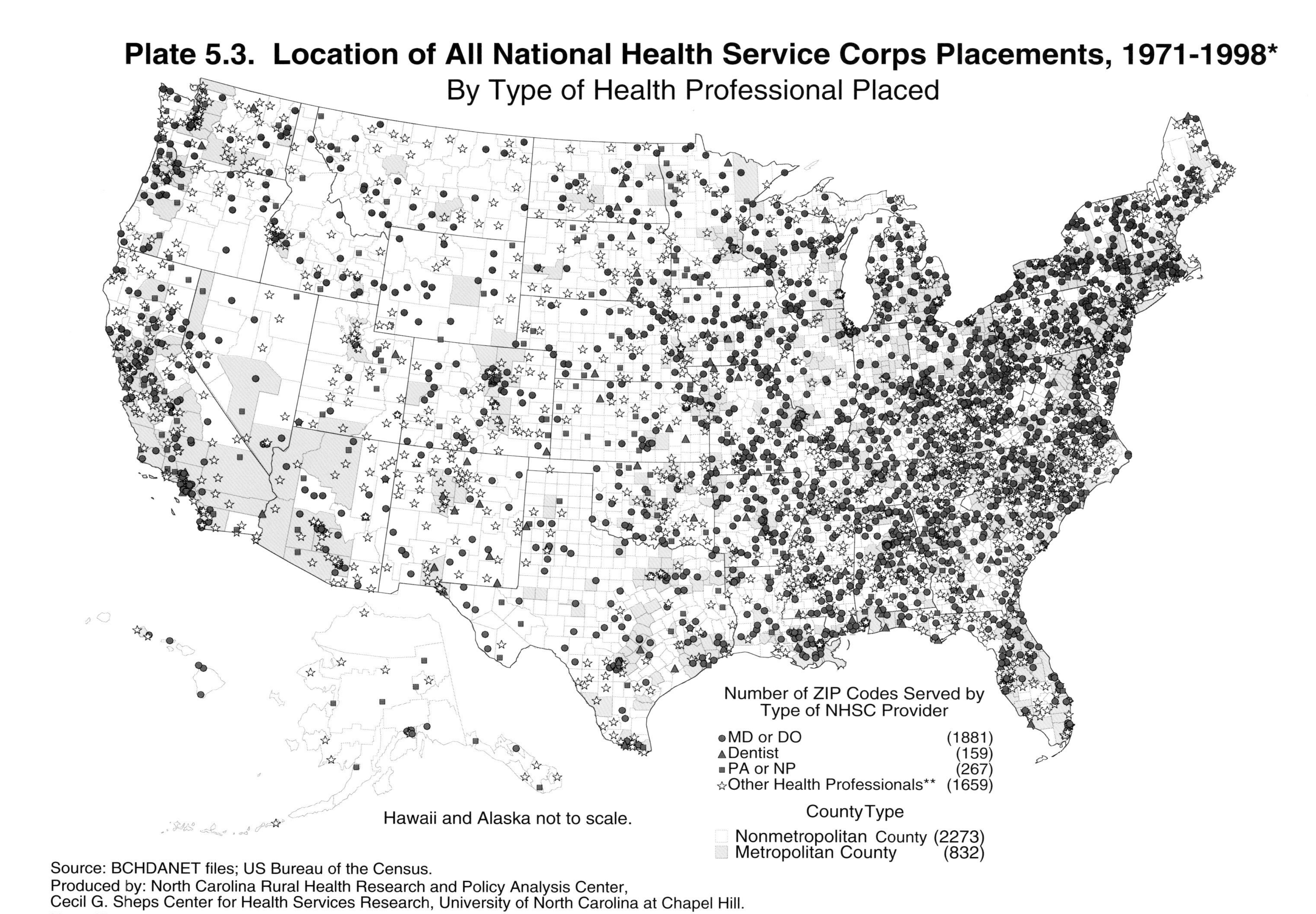

Source: BCHDANET files; US Bureau of the Census.
Produced by: North Carolina Rural Health Research and Policy Analysis Center,
Cecil G. Sheps Center for Health Services Research, University of North Carolina at Chapel Hill.
Note: *Data are cumulative for the years 1971 to 1998;
**Other Health Professionals include certified nurse midwives, nurse midwives, therapists, nurses, social workers, and multiple types of providers.
Not shown on this map are American Samoa, Micronesia, Guam, the Marshall Islands, the Mariana Islands, Puerto Rico, Palau and the Virgin Islands, which also were served by the NHSC.

Plate 11.1. Rural Health Networks by State, 1997

Location of Administrative Office

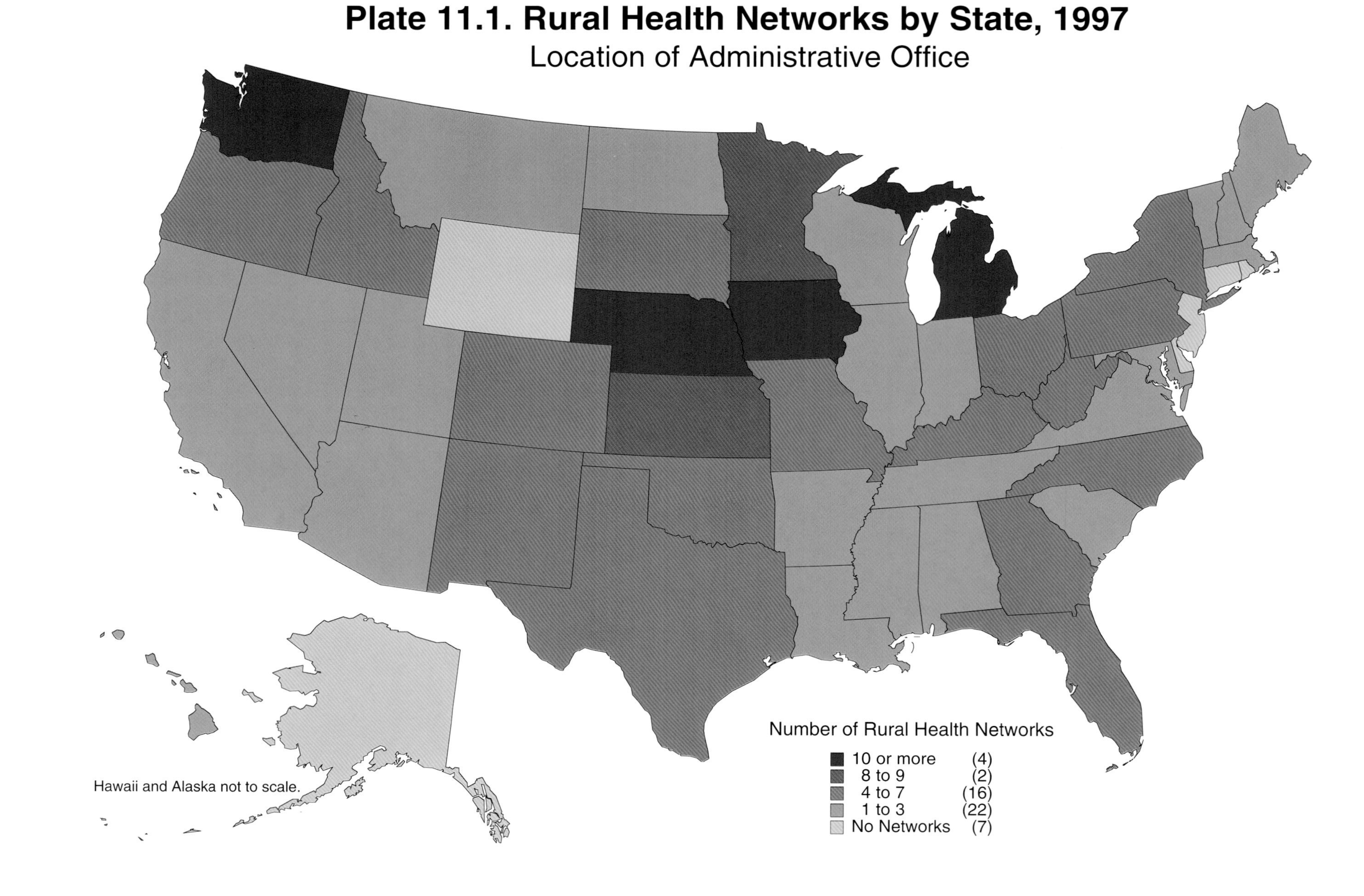

Source: Moscovice, Wellever and Krein, 1997.
Produced by: North Carolina Rural Health Research and Policy Analysis Center,
Cecil G. Sheps Center for Health Services Research, University of North Carolina at Chapel Hill.

Plate 12.1. Infant Mortality Rate, 1991-1995

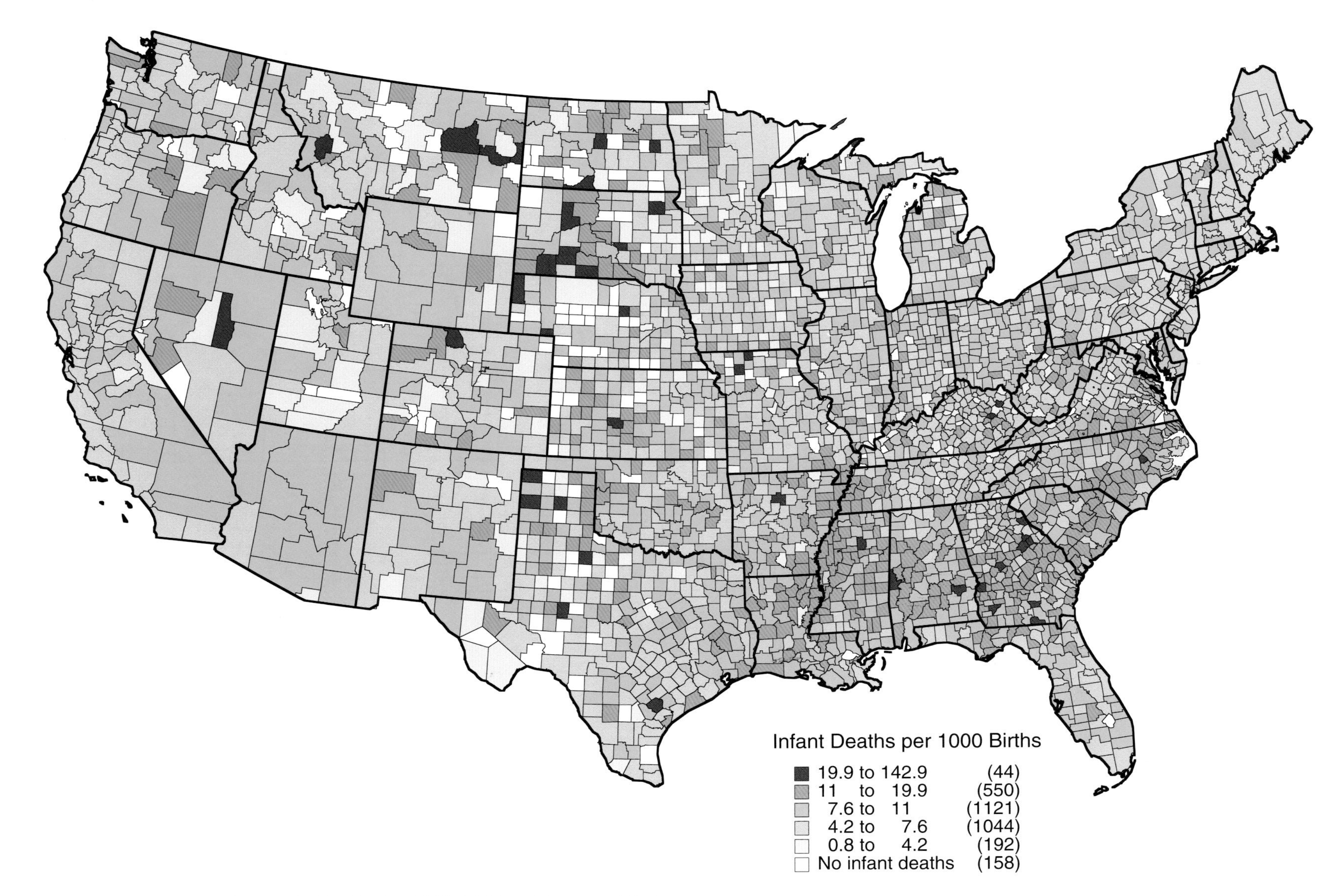

IMR is a five year average for 1991-1995

Source: Area Resource File, ODAM, BHPr, HRSA, PHS, DHHS, February, 1997.

Produced by: North Carolina Rural Health Research and Policy Analysis Center, Cecil G. Sheps Center for Health Services Research, University of North Carolina at Chapel Hill.

Plate 12.2. Low Birth Weight Rate, 1993-1995

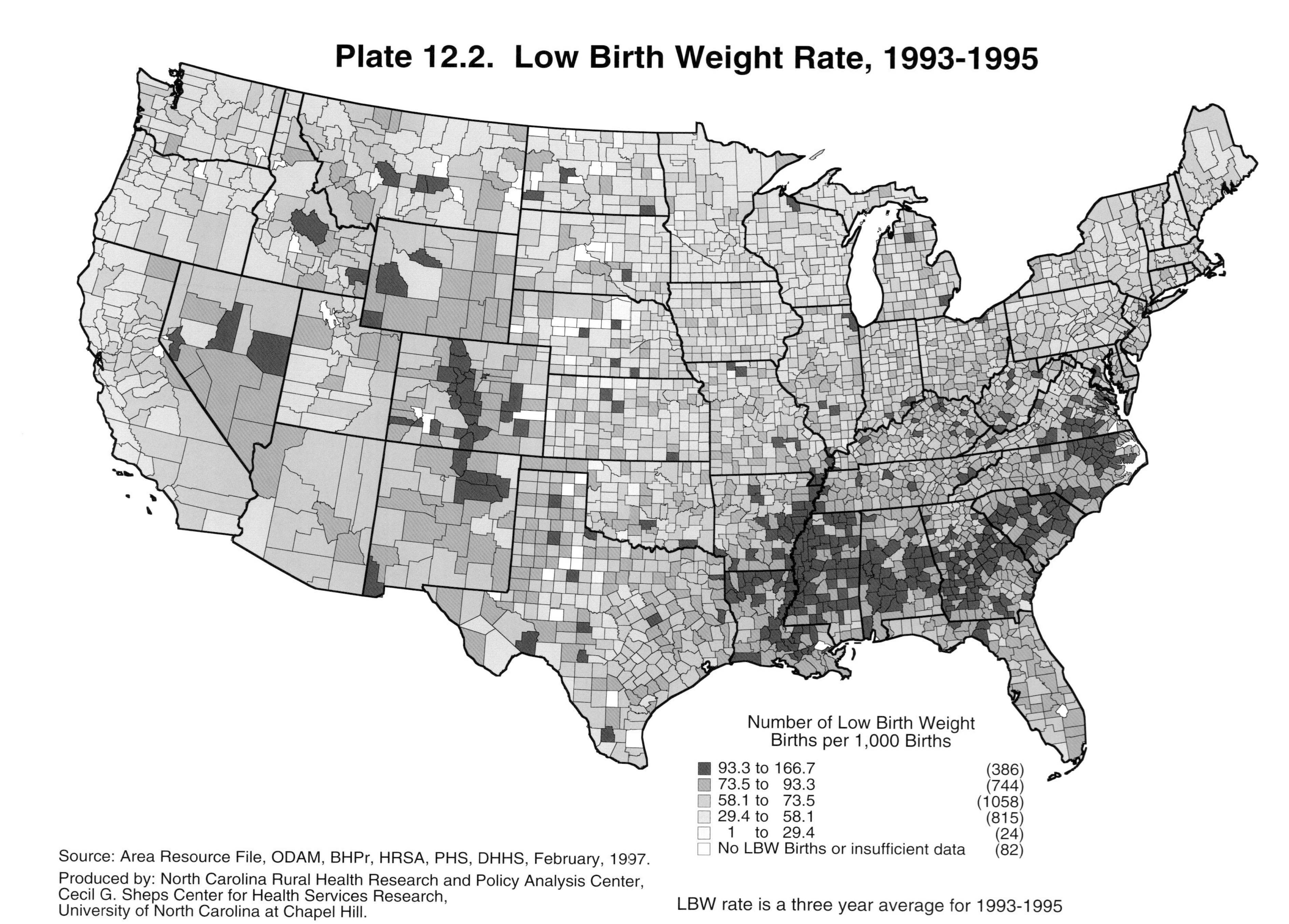

Source: Area Resource File, ODAM, BHPr, HRSA, PHS, DHHS, February, 1997.

Produced by: North Carolina Rural Health Research and Policy Analysis Center, Cecil G. Sheps Center for Health Services Research, University of North Carolina at Chapel Hill.

LBW rate is a three year average for 1993-1995

Plate 14.1. Mental Health Professional Shortage Areas, 1997

Nonmetropolitan Counties

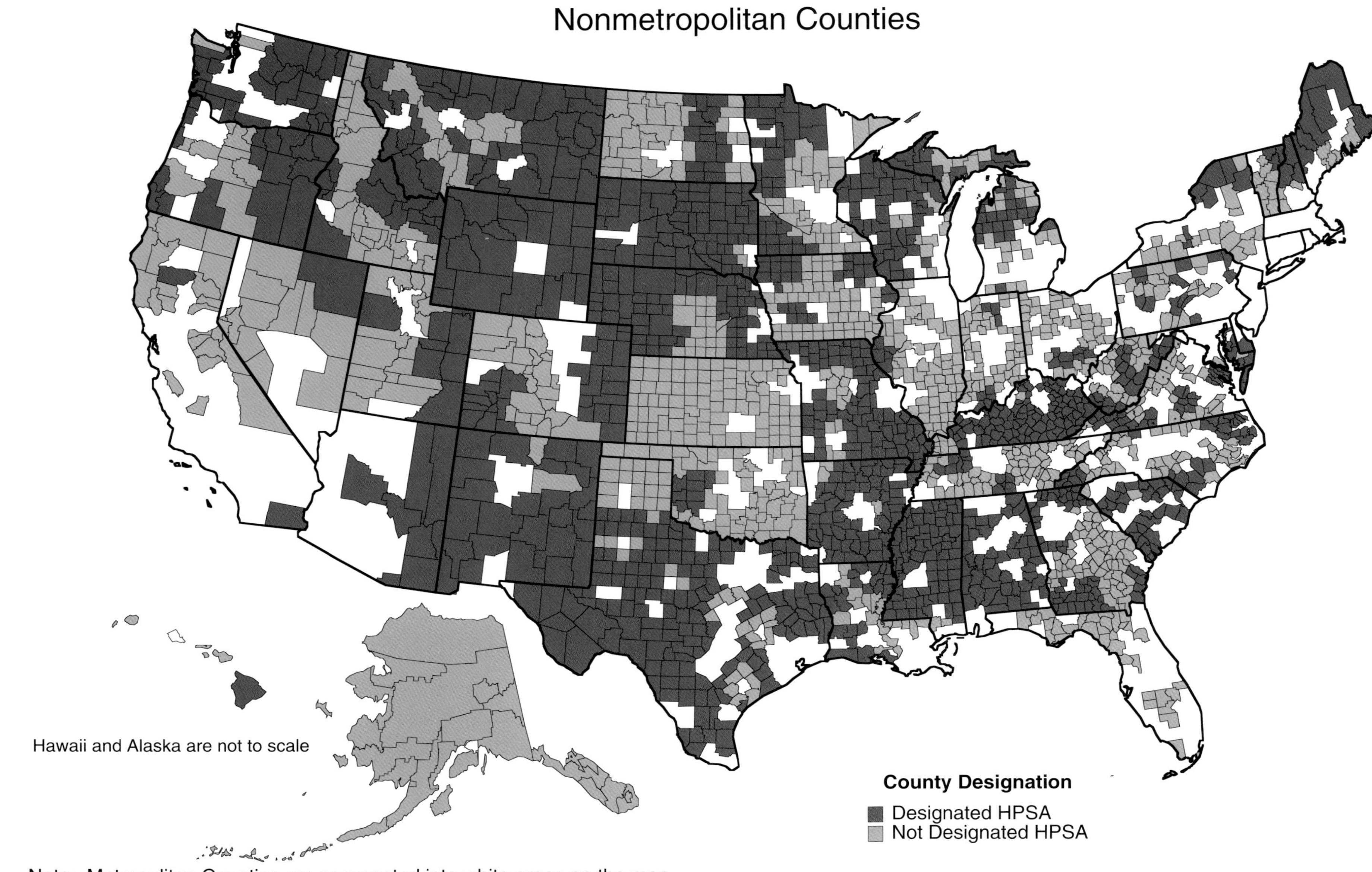

Note: Metropolitan Counties are aggregated into white areas on the map.
Source: Division of Shortage Designations, BPHC, HRSA, DHHS, 1997.
Produced By: North Carolina Rural Health Research and Policy Analysis Center,
Cecil G. Sheps Center for Health Services Research,
University of North Carolina at Chapel Hill.

physicals, and eye exams). As of December 1996, 65% of the Medicare risk plans charged no additional premium to enrolled beneficiaries, even when providing enhanced services (PPRC, 1997b). Consequently, because beneficiaries in most urban areas have access to one or more Medicare HMOs they also have access to enhanced benefits, whereas beneficiaries in most rural areas do not.

Payment Methodology Legislated by the Balanced Budget Act (BBA) of 1997

The 1997 BBA replaced the AAPCC methodology with one under which each county's base payment rate is set as the higher of (1) a local/national blended rate, (2) a national "floor," or (3) a "hold harmless" or "minimum update" rate, set 2% above the previous year's rate for the county. The resulting county base rates will continue to be adjusted for risk factors of the individual HMO enrollee when computing the actual capitation payments made to Medicare risk plans. For 1998 and 1999, the individual risk adjustment factors were the same as had been used under the AAPCC methodology. The BBA calls for a new risk adjustment methodology to be implemented beginning with year 2000 payments. Initially this risk adjustment will be based on diagnostic information for patients who had an inpatient hospital stay.

For 1998, the national payment floor was set at $367 per month for all counties in the United States increasing in subsequent years by the national per capita growth rate for Medicare expenditures, which is to be projected each March by the Secretary of DHHS. A 4% growth rate was projected for 1999, which when combined with the 0.5 percentage point offset mandated by the BBA resulted in a 3.5% growth rate and a 1999 floor amount of approximately $380.

The blended rates are computed as a weighted average of the county's own local rate from 1997 and a national rate that has been adjusted to reflect county-by-county differences in physician and hospital input prices. Prior to blending, Medicare's expenditures related to direct and indirect graduate medical education (GME) are to be removed from the local component. In 1998, 20% of the GME costs in the county were "carved out," and this percent will increase by 20 percentage points each year until all GME costs are removed in the year 2002.*

*Medicare's direct GME payments have increased from $1.3 billion in fiscal year (FY) 1990 to approximately $2.0 billion in FY 1995, an increase of 50% according to Bruce C. Vladeck, Ph.D. Administrator, Health Care Financing Administration, in his testimony on "Graduate Medical Education" before the Senate Finance Committee, March 12, 1997. In addition, Medicare essentially pays twice for high-priced teaching facilities both in GME and the hospital wage index.

The GME-adjusted local rate is combined with the input-price adjusted national rate to derive the county's blended rate, using the local/national blending percentages that are in effect for the given year. The blending weights for 1998 were set at 90% of the local rate and 10% of the national rate. These relative weights shift by 8 percentage points each year, until a 50/50 blend is reached in the year 2003.

The resulting blended rate is then compared with the relevant floor and hold-harmless rates for the county for the year, and the county is provisionally assigned the highest of these three rates. Finally, a budget neutrality adjustment is made to ensure that total payments under the new system are equal to the payments that would have been made if every county had been paid using only local rates. As legislated by the BBA, any payment reductions needed to achieve budget neutrality must be taken only from counties receiving the blended rates. If the budget neutrality adjustment causes a county's blended rate to fall below either the floor or the hold-harmless rate, the county is assigned the higher of these two alternative rates. The budget neutrality calculation is then repeated, and payments to counties still assigned blended rates are adjusted as needed. The process continues until either the blended rates are reduced sufficiently to achieve budget neutrality across all counties, or no blended-rate counties remain and no further steps to budget neutrality could be taken without reducing the floor and/or hold harmless rates.

The BBA also permits governors to request that payment rates be computed over geographic areas other than counties. Examples of these alternative areas include statewide payment areas, areas that encompass all counties of a single MSA or PMSA, and consolidation of all of the state's nonmetropolitan counties into a single payment area. Such changes might change the relative distribution of Medicare HMO payments *within* a state (e.g., urban vs. rural counties) but would be subject to an additional budget neutrality constraint designed to ensure that the state as a whole receives no more Medicare payments under the new payment area configuration than it would have received under the county-based system.

Impact of the BBA on Risk Plan Payment Rates

This section shows the likely impact of the BBA changes on payment rates for rural and urban areas. These simulations are based on work completed by the Project HOPE's Walsh Center for Rural Health Analysis under contract to the Office of Rural Health Policy. The simulation model replicates the 1998 and 1999 payment rates already computed by HCFA, and projects rates through the year 2003, when the BBA will be fully implemented. The simulations incorporate actual U.S. DHHS growth rate projections through 1999, and use Congressional Budget Office projections for later years. The model makes no attempt to incorporate changes arising from the still-to-be defined risk-adjustment methodology that will take effect in the year 2000, and assumes that all states will continue to use county payment areas throughout the implementation period. Complete details on the simulation methods are available in Schoenman (1997 and 1999).

Mean payment rates in 1997 and 1998 for various types of urban and rural counties (grouped by urban influence code) show clearly that urban rates are consistently above rural rates in both years, but that the differences are slightly less striking in 1998 due to the larger percentage increases experienced in rural areas as a result of the BBA (Fig. 6.5). Among rural counties, the payment increases were generally greater for areas that are not adjacent to a metropolitan area, especially if they have no city of more than 10,000 people. Counties in large metropolitan areas experienced the smallest increase in payment rates between 1997 and 1998, with most receiving only the 2% minimum update.

Rate changes between 1997 and 1998 for county groupings based on 1997 AAPCC payment rates and for groupings defined by 1995 Medicare HMO enrollment rates among aged beneficiaries show that all counties in the lowest quartile of payment rates for 1997—92% of which were rural—were brought up to the floor rate in 1996 (Table 6.8). This change represented an average payment increase of nearly 21% for these counties. Thus, for 1998, the floor was particularly important for increasing payments in the lowest paid and rural areas.

All counties in the top half of the 1997 payment rate distribution (all of whom had 1997 payment rates above $367), saw their rates increase by the 2% minimum update in 1998. These counties were more likely to be urban.

A similar story can be told for groups of counties defined by their 1995 Medicare HMO penetration rates. The greatest increases in rates from 1997 to 1998 occurred in counties where there was little or no Medicare HMO enrollment in 1995. These counties were overwhelmingly rural, and the payment floor was disproportionately responsible for the large rate increases. Conversely, counties with relatively high rates of Medicare HMO enrollment, which were disproportionately urban, saw smaller-than-average increases in their payment rates, and were more dependent on the 2% minimum update than on the payment floor.

The projected trends in mean payment rates through the year 2003, expressed in 1998 dollars, shows a slight slowing in the projected growth rate for risk plan payments after the beginning of the BBA implementation in 1998 (Fig. 6.6). Importantly, however, the trend lines for urban and rural areas do not converge appreciably over the time period considered, with rural payment rates remaining consistently lower than urban payment rates.

Figure 6.7 shows the minimum and maximum change in payment rates for each year from 1997 to 2003 for urban versus rural counties. With the exception of the 1997 to 1998 period, when some counties in rural and urban areas alike received a significant increase in payment rates thanks to the new payment floor, the BBA will greatly decrease rate volatility. After 1998, rates for rural areas will be only slightly more volatile than rates for urban areas. Of course, because

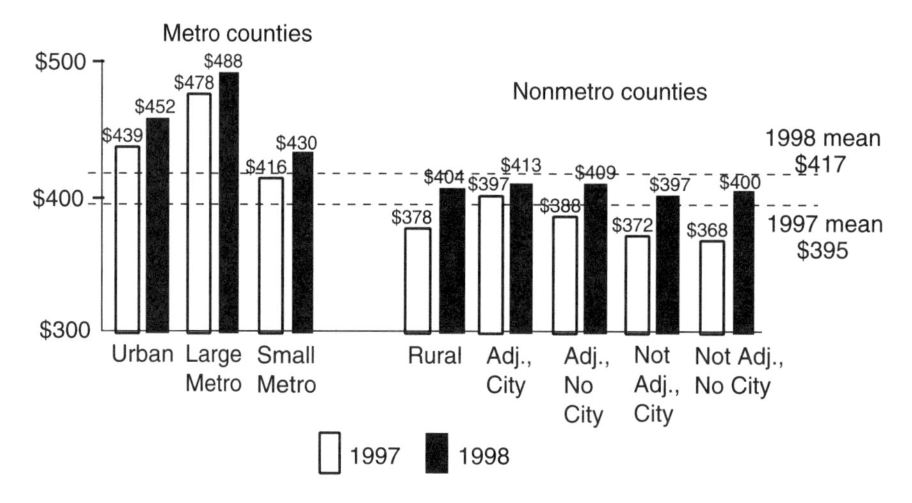

Figure 6.5. Mean AAPCC payment rates by county type.

Table 6.8 Risk Plan Payment Changes in 1998 by 1997 Payment Rate and 1995 HMO Enrollment Percent

Categories of Counties	*Number of Counties*	*Percent Rural*	*Mean Rate*	*Percent Change 1997–1998*	*Percent at Floor*	*Percent at 2% Up*
1997 AAPCC RATE (QUARTIES)						
$221–$341	776	92.3	$367.00	20.5	100	0.0
$342–$385	777	77.7	$374.64	3.1	40.7	59.3
$386–$437	778	71.6	$418.66	2.0	0.0	100.0
$438–$721	785	51.5	$506.45	2.0	0.0	100.0
1995 HMO ENROLLMENT						
None	149	99.3	$403.39	11.6	47.7	52.3
< 1%	2,014	79.9	$408.31	7.2	37.9	62.1
1%–5%	520	63.5	$425.65	5.9	30.2	69.8
5%–10%	184	53.3	$447.51	4.4	20.1	79.9
> 10%	249	43.8	$454.02	5.1	25.3	74.7
All Counties	3,116	73.2	$416.93	6.9	35.0	65.0

of the hold harmless provision of the BBA, the smallest annual rate change that any county will ever see is always a 2% *increase*. The wide upward and downward swings in payment rates that plagued many rural counties in the past will no longer occur. Thus, when a rural county experiences an especially large change in payment rates from one year to the next, it will always be in the upward direction, a fact that should be attractive to managed care companies considering a move into new market areas.

The relative importance of each payment method throughout the implementation period for urban versus rural counties shows that no county received a blended payment rate in 1998, and this situation will persist in 1999 (Fig. 6.8). In both years, the floor payments will be more important to rural counties, and the 2% minimum updates will be more important for urban counties. Blended rates are expected to begin to appear in the year 2000. The importance of this payment mechanism will grow dramatically over time, and will be consistently more important for urban areas than for rural areas. The payment floors will play an increasingly smaller role in the payments to urban areas, but will remain very important for rural counties. Finally, the importance of the hold-harmless provision will diminish over time for all types of counties.

The fact that no counties receive the blended rate in 1998 or 1999 signals the failure to achieve budget neutrality in these years. In essence, to pay for the higher rates given to floor and minimum update counties, rates

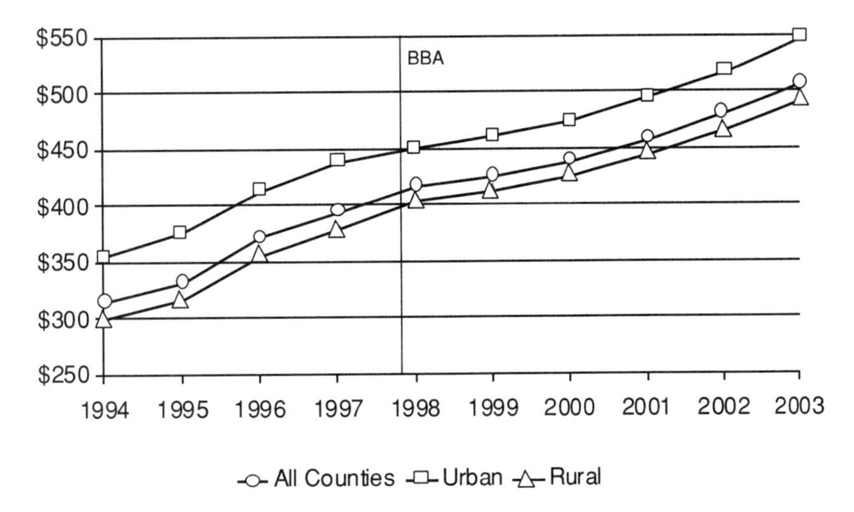

Figure 6.6. Mean payment rates by county type, 1994 to 2003.

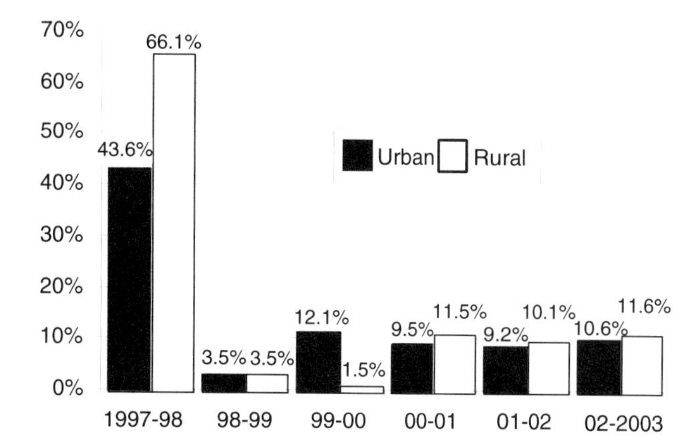

Figure 6.7. Estimated annual AAPCC rate volatility due to BBA 1997. *The lowest increase in any year is set to 2%.

for counties that were provisionally assigned a blended rate were continuously ratcheted downward through successive budget neutrality iterations until no blended rate counties remained and no further movement toward budget neutrality could occur. As long as the floor payment level and minimum updates are protected by statute, the BBA budget neutrality provision is not necessarily a binding constraint. Additionally, since the BBA contains no "look-back" provision to correct for failure to achieve budget neutrality in a prior year, the higher Medicare expenditures arising from this situation will not be recouped in future years. In the BBA implementing regulations published by U.S. DHHS in late June 1998, HCFA indicated that it was considering seeking a statutory change to address the budget neutrality shortcoming of the BBA.

In sum, these simulations indicate that the BBA changes to the methodology for paying Medicare risk plans will improve capitation payments made for beneficiaries living in rural areas. The floor payments and, in later years, the blended rates will help to bring rural payments closer to the national mean. Year-to-year volatility in payments will also be reduced, and payment decreases will be eliminated. These changes should make rural areas more attractive markets for managed care plans wishing to serve Medicare beneficiaries. Even with these improvements, however, rural rates will continue to lag below urban payment rates. Whether the BBA changes are sufficient to bring about the desired entry into rural markets by managed care plans remains to be seen. Additionally, there is some anecdotal evidence that existing (urban) Medicare HMOs are streamlining their benefit package in response to receiving only a 2% increase in payment rates. Most observers agree that these expanded benefit packages have been responsible for attracting Medicare beneficiaries to managed care plans. If HMOs enter rural markets in response to the payment increases, yet do not offer the expanded benefit packages that have traditionally been available, it is an open question whether rural beneficiaries will find the managed care option attractive.

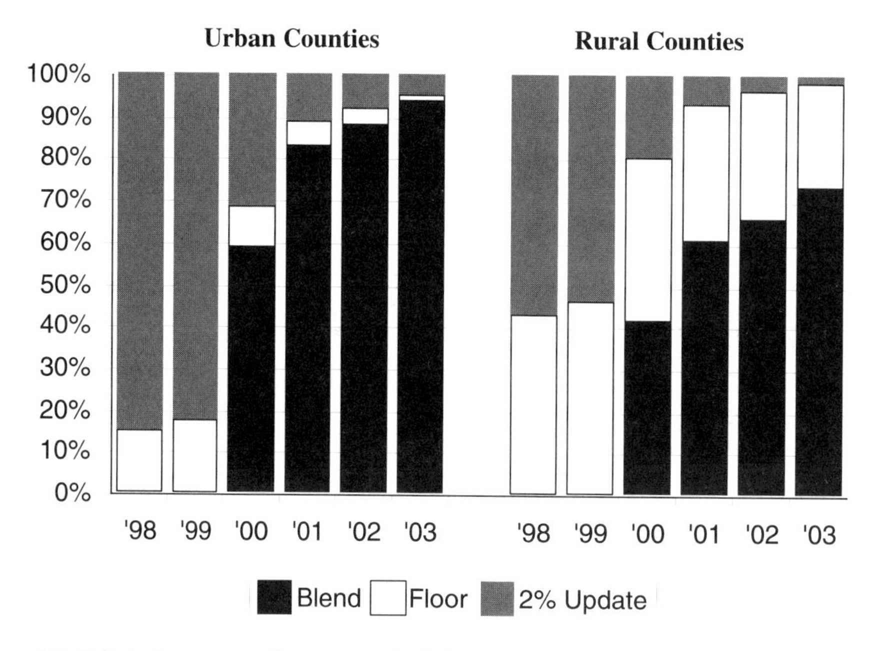

Figure 6.8. Relative importance of payment method alternatives, rural and urban counties, 1998 to 2003.

REFERENCES

Casey M. 1997. Serving Rural Medicare Risk Enrollees: HMO's Decisions, Experiences, and Future Plans. University of Minnesota Rural Health Research Center, Working Paper #19.

Committee on Ways and Means, U.S. House of Representatives. 1990. Overview of Entitlement Programs "Green Book"), June 5, 1990.

Davis K, Anderson G, Rowland D, et al. 1990. Health Care Costs Containment. The Johns Hopkins University Press.

Laschober M. 1997. Health and health care of the medicare population: data from the 1993 Medicare Current Beneficiary Survey. Westat.

Medicare Payment Advisory Commission (MedPAC). 1998b. Health Care Spending and the Medicare Program: A Data Book. Washington, DC: MedPAC.

Medicare Payment Advisory Commission (MedPAC). 1998a. Report to the Congress: Contest for a Changing Medicare Program. Washington, DC: MedPAC.

Moon M. 1996. Medicare Now and in the Future, 2nd ed. Washington, DC: The Urban Institute Press.

Physician Payment Review Commission (PPRC). 1997a. Annual Report to Congress. Washington, DC: PPRC.

Physician Payment Review Commission (PPRC). 1997b. Medicare Managed Care: Premiums and Benefits. Basics No. 4, Washington: PPRC.

Physician Payment Review Commission (PPRC). 1996. Monitoring Access of Medicare Beneficiaries. Washington, DC: PPRC.

Physician Payment Review Commission (PPRC). 1992. Monitoring Access of Medicare Beneficiaries. Washington, DC: PPRC.

Prospective Payment Assessment Commission (ProPAC). 1997. Medicare and the American Health Care System: Report to the Congress. Washington, DC: ProPAC.

Ricketts TC, Johnson-Webb KD. 1997. Definitions of Rural: A Handbook for Health Policy Analysis. FORHP.

Schoenman J. 1997. Impact of the Balanced Budget Act of 1997 on Medicare Risk Plan Payment Rates for Rural Areas. Final Report submitted to the Office of Rural Health Policy.

Schoenman J. 1999. Impact of the BBA on Medicare HMO Payments for Rural Areas. Health Affairs 18: 244–254.

Serrato C, Brown R, Bergeron J. 1995. Why do so few HMOs offer medicare risk plans in rural areas? Health Care Financing Review 17: 85–97.

Stearns SC, Slifkin RT, Walke T. 1997. Using the Medicare Current Beneficiary Survey for Analysis of Rural Health Policy Issues. Chapel Hill, NC: North Carolina Rural Health Research Program, the University of North Carolina at Chapel Hill.

7

State Laws and Programs That Affect Rural Health Delivery

REBECCA T. SLIFKIN

Many government programs and regulations, both state and federal, affect the health care infrastructure of rural areas. Unlike the federal government, states are in the unique position of being able to respond to the specific needs of their communities, and many of the new government programs that focus on improvement of the health of rural populations have been state-initiated. These initiatives have both a direct benefit to states, in terms of improvement of their populations' health, and also an indirect benefit, as the presence of a health care delivery system is critical to the economic development of rural areas (McCloskey and Luehrs, 1990).

States have designed, funded, and implemented a variety of programs to support rural health care systems and improve access to care for rural residents. By far the most prevalent are programs that focus on the recruitment and/or retention of practitioners. Other state programs seek to improve access to specialized services or improve the technical and data support necessary for rural health care systems planning. In addition, some state programs, such as high-risk insurance programs and the Medicaid program (covered in Chapter 8, Medicaid Managed Care in Rural Areas), are important to rural populations, even though their focus is statewide.

State regulations can also support the development of rural health care delivery systems. Although not specifically focused on rural areas, antitrust immunity and J-1 visa waivers are examples of state regulations that can have an important positive effect on rural health care delivery. Other legislation, such as certificate of need laws and licensure and practice acts, can either support or hinder rural health delivery systems, depending on how the legislation is framed and implemented.

PROGRAMS TO INCREASE PRIMARY CARE PRACTITIONER SUPPLY IN RURAL AREAS

Access to health care services remains a major problem for rural populations, who are much more likely than urban residents to live in areas with a shortage of primary care practitioners. States have initiated a number of programs designed to improve the supply of primary care practitioners in rural and underserved areas by increasing the overall primary care practitioner supply in the state, recruiting practitioners to rural and underserved areas, and retaining practitioners once they are there.

Increasing the Overall Primary Care Practitioner Supply

A number of states have instituted policies to increase the overall supply of primary care practitioners through changes in their medical education systems. States exert control over medical education through appropriations to schools, by creating and supporting specific primary care training programs, and by mandating that schools support state policies (Weissert, Knott, and Stieber, 1994). Although some of these initiatives were not stimulated from rural health needs, rural areas benefit from these strategies as the need for primary care practitioners in rural areas is great. In the past decade, states have passed legislation that specifically encouraged or mandated the creation of departments of family medicine (at least 13 states); created special grant programs for family physician training (over 40 states); reformed curricula and emphasized community-based education; and promoted preferential admissions and early intervention in secondary schools to encourage health careers for minority students and students from underserved communities (Henderson, 1994). As of 1997, 85 nurse practitioner and physician assistant training programs received state funds. These funds account for 67% of the nurse practitioner programs' budget, on average, and 36% of the physician assistant training program budgets. In general, state funds constitute an important source of revenue for the programs that receive them (Henderson and Fox-Grage, 1997b).

Scholarship and Loan Repayment Programs

Almost all states now fund programs to increase the practitioner supply in rural and underserved areas through tuition payment programs (Fig. 7.1). These programs assist health care practitioners in paying for their education in exchange for service for a specified period of time in an underserved area. Programs that cover educational costs are generally one of two types: scholarship or loan programs. In scholarship programs, the student enters into an agreement with the program prior to educational training and agrees to work in a health professions shortage area or underserved community after graduation in exchange for payment of tuition. Loan programs differ by timing: health care professionals who have completed their training agree to practice in underserved areas in exchange for payment of student loans.

Both types of programs have a required length of service for each year of tuition paid. If an individual does not meet the service obligation, penalties (the level of which ranges across programs) are imposed. State-supported tuition payment programs are generally funded by the state, but some programs are financed in part by federal grants. Approximately one third of state-supported tuition payment programs receive 40% to 50% of program costs from the National Health Service Corps. Additionally, an increasing number of local communities and private organizations contribute financial support to tuition payment programs (Henderson and Fox-Grage, 1996).

Loan repayment and scholarship programs exist for allopathic and osteopathic physicians, dentists, nurses, nurse practitioners, physician assistants, and midwives. In five states, programs are specifically targeted at minority students. By 1996, at least 102 state-funded tuition payment programs operated in 47 states. In addition, at least nine more programs were administered by state agencies, even though funds came from other sources. State loan repayment and scholarship programs are relatively new: 63 of these programs have been in existence for 5 years or less (Henderson and Fox-Grage, 1997a). Loan repayment programs are much more common than scholarship programs (Fig. 7.1).

States use a variety of methods to determine where to place health care practitioners who participate in state-funded service-contingent programs. Among 34 states that responded to a survey regarding their programs, 75% of programs used more than one designation method. Across the respondents, 60% used a state-specific method for designating areas to be served, 50% used the federal Health Professional Shortage Area (HPSA) designation, and 25% made use of the federal Medically Underserved Area (MUA) designation in order to identify areas eligible to receive practitioners from the program. One state allowed practitioners to locate anywhere within the state (Taylor and Pathman, unpublished).

Other Recruitment and Retention Programs

A number of states have instituted programs that expose health care professionals in training to rural practice, in hopes that the exposure from rural rotations will increase the likelihood that graduates will choose to practice in rural areas. As of 1995, 38 states had programs of this type for medical students or residents, and 34 states had programs for physician assistants, nurse practitioners, certified nurse midwives, and social workers (Table 7.1) (Orloff and Tymann, 1995).

In addition to increasing the overall number of primary care practitioners trained, states have initiated programs to channel these practitioners to rural areas. These initiatives, which match professionals to sites, use a variety of methods such as recruitment fairs, salaried recruiters, and the maintenance of databases to link available practitioners to rural sites with shortages (Orloff and Tymann, 1995).

Another series of state strategies address the fact that practitioners in rural areas often earn less than their urban counterparts, and although the cost of living may be lower in rural areas, large student loans or prohibitive medical malpractice premiums may act as barriers preventing practitioners from locating in rural areas. A variety of financial incentive programs are used as mechanisms to make rural practice more attractive, by offering

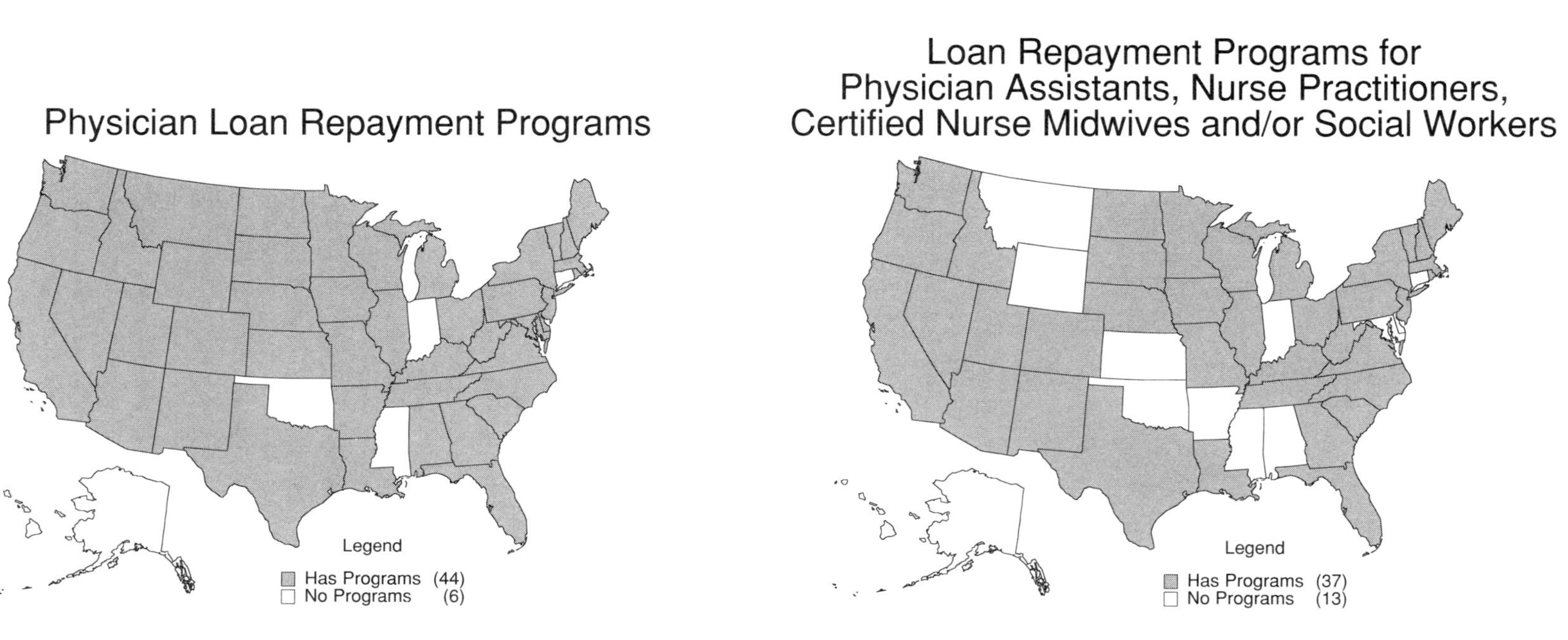

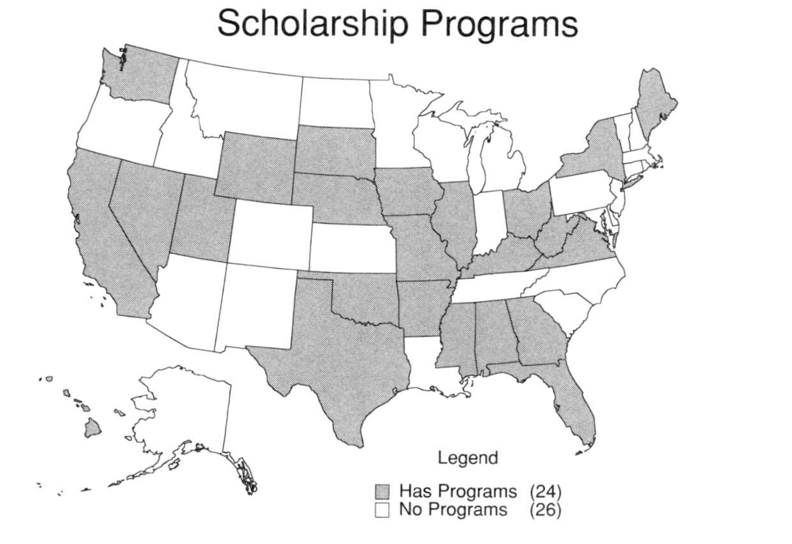

Figure 7.1. States with health care professional scholarship and loan repayment programs, 1995. Source: Orloff TM, Tyman B. 1995. Rural Health: An Evolving System of Accessible Services. National Governors' Association. Produced by North Carolina Rural Health Research and Policy Analysis Center, Cecil G. Sheps Center for Health Services Research, University of North Carolina at Chapel Hill.

Table 7.1 States with Recruitment and Retention Programs

	Medical Student/ Resident Rural Rotation	*Other Practitioner Rural Rotation*	*Site Match Program*	*Secondary or Undergrad Rural Health Education Rotation*	*Technical and Training Assistance*	*Financial/ Tax Incentives*	*Locum Tenens Program*
AL	✓	✓	✓	✓		✓	
AK	✓	✓				✓	
AZ	✓	✓	✓	✓	✓	✓	✓
AR	✓	✓			✓	✓	
CA	✓	✓	✓		✓		
CO	✓		✓	✓	✓		✓
FL	✓	✓			✓		
GA	✓	✓			✓		
HI	✓	✓		✓			
ID	✓	✓	✓		✓		✓
IL	✓			✓		✓	
IN	✓	✓			✓		
IA	✓	✓			✓		
KS					✓		
KY	✓	✓	✓	✓	✓		✓
LA	✓		✓	✓		✓	✓
ME	✓	✓				✓	✓
MD	✓	✓			✓		
MA	✓	✓	✓		✓		
MI		✓	✓		✓		
MN	✓	✓			✓		
MS				✓			
MO	✓	✓		✓	✓		
MT	✓	✓			✓		
NE	✓	✓	✓	✓			
NV	✓	✓			✓		
NH	✓	✓	✓		✓		✓
NM		✓			✓	✓	✓
NY			✓		✓	✓	
NC	✓	✓	✓	✓	✓	✓	✓
ND	✓	✓	✓	✓			
OH	✓	✓					
OK	✓		✓	✓		✓	
OR			✓		✓	✓	
PA			✓	✓	✓		
RI	✓						
SC	✓	✓			✓	✓	✓
SD	✓	✓					
TN	✓	✓			✓	✓	✓
TX	✓	✓	✓	✓			✓
UT		✓	✓				
VT	✓		✓		✓	✓	
VA	✓	✓					
WA	✓	✓	✓				✓
WV	✓	✓	✓	✓	✓		
WI			✓		✓		
WY	✓		✓		✓		
Total	38	34	24	16	29	16	13

Source: Orloff TM, Tymann B. 1995. Rural Health: An Evolving System of Accessible Services. National Governors' Association.

practitioners who are willing to locate in rural or underserved areas bonuses or income tax credits. As of 1995, six states offered income tax credits to practitioners in rural practice (Henderson and Fox-Grage, 1996).

States also offer financial incentives to practitioners in the form of malpractice premium subsidies in hopes of either making rural practice more attractive or allowing practitioners already in rural practice to broaden the array of services offered. Rising malpractice premiums, particularly for high-risk care such as obstetrics, has resulted in a decrease in the provision of obstetric services by primary care practitioners (Ricketts et al., 1995). In many rural areas, which often do not have the population base to support an obstetrician, the primary care practitioner may be the only source of these services. Malpractice premium discounts or subsidies enable rural primary care practitioners to financially afford to provide obstetric services.

Finally, 13 states have *locum tenens* programs to address the long-standing problem faced by rural practitioners of not having sufficient professional support to permit time off for pursuit of continuing education or personal leave time (Orloff and Tymann, 1995). Although individual programs use different mechanisms, the goals of these programs are the same: to provide a pool of health care professionals that can provide substitute services for rural practitioners who need a break. *Locum tenens* programs are available for a variety of health care professionals, including physicians, physician assistants, pharmacists, and nurse practitioners.

PROGRAMS THAT IMPROVE ACCESS TO SPECIALIZED SERVICES

Inadequate health care services in rural areas can often create access problems that are more pronounced for certain segments of the population. States have initiated a variety of programs to increase access to specific types of services in rural areas. These programs may focus on the provision of particular specialized medical services and/or target a subset of the population. Many of these programs are run through the states' Office of Rural Health (described in greater detail below and in Chapter 5, Federal Programs and Rural Health).

The most common type of specialized service programs are those that target mothers and children. Sixteen states have programs that provide perinatal, obstetric, and/or pediatric services, or focus on immunization delivery (Fig. 7.2) (Orloff and Tymann, 1995). The focus on maternal and child health is the result of several factors. First, rising malpractice premiums for physicians who provide obstetric care has driven many family practitioners away from offering these services. In rural areas, these physicians may be the only source of obstetric care within a reasonable distance. Second, there are few easily measurable population-based indicators of health status: two maternal and child health indicators that can be measured are infant mortality and immunization rates. When infant mortality is too high or immunization rates too low, the appropriate legislative response is programs that target pregnant women and children.

A number of state programs address other specialized service needs in rural areas. These programs vary across states and reflect state-specific responses to a perceived need. These programs focus on supporting emergency medical services, providing mental health and substance abuse services, delivering migrant health services, increasing access to primary care services through community health services development or the use of mobile clinics, and providing HIV/AIDS education and services (Orloff and Tymann, 1995).

STATE HIGH RISK HEALTH INSURANCE PLANS

State high risk health insurance plans (risk pools) were developed to provide health care coverage to a portion of the uninsured population. Risk pools serve as a source of health insurance for people who have been denied coverage due to a preexisting medical condition or who cannot find health insurance at a rate lower than is offered by the risk pool. Although not specifically targeted at rural populations, risk pools may be a viable insurance option for rural residents, who are more likely than urban residents to be unemployed. In 1996, the unemployment rate was 6.44% in nonmetropolitan counties, as compared to 5.16% in metropolitan counties (Area Resource File, 1998). Nonmetropolitan residents are also less likely than urban residents to have coverage from an employer, making this population particularly vulnerable to rapidly increasing premiums or loss of coverage due to a medical condition.

Since 1976, 28 states have enacted legislation forming risk pools and as of 1997, active pools operate in 26 states. Only seven states provided an alternative to risk pools through open enrollment for individuals in Blue Cross/Blue Shield associations, and it is likely that the recent trend toward conversion of the Blues to for-profit entities will further decrease the number of states with open enrollment at affordable premiums (Communicating for Agriculture, 1997). As of December 1996, over 90,000 persons were enrolled in risk pools, but data do not exist on how many of the enrollees are rural resi-

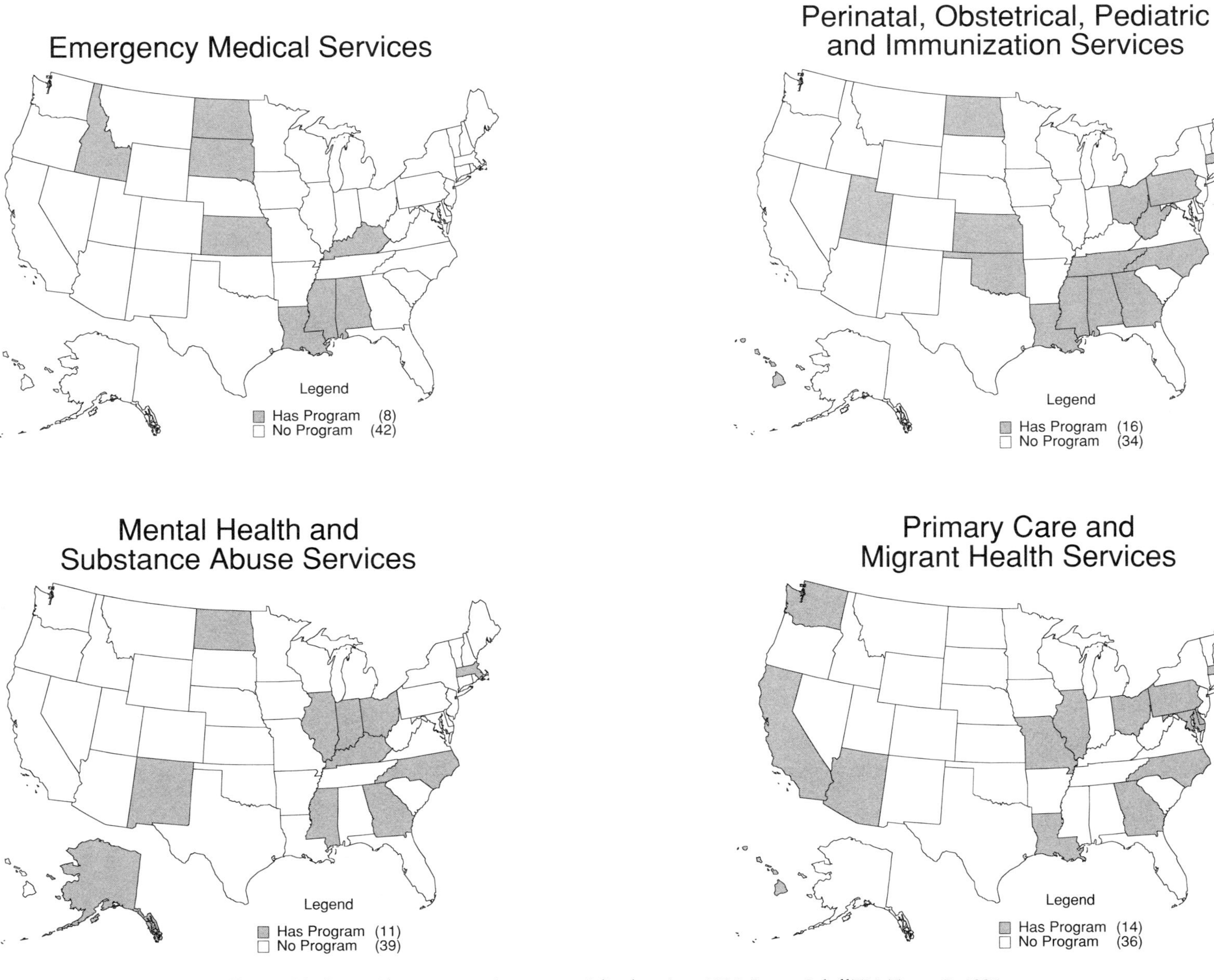

Figure 7.2. State with programs to increase specialized services, 1995. Souce: Orloff TM, Tyman B. 1995. Rural Health: An Evolving System of Accessible Services. National Governors' Association. Produced by North Carolina Rural Health Research and Policy Analysis Center, Cecil G. Sheps Center for Health Services Research, University of North Carolina at Chapel Hill.

dents. The risk pools are typically independent entities governed by a board and administered by an insurance carrier selected by the board. Limits on premiums for coverage typically range from 125% to 200% of the state's average premium for a healthy individual (Communicating for Agriculture, 1997). Because premiums collected do not always meet program costs, most states have covered pool losses through private insurer member assessments.

DATA SYSTEMS

Effective program planning and implementation, resource allocation, and practice management rely on access to pertinent information and data management systems. Rural communities often do not have their own data systems, but a number of states have data systems that can support the provision of rural health care. The information contained in these systems can be used to more effectively target funds, manage limited resources, and plan programs. The types of data systems and the uses to which they are put are diverse. Databases may contain health and demographic data on populations and/or information on health professionals. In some states, rural communities or providers are linked to sources with general information on state resources, patient visit coding support services, or centralized billing systems. Databases can be used to analyze the needs of local communities, determine areas with unmet need, and target areas that need technical assistance in recruitment and retention of practitioners. For example, 14 states "use data systems to support needs assessments and strategic planning activities in rural areas (and) 12 states are also sharing information found in statewide databases as a cost-effective strategy for providing rural communities with the data they need to increase access to care and extend limited resources" (Orloff and Tymann, 1995).

STATE OFFICES OF RURAL HEALTH

The mission of state offices of rural health (SORH) is to initiate, support, and/or sustain many state and local programs that aim to improve the delivery of health care services to rural residents. The oldest SORH started in North Carolina in 1973. Other states that began SORHs in the 1970s include Wisconsin (1976), Nevada (1977), Oregon (1979), and Arkansas (1979). Ten states started SORHs in the 1980s (Arizona, North Dakota, Utah, Nebraska, South Dakota, Illinois, Kansas, Texas, Washington, and Kentucky). In 1991, a federal grant program was established for the purpose of supporting the creation of SORHs (described in more detail in Chapter 5, Federal Programs and Rural Health). As a result of this initiative, there is now an SORH in every state. SORHs are typically located in the state health department (35 states), but sometimes are housed in universities (10 states) or are independent not-for-profit organizations (five states) (Table 7.2).

The offices are involved in a wide range of activities that support rural health care. Almost all SORHs function as information clearinghouses, providing a centralized source of data, literature, and other resources for those interested in the betterment of rural health. Many SORHs publish a newsletter, and over half sponsor an annual conference on rural health. The majority of SORHs provide technical assistance to rural providers in hospitals, clinics, communities, or networks. Among the numerous types of technical assistance offered are help with grant applications, practice management, clinic and network development, shortage designation applications, planning, and evaluation (Office of Rural Health Policy, 1997).

STATE LAWS THAT HELP OR IMPEDE RURAL HEALTH

A number of state laws affect the rural health care delivery system. Some state laws are specifically intended to improve access to health care services (for example, Freedom of Choice laws or waivers of J-1 visa requirements). Others, such as licensure and practice acts, have the potential to restrict access to services, depending on how the regulations are framed.

Licensure and Practice Acts

Licensure of health professionals is a function performed by all states. Licensing of professionals is usually controlled by a "professional practice act," in which the state outlines the scope of practice for health care professionals, defining who can practice and what health care services they are allowed to provide. In rural areas that rely on nonphysician practitioners (physician assistants, nurse practitioners, and midwives) for the provision of primary care, state laws dictating the scope of practice for these practitioners can either support or impede the provision of health care.

Mid-level practitioners can be seen as either physician extenders or as labor substitutes. The extent to which

Table 7.2 Characteristics of State Offices of Rural Health

State	*Organizational Location*	*Information Clearinghouse*	*Annual Conference*	*Newsletter*	*J-1 Visa Clearance*	*Technical Assistance*
AL	Health Dept.	✓	✓	✓	✓	
AK	Not-for-Profit	✓	✓	✓		✓
AZ	University	✓				✓
AR	Health Dept.	✓		✓		✓
CA	Health Dept.	✓				✓
CO	Not-for-Profit	✓	✓	✓		✓
CT	Health Dept.	✓				
DE	Health Dept.	✓		✓	✓	✓
FL	Health Dept.	✓	✓	✓		✓
GA	Health Dept.	✓	✓	✓		✓
HI	Health Dept.	✓		✓	✓	✓
ID	Health Dept.	✓		✓	✓	✓
IL	Health Dept.	✓	✓	✓	✓	✓
IN	Health Dept.	✓	✓	✓		✓
IA	Health Dept.	✓	✓	✓		✓
KS	Health Dept.				✓	✓
KY	University	✓		✓		✓
LA	Health Dept.	✓		✓		✓
ME	Health Dept.	✓		✓		✓
MD	Health Dept.	✓	✓	✓		✓
MA	Health Dept.	✓		✓		✓
MI	University	✓		✓		✓
MN	Health Dept.	✓		✓		✓
MS	Health Dept.	✓		✓	✓	✓
MO	Health Dept.	✓	✓			✓
MT	University	✓		✓		✓
NE	Health Dept.		✓	✓		✓
NV	University	✓				✓
NH	Health Dept.	✓				✓
NJ	Not-for-Profit	✓		✓		✓
NM	Health Dept.	✓		✓	✓	✓
NY	Health Dept.	✓		✓		✓
NC	Health Dept.					✓
ND	University	✓	✓	✓	✓	✓
OH	Health Dept.	✓		✓	✓	✓
OK	Health Dept.	✓	✓	✓	✓	✓
OR	University	✓		✓		✓
PA	University	✓	✓	✓	✓	✓
RI	Health Dept.	✓		✓		✓
SC	Not-for-Profit	✓	✓	✓		✓
SD	University	✓	✓	✓		✓
TN	Health Dept.	✓		✓		✓
TX	Not-For-Profit					✓
UT	Health Dept.	✓	✓	✓		✓
VT	Health Dept.	✓		✓		✓
VA	Health Dept.	✓				✓
WA	Health Dept.	✓			✓	✓
WV	Health Dept.	✓		✓		✓
WI	University	✓		✓		✓
WY	Health Dept.	✓				

Source: Office of Rural Health Policy. 1997. State offices of rural health: helping communities through federal, state, and local partnerships. Health Resources and Services Administration, U.S. Department of Health and Human Services, Rockville, MD.

mid-levels can fill primary care practitioner roles in rural areas depends in part on the degree of independence from physicians that they are granted by state law: when less supervision is required, mid-level practitioners are more able to function as physician substitutes in areas with few or no physicians.

Of particular importance to rural areas is the degree of prescriptive authority granted to mid-level practitioners. States with a more favorable practice environment with regard to prescriptive authority have significantly higher numbers of mid-level practitioners as compared with states with more restrictive laws (Sekscenski et al., 1994). Most states allow at least minimal prescriptive authority to mid-level practitioners (Sage and Aiken, 1997). As of 1997, physician assistants had prescriptive authority in 42 states, but the restrictions placed on this privilege vary considerably across the states. While 33 states grant nurse practitioners prescriptive authority with the collaboration of a physician, these practitioners have independent prescriptive authority in only 15 states (Rothouse, 1998a).

The advent of telemedicine has created a new limiting role of practice acts—one that may have adverse consequences for rural areas whose closest urban center is across state lines. The central issue is whether physicians who are located out-of-state, but provide services to in-state patients through telemedicine, should be licensed in the state where the patient is located. The requirement of licensure can be a barrier to practice, as the licensing process can be expensive and time-consuming (in 80% of states, physicians are required to appear in-person before the licensing board). Between 1995 and 1998, 19 states passed legislation extending licensure requirements to physicians who practice interstate medicine and one state has written an administrative rule. In addition, 10 state medical boards have issued rulings requiring full licensure, and since January 1998 legislation concerning licensure of out-of-state physicians has been introduced in 15 states (Rothouse, 1998b). In Texas, for example, physicians cannot treat Texas citizens unless they hold a Texas license to practice medicine. As a consequence, telemedicine linkages with medical centers located in adjoining states are constrained (Jones, 1996).

Immunity from Antitrust Laws

Antitrust laws were established to prevent businesses from gaining an unfair economic advantage through agreements with other entities. These federal laws are enforced by the Federal Trade Commission and the Department of Justice (Ross-Lee, Kiss, and Weiser, 1995). The intent of antitrust laws is to maintain a competitive market but not to assure that any given individual business remains competitive (Greaney, 1997). As rural providers respond to the increasing presence of managed care, the formation of networks, although often necessary for the economic survival of the providers involved, can also violate antitrust laws. In sparsely populated rural areas, there may not be enough providers to support more than one network, and providers who participate in a sole rural health network may be in violation of antitrust laws (Casey, Wellever, and Moscovice, 1997; Teevans and Rosenberg, 1997). In response to the growing consensus that collaborative arrangements among health care providers are one mechanism to reduce the cost of care and also ensure the economic survival of the collaborating members, some states have passed legislation to provide network participants with immunity from antitrust liability. Private party activities can receive state action immunity from antitrust laws when the anticompetitive activity falls under state regulation (Ross-Lee, Kiss, and Weiser, 1995). Some state laws cover specific hospitals whereas others are more broad—covering hospital, physicians and other health care providers (Teevans and Campion, 1995). A number of states "have opted to grant antitrust immunity to those merger and joint venture activities that are perceived to save facilities from closing and protect local providers from 'outside ownership.'" As of 1995, 24 states had passed such legislation (Holahan and Nichols, 1996).

One example of state action immunity is in Washington State, where health care providers can apply for immunity from antitrust laws by petitioning a state body, the Health Care Policy Board. To grant immunity, the board, after review of a written application and conduct of a public hearing, must decide that "the benefits of the proposed project outweigh its disadvantages." This same board is then responsible for the oversight of approved projects (Saver et al., 1997).

Certificate of Need

As of 1996, 37 states have certificate of need (CON) regulations, requiring health care institutions to apply to the state for permission before making a new capital outlay in excess of a specified dollar amount or offering a new service or technology (Lamphere et al., 1997). The global purpose of CON legislation is to eliminate costly and unnecessary expansion of the health care infrastructure, and to ensure that resources are geographically distributed across the state. Although the latter purpose should help rural areas, CON laws can also have a negative impact on rural areas, which typically lag behind urban areas in terms of sophistication of health care facilities and services.

Filing a CON is costly in terms of both time and money. For small rural hospitals with low patient volume, finding the resources to file a CON can be difficult. Thus, in states with CON laws, rural hospitals wishing to offer a new service in an attempt to remain financially viable may find it difficult to do so, as they "can neither justify the need nor afford the cost" (Kiel, 1993).

Waivers of J-1 Visa Requirement

Every year, a substantial number of foreign medical school graduates receive J-1 visas, enabling them to pursue postgraduate training in the United States. Under the terms of the J-1 visa, when graduate training is complete, the graduates must return to their home countries for at least 2 years. In 1994, the Amendment of the Immigration and Nationality Act (P.L. 103–416) gave states the authority to request up to 20 waivers of this J-1 visa requirement per year. Under the terms of the amendment, physicians receiving waivers allowing them to remain in the country must serve in areas that are designated as either health professional shortage areas (HPSA) or medically underserved areas (MUA) for at least 3 years. At the end of the required employment term, foreign-born physicians can apply for permanent residency status (General Accounting Office, 1996).

Although it is not known how many of the underserved areas that receive physicians with waivers are rural, the number of these areas receiving physicians through state request is increasing. In fiscal year (FY) 1995, results from a survey by the General Accounting Office indicated that 20 states had requested waivers. By FY 1996, the number had increased to 34 states (that either had already requested waivers or planned to do so within the year).

CONCLUSION

States support, and sometimes hinder, the rural health care delivery system in a number of ways. For states with a large rural population, the coordination of these efforts is enhanced by the presence of a strong State Office of Rural Health. Although little data exist with which to evaluate the success of state-level programs, states remain an important source of rural health policy because they are responsible for developing programs that reflect the specific needs of their rural communities.

REFERENCES

Area Resource File. 1998. Office of Research and Planning, Bureau of Health Professions, Health Resources and Services Administration, Department of Health and Human Services.

Casey MM, Wellever A, Moscovice I. 1997. Rural health network development: public policy issues and state initiatives. J of H Politics, Policy and Law 22(1): 23–27.

Communicating for Agriculture. 1997. Comprehensive health insurance for high-risk individuals. Fergus Falls, MN: Communicating for Agriculture, Inc.

General Accounting Office. 1996. Foreign physicians: exchange visitor becoming major route to practicing in US underserved areas. Washington, DC: GAO/HEHS-97-26.

Greaney TL. 1997. Public licensure, private certification and credentialing of medical professions: an antitrust perspective. In: Jost TS, ed. Regulation of the Healthcare Professions. Chicago, Ill: Health Administration Press; 149–168.

Henderson TM. 1994. State efforts to increase community-based medical education. Intergovernmental Health Policy Project, George Washington University, Washington, DC.

Henderson TM, Fox-Grage W. 1996. State incentives to improve the practice environment in underserved areas. Intergovernmental Health Policy Project, George Washington University, Washington, DC.

Henderson TM, Fox-Grage W. 1997a. Evaluation of state efforts to improve the primary care workforce. Washington: National Conference of State Legislatures [Pew Charitable Trust].

Henderson TM, Fox-Grage W. 1997b. Training nurse practitioners and physician assistants: how important is state financing?. Washington: National Conference of State Legislatures [Pew Charitable Trust].

Holahan J, Nichols L. 1996. State health policy in the 1990s. In: Rich RF, White WD. eds. Health Policy, Federalism and the American States. Washington, DC: Urban Institute Press: 39–70.

Jones TL. 1996. Don't cross that line. Texas Med Mar: 28–32.

Kiel JM. 1993. How state policy affects rural hospital consortia: the rural health care delivery system. The Milbank Quarterly 71(4): 625–643.

Lamphere J, Holihan D, Brangan N, Burke R. 1997. Reforming the health care system: state profiles 1997. Washington, DC. AARP.

McCloskey AH, Luehrs J. 1990. State initiatives to improve rural health care. Washington, DC: National Governors' Association, Health Policy Studies Division.

Office of Rural Health Policy. 1997. State offices of rural health: helping rural communities through federal, state and local partnerships. Rockville, MD: HRSA, DHHS.

Orloff TM, Tymann B. 1995. Rural health: an evolving system of accessible services. Washington, DC: National Governors' Association, Center for Best Practices, Health Policy Studies Division.

Ricketts TC, Tropman S, Slifkin RT, Konrad TR. 1995. Migration of obstetricians-gynecologists into and out of rural areas, 1985–1990. Med Care 34(5): 428–438.

Ross-Lee B, Kiss LE, Weiser MA. 1995. Impact of antitrust laws on physician networking and rural communities. J of Am Osteopathic Assoc 95(11): 670–675.

Rothouse M. 1998a. Scope of practice/Prescriptive privileges. Washington: National Conference of State Legislatures [Pew Charitable Trust].

Rothouse M. 1998b. Telemedicine. Washington: National Conference of State Legislatures [Pew Charitable Trust].

Sage WM, Aiken LH. 1997. Regulating interdisciplinary practice. In:

Jost TS, ed. Regulation of the Healthcare Professions. Chicago, Ill: Health Administration Press: 71–102.

Saver B, Casey S, House P, Lishner D, Hart G. 1997. Antitrust and state action immunity in rural Washington state. Rural Health Working Paper Series #42. Seattle, WA.

Sekscenski ES, Sansom S, Bazell C, Salmon ME, Mullan F. 1994. State practice environments and the supply of physician assistants, nurse practitioners and certified midwives. N Engl J Med 331: 1266–1271.

Taylor D, Pathman D. Site eligibility and physician allocation procedures of state service contingent programs. Unpublished paper.

Teevans JW, Campion DM. 1995. State-action immunity: immunizing health care cooperative agreements. Washington, DC: Alpha Center.

Teevans JW, Rosenberg S. 1997. Health care antitrust enforcement in rural America: a recommended safety zone. Oakland, California: Rosenberg & Associates.

Weissert CS, Knott JH, Stieber BE. 1994. Explaining policy choices among the states. J of H Policy, Politics and Law 19(2): 361–393.

8

Medicaid Managed Care in Rural Areas

REBECCA T. SLIFKIN AND MICHELLE M. CASEY

Medicaid is a government-sponsored health insurance program for eligible individuals. States determine their own eligibility requirements and benefits, working within guidelines set by the federal government. The cost of the Medicaid program is borne by both state and federal governments, with the federal contribution determined by relative indicators of state wealth. In 1996, for every dollar spent on Medicaid, the federal government paid 60 cents, on average, and states contributed 40 cents (Lamphere et al., 1997).

Eligibility requirements for Medicaid vary across the states. In most states, people receiving cash assistance under SSI or Temporary Assistance to Needy Families program automatically qualify for Medicaid. In addition, others can qualify if they meet certain income, resources, and category requirements (for example, children under age 21, pregnant women, elderly or disabled). Income standards vary across states and categories of people. Usually the states have established more liberal income rules for pregnant women and children. Thus, a state may allow pregnant women or infants under age one to qualify for Medicaid with family incomes up to 185% of the federal poverty level; the same state may set its income eligibility threshold for elderly and disabled at 75% of the federal poverty level. Resource limits (such as savings or other assets that could be converted to cash) also vary across states and program categories.

Across the United States, approximately 37 million people were enrolled in Medicaid at some point during 1996. Data are not available as to the percentage of these people who reside in rural areas. In 1996, $158.5 billion was spent nationally for the Medicaid program, accounting for 20% of state expenditures (National Association of State Budget Officers, 1997). Historically, Medicaid has paid physicians fee-for-service, based on a state-specific rate schedule. The first half of the 1990s saw a change in this payment methodology, as states turned increasingly to managed care programs.

MEDICAID MANAGED CARE

The number of Medicaid recipients who are enrolled in some type of managed care program increased dramatically in the first half of the 1990s: from 2.7 million beneficiaries in 1991 (9.5%) to 15.3 million (43% of all beneficiaries) in 1997 (National Association of State Budget Officers, 1997; Health Care Financing Administration, 1997). Enrollment is disproportionately higher among women and children; very few Medicaid managed care programs include the aged, blind, or disabled. Although the growth of some forms of managed care, particularly full-risk managed care, has more often been focused in urban areas, a substantial number of rural Medicaid beneficiaries are now enrolled in some type of managed care program. Section 1115 and Section 1915(b) waivers from the Health Care Financing Administration (HCFA) have allowed states to implement Medicaid managed care programs that in the past would have been prohibited under federal Medicaid requirements; for example, they allow states to mandate enrollment in managed care plans and the use of primary care gatekeepers.

Medicaid managed care programs have both potential benefits and risks for rural areas (Wysong et al., 1997). The coordination of care and preventive emphasis of managed care might improve outcomes for rural populations. However, closed provider panels could result in the narrowing of already restricted provider choices and the weakening of the health care infrastructure in rural areas, through exclusion of local providers. Opportunities to reduce Medicaid costs by implementing managed care in rural areas may be limited because rural areas have historically had lower costs and relied more heavily on primary care providers than urban areas. As there has been very little research to date that evaluates the benefit of Medicaid managed care for rural populations, this chapter will focus on what is known about the implementation of Medicaid managed care.

TYPES OF PROGRAMS IN RURAL AREAS

Medicaid managed care models range from primary care case management (PCCM) programs, in which providers receive a nominal case management fee and are reimbursed on a fee-for-service basis, to fully capitated programs that pay health plans to provide comprehensive Medicaid services for a fixed monthly per capita rate. Although in fully capitated programs the contracted health plan receives a capitated payment from Medicaid, the provider may or may not receive a capitated payment from the health plan. A third Medicaid managed care model, partial risk programs, generally pay for primary care and case management on a capitated basis but maintain specialty and inpatient services under fee-for-service arrangements. Many states use multiple ("mixed") models, combining fully capitated and PCCM programs, to achieve statewide Med-icaid managed care coverage. Most commonly, capitated plans cover beneficiaries in urban areas and PCCM programs cover rural beneficiaries (Freund and Hurley, 1995).

In some states, mental health services are included in Medicaid managed care programs; in others, these services are "carved out" to be either reimbursed on a fee-for-service basis or covered under a separate managed care program. For a more detailed discussion of state mental health services, refer to Chapter 14, Rural Mental Health and Substance Abuse.

As of May 1997, Medicaid managed care programs were operating in just over half of all nonmetropolitan counties. In comparison, nearly three fourths of urban counties were covered. Urban counties were much more likely to be covered by mandatory fully capitated programs, whereas PCCM programs were more often found in rural counties (Fig. 8.1).

The type of program found in rural counties appears to be related to proximity to a metropolitan county. Rural counties that are adjacent to metropolitan counties were more likely to have fully capitated programs when

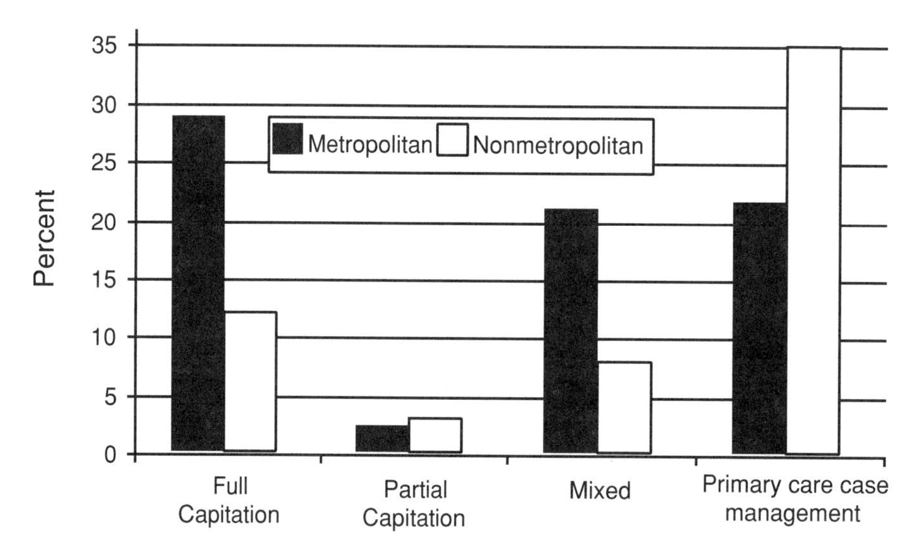

Figure 8.1. Percent of metropolitan and nonmetropolitan counties participating in Medicaid managed care as of May, 1997. Nonmetropolitan counties are defined using the June 1997 Office of Management and Budget designation. According to that designation, there are 833 metropolitan and 2,249 nonmetropolitan counties in the United States. Mixed programs include some combination of full capitation, part capitation, and PCCM. Source: Slifkin R, Hoag S, Silberman, P, Felt-Lisk S, Popkin B, 1998.

compared to nonadjacent rural counties (Fig. 8.2). In contrast, nonadjacent rural counties were more likely to have PCCM programs than either metropolitan counties or the adjacent rural counties.

Geographic differences in the type of programs offered are most apparent in states that use several types of managed care and make enrollment mandatory for some populations and voluntary for others. Among these states, almost all mandatory HMO programs began, and often have remained, in urban areas. When rural counties were included in fully capitated programs, participation was often voluntary.

Despite the fact that fully capitated programs are less common in rural than in urban areas, there are still a substantial number of rural enrollees. As of 1995–96, over 700,000 rural Medicaid recipients, or about 10.5% of rural recipients nationally, were enrolled in full-risk HMOs and prepaid health plans that covered general medical services (Moscovice, Casey, and Krein, 1998). Seven states had more than half of their rural Medicaid recipients enrolled in these plans; 26 states had no rural Medicaid HMO or prepaid health plan enrollment (Fig. 8.3). By May 1997, nine states had mandatory fully capitated programs that were statewide or virtually statewide, and so covered all rural areas.

Rural enrollment in fully capitated Medicaid programs is concentrated in a small number of states. Eighty-six percent of all rural Medicaid HMO/prepaid health plan enrollees live in just five states: Tennessee, Oregon, Washington, Hawaii, and Arizona (Table 8.1). Four of these states (Tennessee, Oregon, Hawaii, and Arizona) have implemented statewide Medicaid managed care initiatives under Section 1115 waivers.

Medicaid HMO/prepaid health plan enrollment rates vary considerably by county population and adjacency to a metropolitan area. Rural counties with Medicaid HMO/prepaid health plan enrollees have larger populations and higher population density than rural counties without enrollees (Table 8.2). Rural counties with Medicaid HMO/prepaid health plan enrollees have a higher number of physicians per capita, but a smaller number of community hospital beds per capita. They also have higher percentages of their population employed in manufacturing, construction, and white collar employment, and a lower percentage employed in agriculture.

HOW RURAL PROGRAMS HAVE BEEN IMPLEMENTED

States include rural areas in managed care programs for a number of reasons: cost savings, increased access to care (for example, by increasing the number of participating providers through the use of financial incentives such as the monthly case management fee), to improve quality, and for the simplicity of having to operate only one statewide program (Slifkin et al., 1998).

Although reduced reliance on the emergency department is typically a major motivation for the implemen-

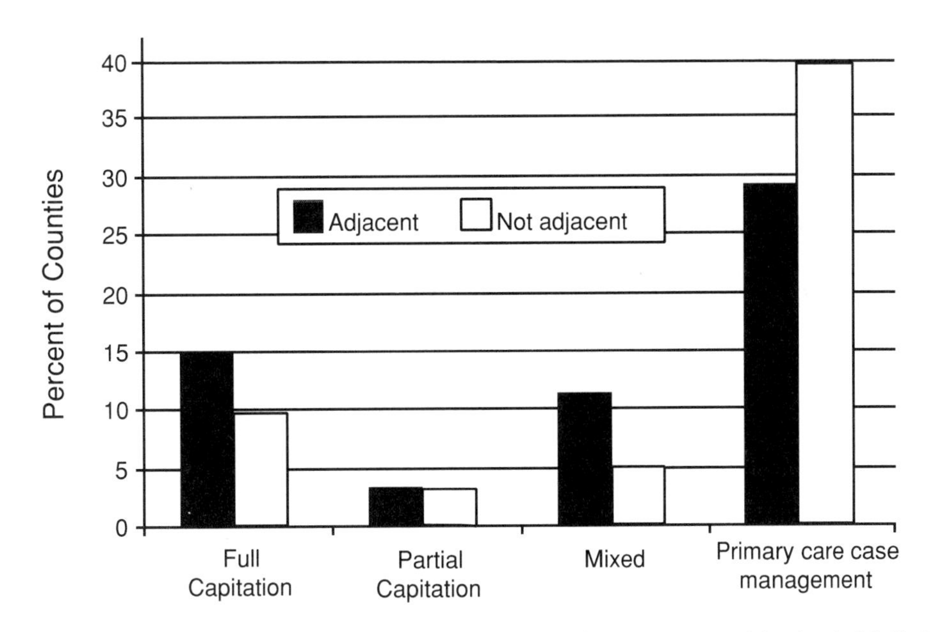

Figure 8.2. Percent of adjacent and nonadjacent nonmetropolitan counties participating in Medicaid managed care as of May 1997. Source: Slifkin R, Hoag S, Silberman P, Felt-Lisk S, Popkin B, 1998.

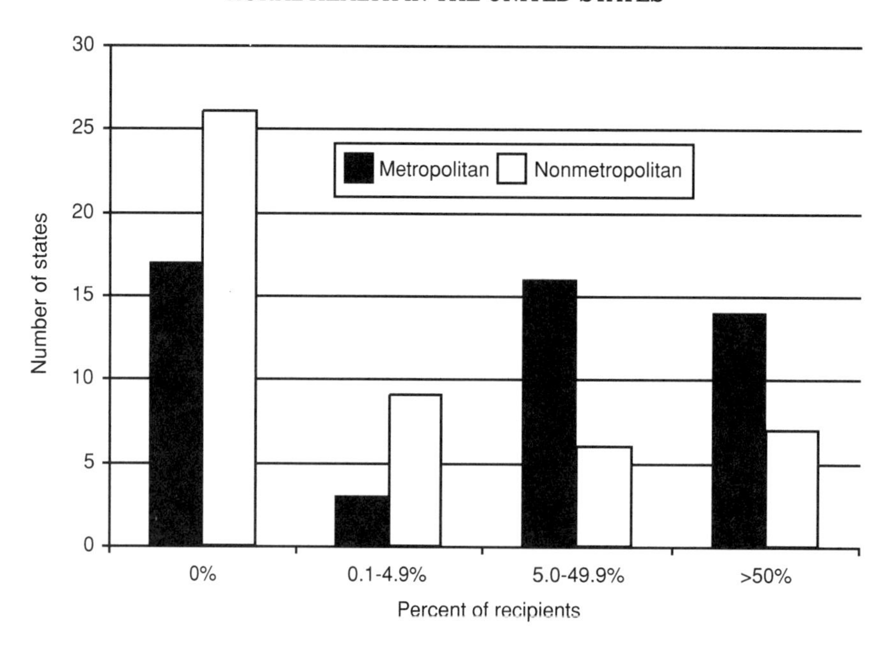

Figure 8.3. Percent of states' metropolitan and nonmetropolitan recipients in medicaid HMOs and prepaid health plans, 1995 to 96. Source: University of Minnesota Rural Health Research Center, 1997.

tation of Medicaid managed care, in general it was not noted as a reason for the inclusion of rural populations in managed care programs.

Equally varied are the ways that Medicaid managed care has been implemented in rural areas. Some states include rural areas in statewide fully capitated programs; others have implemented fully capitated programs in some areas, usually urban, and PCCM programs in others. Among states that have instituted PCCM programs, there is diversity in the ultimate goal—some states intend to remain with PCCM programs, others use this type of program to prepare consumers and providers for full capitation.

There is also broad diversity across states in whether and where managed care programs are mandatory for Medicaid recipients—although, as noted above, some states include rural areas in mandatory fully capitated programs. In other states, either enrollment in managed care is mandatory but the enrollee has a choice between a PCCM or fully capitated plan, or participation in any sort of managed care is completely voluntary. The latter strategies have generally been seen in states where rural areas were perceived not to be ready for managed care, or where they did not have the infrastructure to support such a delivery system.

Table 8.1 Distribution of Rural Medicaid HMO/ Prepaid Health Plan Enrollment, 1995–96

State	*Percent of Enrollment Nationally*
Tennessee	43
Oregon	13
Washington	13
Arizona	8
Hawaii	8
All other states	14

Source: University of Minnesota Rural Health Research Center, *Rural Managed Care: Patterns and Prospects*, 1997, analysis of data from Medicaid agencies in the 50 states.

Where totally voluntary programs exist in rural areas, enrollment tends to be low. Similarly, when offered a choice between HMOs and PCCM programs, rural residents tend to choose PCCM. Although in some rural areas fewer plans are available when compared with urban places, in other places rural residents have the same number of plans to chose from as urban residents do but are still much more likely to choose PCCM. It is not known whether this is because of a preference for this model of care, or because the providers that participate in the available fully capitated plans are less accessible to rural residents than PCCM program providers.

OBSTACLES FACED AND HOW THEY HAVE BEEN HANDLED

Implementing Medicaid managed care in rural areas has not always been easy. The most significant barrier states have faced is the absence of health plans willing to par-

Table 8.2 Characteristics of Rural Counties with and without Medicaid Prepaid Health Plan Enrollees (n = 47 states)[a]

	Counties with Enrollees (n = 330)	*Counties without Enrollees (n = 1,924)*
COUNTY CHARACTERISTICS		
Population, 1994	31,423	21,476
Population density, 1994 (per square mile)	47.5	35.0
Unemployment rate, 1992 (number unemployed/ number civilian labor force)	8.3%	7.6%
College Educated, 1990 (percent of population 25 years and older)	14.3%	16.4%
Income per capita, 1993 (1,000s of 1993 dollars)	$16.4	$15.8
Percent of population 65 years and older, 1994	15.2%	16.0%
Community hospital beds, 1993[b] (per 1,000 residents)	3.1	4.1
Hospital occupancy rates, 1993[b] (community hospital beds)	0.51%	0.50%
Physicians per capita, 1994[c] (per 1,000 residents)	0.9	0.8
PERCENT OF 1990 POPULATION IN DIFFERENT OCCUPATIONS		
Agriculture	8.0%	11.3%
Construction	7.1%	6.8%
Health services	7.3%	7.5%
White collar jobs	43.5%	41.6%
Manufacturing	21.1%	17.9%

[a] Alaska is excluded because Area Resource File data on Alaska are only available on the state level. New Jersey and Rhode Island do not have any counties designated by OMB as nonmetropolitan.
[b] Counties without hospitals are not included.
[c] Includes MDs and DOs.
Source: University of Minnesota Rural Health Research Center, *Rural Managed Care: Patterns and Prospects*, 1997, analysis of data from Medicaid agencies in the 50 states, 1995–96; Area Resource File, 1996; HCFA (AAPCC rates), 1996.

ticipate in rural areas and/or lack of providers. The lack of sufficient covered lives to make prepayment feasible is likely to be a factor in plans' avoidance of rural areas. There are also real concerns as to whether plans can reduce utilization enough to outperform low capitation rates. An inadequate supply of providers may also result from resistance to managed care among local providers or a limited number of providers who can meet HMO credentialing requirements. The latter stems from the use of mid-level practitioners in some rural areas. These types of practitioners may not be eligible primary care providers under certain plans. The limited number of providers in rural areas can also be a barrier to PCCM programs becauses these programs require 24-hour telephone access to a primary care provider. A provider who does not have a sufficient number of colleagues with whom to share after-hours on-call duty may feel unable to meet the requirements.

States have used a number of strategies to secure provider and plan participation in rural areas, ranging from mandates to incentives for voluntary participation. Several states with fully capitated programs have used regional contracting strategies, in which HMOs that wish to participate must contract to serve an entire region, which often encompasses both urban and rural areas. One state counteracted the reluctance of HMOs to enter rural markets by sharing a certain portion of risk with the plans. In areas where a commercial HMO does not exist, some states have assisted with the development of community-sponsored HMOs.

In order to facilitate inclusion of rural areas into Medicaid managed care programs, states have also shown flexibility in program requirements. Many states have allowed a wide range of providers to function as primary care case managers, including specialist physicians, federally qualified health clinics (FQHCs), rural health clinics (RHCs), Indian health clinics (IHCs), public health clinics, and mid-level practitioners (physician assistants and nurse practitioners). States have also responded to one of the greatest barriers to rural practitioner participation—the federal Medicaid statute requirement that primary care case managers offer 24-hour coverage—by allowing hospital emergency rooms to share coverage with providers who do not have a usual source of back-up (Felt-Lisk et al., 1999).

Another way that states have dealt with low rural provider supply is by easing travel standards. Most states with Medicaid managed care programs have instituted minimum travel and distance standards to a primary care provider (typically 30 minutes or 30 miles), but some do not impose such restrictions in rural areas, or they increase the travel times and distances for rural areas. Although this strategy improves the feasibility of program implementation in rural areas, it is not yet know whether it will have an impact (either positive or negative) on access to care for rural residents.

State Medicaid agencies have also used other, less common, creative strategies for promoting rural implementation of Medicaid managed care. These include working closely with the State Office of Rural Health to ease implementation; developing rural task forces to get provider and consumer input on the design of the program before implementation; training rural residents to act as lay health advisers, who in turn help other rural residents negotiate the new system; and conducting extensive meetings with community providers before implementation to increase readiness for managed care.

CONCLUSION

The Balanced Budget Act (BBA) of 1997 is expected to further promote the growth in Medicaid managed care in rural areas. Where previously states were required to receive a waiver from federal Medicaid requirements before implementing mandatory managed care programs, in some instances this is no longer the case. For example, prior to the BBA, states were required to offer Medicaid beneficiaries the "freedom of choice" to receive care from any participating provider. States could restrict choice to managed care plans only through the use of a waiver. Under a 1915(b) waiver, states were still obligated to offer enrollees in Medicaid managed care a choice of at least two plans. Under the BBA, states can mandate managed care for most populations without a waiver, and, under a managed care program, choice of plans is no longer required in rural areas, although every individual must have a choice of at least two primary care providers. This change in requirements is likely to provide impetus for plans to do sole source contracting with regional health systems, as long as choice among providers within the system is available.

To date, research on Medicaid managed care in rural areas has focused on the implementation process, not on outcomes. It remains to be seen whether Medicaid managed care is positively or negatively affecting Medicaid costs, access to care, and health outcomes of low-income rural populations. Such analysis is essential to determine whether there are sufficient benefits to justify moving rural populations to Medicaid managed care systems.

REFERENCES

Felt-Lisk S, Silberman P, Hoag S, Slifkin R. 1999. Medicaid managed care in rural areas: a ten–state follow-up study. Health Affairs 18(2): 238–245.

Freund D, Hurley R. 1995. Medicaid managed care: contribution to issues of health care reform. Annual Review of Public Health. 16: 473–95.

Health Care Financing Administration. 1996. Medicaid managed care enrollment report. Summary statistics, June 30, 1996. Internet. URL: http://www.hcfa.gov/medicaid/omc1996.htm. Health Care Financing Administration.

Health Care Financing Administration. 1997. Medicaid managed care enrollment report. Summary statistics, June 30, 1997. Internet. URL: http://www.hcfa.gov/medicaid/plansum7.htm. Health Care Financing Administration.

Lamphere J, Holahan D, Brangan N, Burke R. 1997. Reforming the health care system: state profiles 1997. Washington, DC: American Association of Retired Persons.

Moscovice I, Casey M, Krein S. 1998. Expanding rural managed care: enrollment patterns and prospects. Health Affairs 17(1): 172–179.

National Health Association of State Budget Officers. 1998. www.nasbo.org/resource/medicaid/ medicaid.htm

Slifkin R, Hoag S, Silberman P, Felt-Lisk S, Popkin B. 1998. Medicaid managed care programs in rural areas: a fifty state review. 17(6): 217–227.

Wysong JA, Rosenthal TC, James PA, Bliss MK, Horwitz ME, Danzo A. 1997. Introducing Medicaid managed care in rural communities: guidelines for policymakers, planners, and state administrators. National Rural Health Association.

9

Hospitals in Rural America

THOMAS C. RICKETTS III AND PAIGE E. HEAPHY

The role of hospitals in the American health care system is changing very rapidly. Indeed, there are some who see hospitals as disappearing from the scene, to be replaced by networks of professionals and institutions tied together through a variety of contractual arrangements to coordinate care and promote health—the so-called virtual hospital. For many rural communities, however, it is the hospital that has served as the focus of health care delivery in the community and that remains as the most prominent—and effective—institution to organize the delivery of health care.

In the 1980s, as the number of rural hospitals closing their doors grew every year, expert observers of the health care sector believed that rural hospitals were perhaps an anachronism and that only those institutions that were very large and integrated with other parts of the health care system would survive (Lillie-Blanton et al., 1992; Mullner, Rydman, and Whiteis, 1990). The leading proposals for national health care financing reform from the White House and the Congress in 1993 and 1994 did not provide much comfort for rural hospitals. Rural areas were seen as part of the nation where managed competition and vertically integrated networks would have trouble catching on (Kronick et al., 1993) and few specific policy recommendations addressed this problem (Rural Policy Research Institute 1994a,b). By 1997, the reality of market changes overtook policy proposals; networks were a growing phenomenon and the cost-saving potential of managed care was being realized. Rural hospitals have survived in the present system partly because federal Medicare payment policies that were discriminatory to rural hospitals have been blunted by legislation and partly because there was a real justification for the location and mission of hospitals in rural places. The number of closings dropped dramatically in 1994 and the dominant theme of rural hospital activities in the last half of the 1990s has been adaptation and innovation to meet the challenges of a changing market. The "exit" option for rural hospitals has not proven popular, despite the fact that rural hospitals are at a disadvantage in many ways compared to urban hospitals, largely because of differences in the resources available to them. The rapid diffusion of new management techniques, new systems of coordination and networking, new information technology, and the adoption of new structures and approaches to health care delivery have enabled rural hospitals to continue in their role as the local and regional centers of health care activity. This chapter will review the numbers, types, and structure of rural hospitals; describe the resources available to them, including staff and financing; and describe special policies and programs that enable rural hospitals to compete in a more interconnected market.

RURAL HOSPITALS IN THE UNITED STATES, THEIR NUMBERS AND DISTRIBUTION

In early 1998, 2,182 nonfederal, acute care, general hospitals in nonmetropolitan counties made up 45% of the total of 4,821 (Fig. 9.1). The nonmetropolitan hospitals were smaller: 72% had fewer than 100 beds and 42% had fewer than 50 beds (Fig. 9.2). Twenty percent (20%) of all hospital beds were in rural hospitals. The median number of staffed beds for nonmetropolitan hospitals

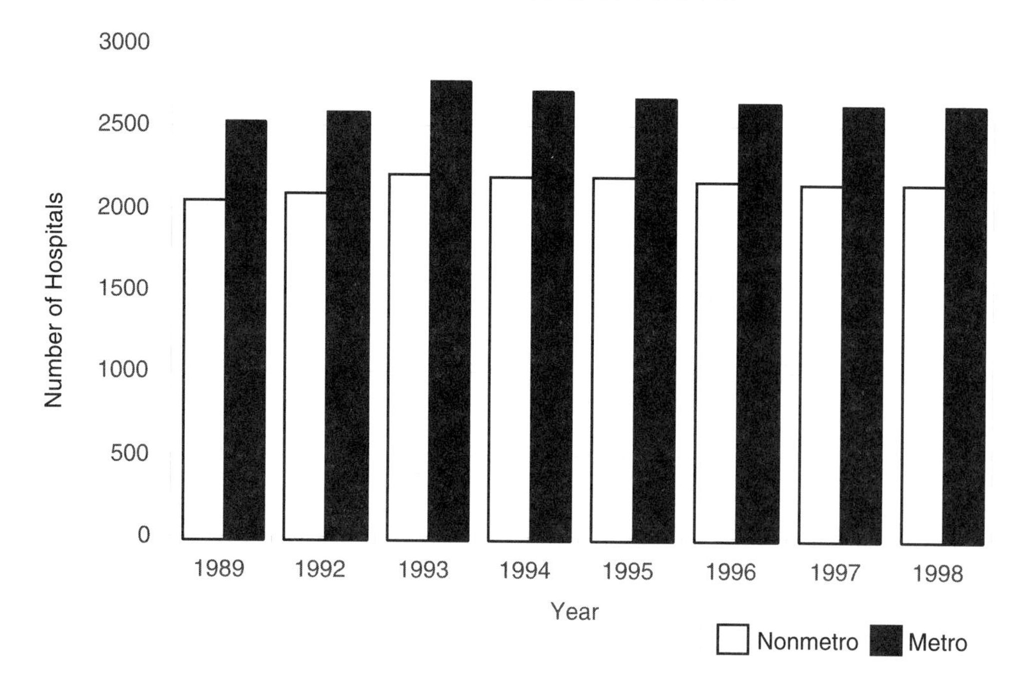

Figure 9.1. Number of hospitals in nonmetropolitan and metropolitan counties, 1989 to 1998. Source: AHA 1991–1997.

was 59 compared with 156 for urban hospitals and the average number of beds per hospital was 82 and 245, respectively. Rural hospital inpatient days accounted for 20% of all hospital inpatient days in the United States.

Medicare and Medicaid are important sources of payment for hospital patients. There are substantial variations in hospital dependence on Medicare payments, but rural hospitals tend to depend more on Medicare and Medicaid patients. Data from 1992–1996 show trends in Medicare patient discharges and patient days for metropolitan and nonmetropolitan hospitals (Fig. 9.3). Medicare pays for almost half of all rural hospital discharges compared with 37% for metropolitan hospitals. However, urban hospitals have higher utilization by

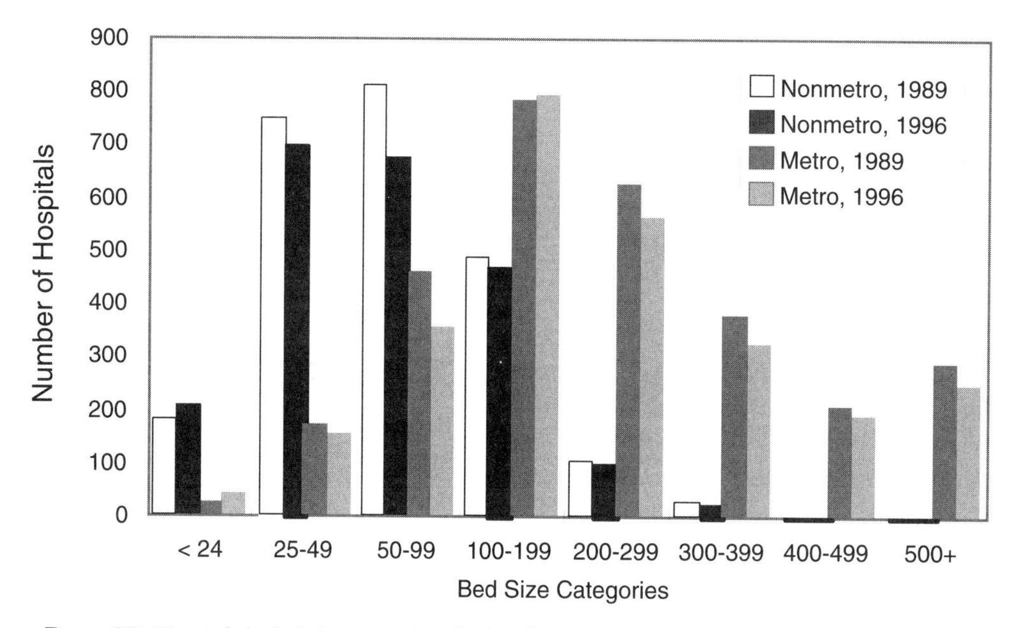

Figure 9.2. Hospitals by bed size categories, 1989 and 1995, nonmetropolitan and metropolitan counties. Source: AHA, 1997.

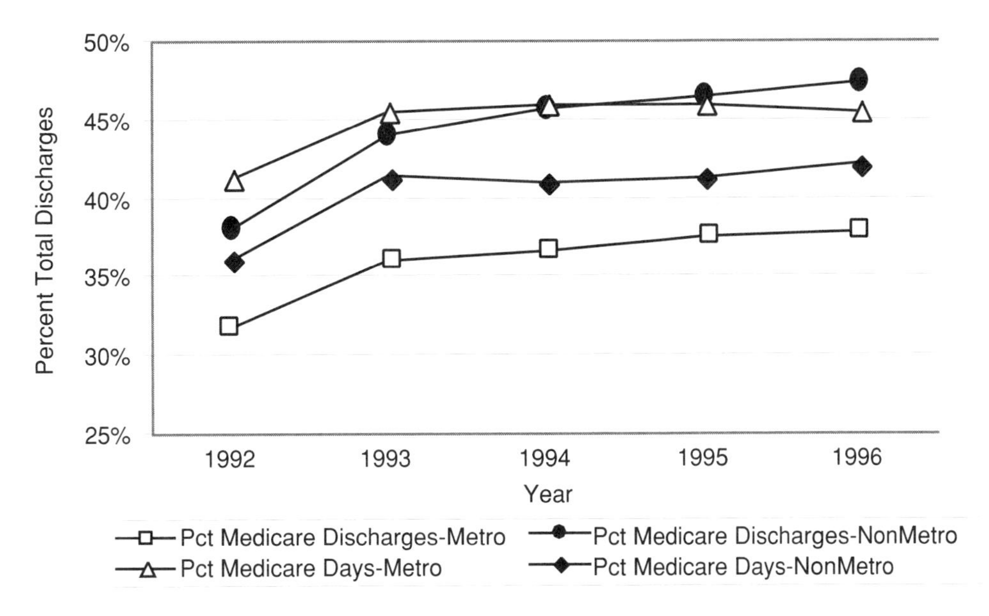

Figure 9.3. Hospital Medicare utilization patterns, metro and non metro, 1992 to 1996. Source: AHA, 1996.

Medicaid patients: 27% of all urban hospital days are for Medicaid patients and only 17% are for rural hospitals.

The utilization of urban and rural hospitals differed in 1996; urban hospitals had higher occupancy rates but shorter lengths of stay (Fig. 9.4).

The distribution and characteristics of rural hospitals varies by geography—larger communities are much more likely to have a hospital than smaller communities. This is reflected in the distribution of hospitals by county type. More hospitals are situated in central city metropolitan counties and in nonmetropolitan counties ad-

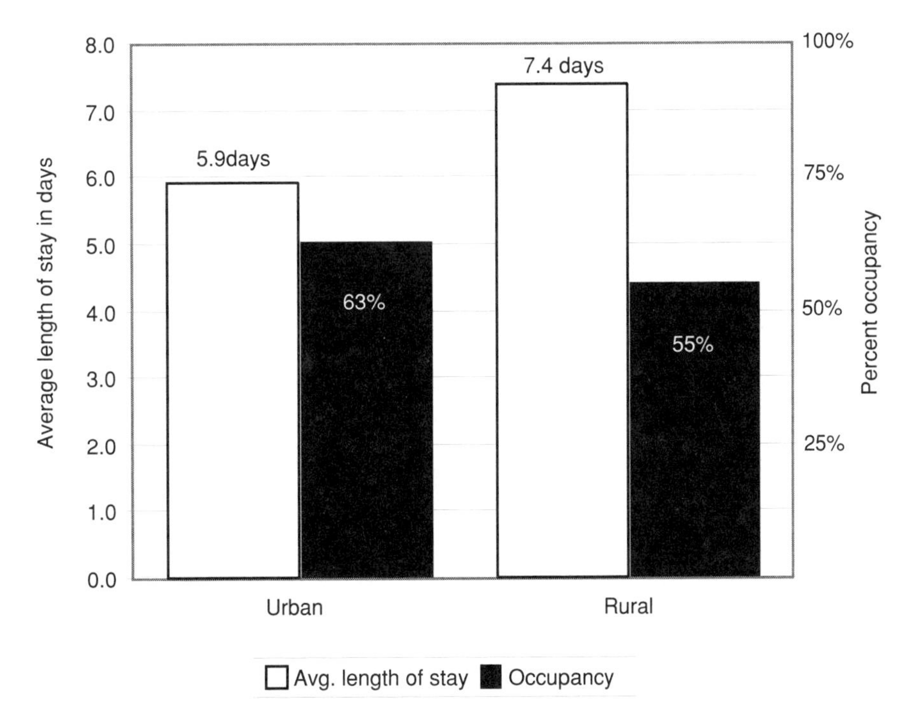

Figure 9.4. Hospital occupancy rate and average length of stay, urban and rural hospitals, 1996. Source: AHA, 1997.

jacent to small metro counties and in nonadjacent counties with smaller towns (Fig. 9.5).

OWNERSHIP AND CONTROL OF RURAL HOSPITALS

Hospital ownership and control are increasingly of interest to policy makers. The majority of rural hospitals are government-owned or fall under some other nonprofit classification; urban hospitals are predominantly other public-sector nonprofit and for-profit hospitals. A larger proportion of rural hospitals (23%) are contract-managed, compared with only 7% in urban areas. The type of government control can range from county to regional authority to state. More than twice the percentage of nonmetropolitan hospitals are controlled by government than are metropolitan hospitals (Table 9.1 and Fig. 9.6). The number of nonmetropolitan hospitals that are organized on a for-profit basis is less than one fourth the number of metropolitan hospitals. Of hospitals controlled by some governmental entity, county government and hospital districts account for the large majority of governmental sponsors (Fig. 9.7). Ownership tends to be associated with size. Government authorities own over 50% of rural hospitals with fewer than 50 beds. As the size of the hospital increases, there is a greater tendency for it to be owned by a nongovernment entity.

RURAL HOSPITAL SURVIVAL

Between 1980 and 1998, the total number of community, general hospitals decreased from 5,842 to 5,153, an 11.8% decrease due to closings, mergers, and conversions. During that period, there were approximately 1,072 closings or conversions to some other form of health care delivery organization, 626 in metropolitan counties and 438 in nonmetropolitan. At the same time, new hospitals were opening or relocating, creating a net reduction of 689 hospitals. The pace of closings slowed after 1990 to the lowest rate in two decades (Fig. 9.8).

The hospitals most vulnerable to closing or conversions were those that had a smaller number of beds and lower occupancy rates, were more often managed as a for-profit concern, were less likely to be accredited by the Joint Commission on Accreditation of Health care Organizations (JCAHO), and had a high percentage of Medicaid inpatient days (General Accounting Office, 1991); also more likely to close among isolated hospitals were those in markets with higher density (Succi, Lee,

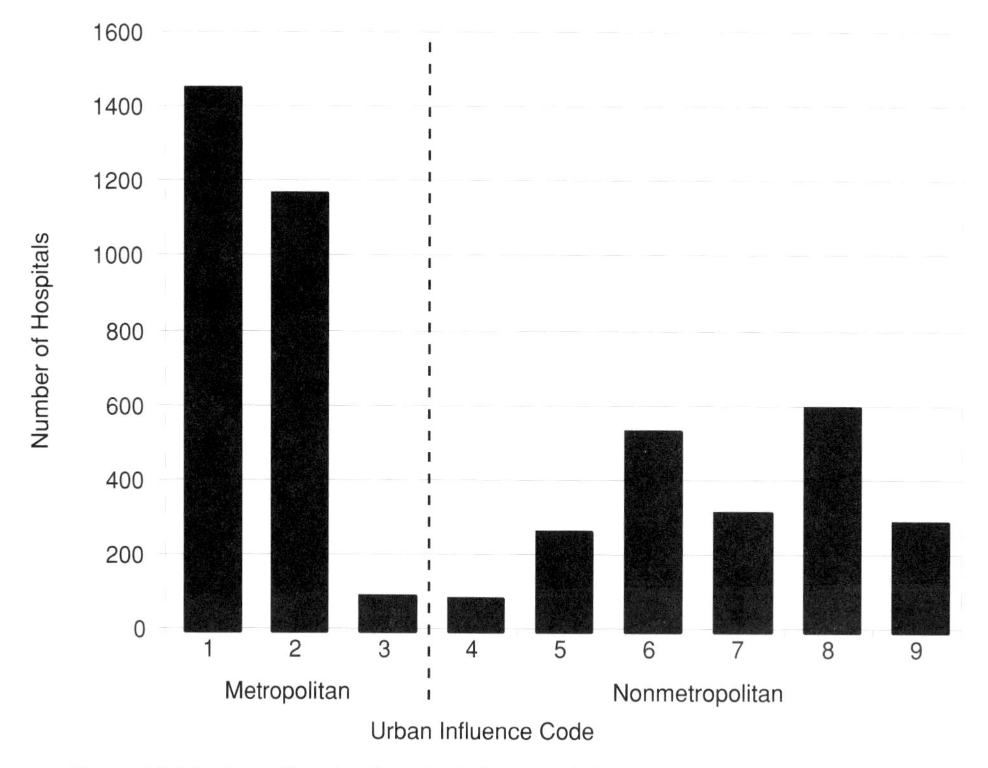

Figure 9.5. Numbers of hospitals by urban influence code location, 1996. Source: BHPr, 1998.

Table 9.1 Hospital Ownership and Control, 1996

	Metro		*Nonmetro*	
Hospital control by	*Number*	*Percent*	*Number*	*Percent*
Government	880	21.9	1110	45.7
Church	447	11.1	160	(6.6%)
Other nonprofit	1740	43.3	939	38.6
For-profit	951	23.7	221	9.1
Total	4018	62.3	2430	37.7

Source: 1995 Annual Survey of Hospitals, American Hospital Association.

and Alexander, 1997). Studies that examined the effects of closed hospitals on local communities found significant changes in utilization and, in one case, health status (Bindman, Keane, and Lurie, 1990; Hadley and Nair, 1991; Rosenbach and Dayhoff, 1995).

The Economic Contribution of Rural Hospitals

One of the key arguments in support of the continued subvention of rural hospitals by government and the removal of differential reimbursement rates for rural hospitals is their contribution to overall rural economies. Gerald Doeksen, Jon Christianson, and others have shown that rural hospitals contribute significantly to local economies and that rural hospitals serve as a source of employment and act as economic engines for many rural communities (Christianson and Faulkner, 1981; Doeksen and Altobelli, 1990; Doeksen, Loewen, and Strawn, 1990; McDermott, Cornia, and Parsons, 1991). Rural hospitals are often the largest or second largest employer in the towns where they are located and they are an important part of the social capital of any community. These economic impact studies estimate the extent of a hospital's financial effects throughout a community's economy using financial models that show how money generated by hospital activity cycles through many hands, supporting more than just the employees and suppliers of a hospital. The value of a rural hospital to its community is much harder to estimate. The immense efforts taken by some communities to keep their hospitals open and operating is a measure of the great value people and communities place on a hospital (Seavey, Berry, and Bogue, 1992).

Strategies for Rural Hospital Survival

The trend toward contraction of the hospital market did not continue through the 1990s. During the period 1994

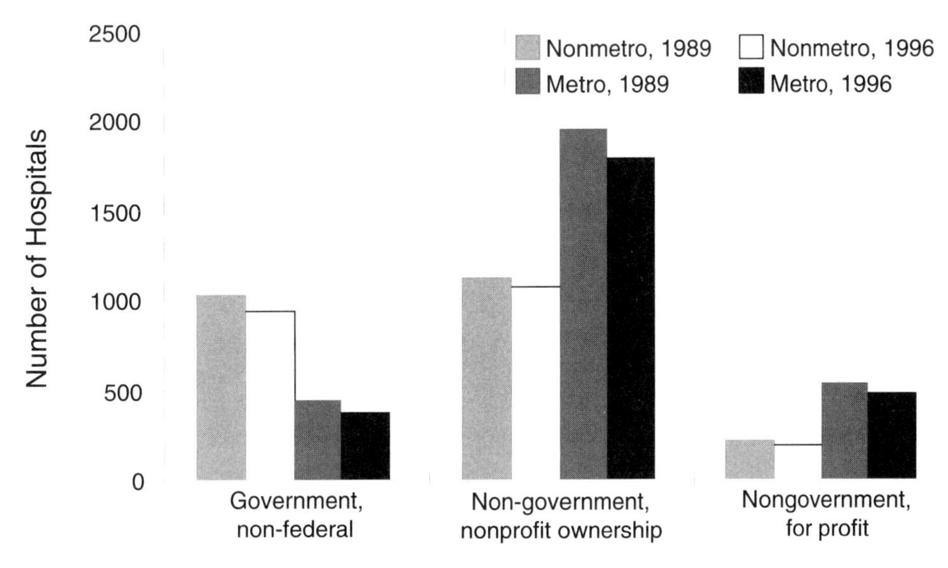

Figure 9.6. Hospital Ownership and Control, metro and nonmetro, 1996. Source: AHA, 1997.

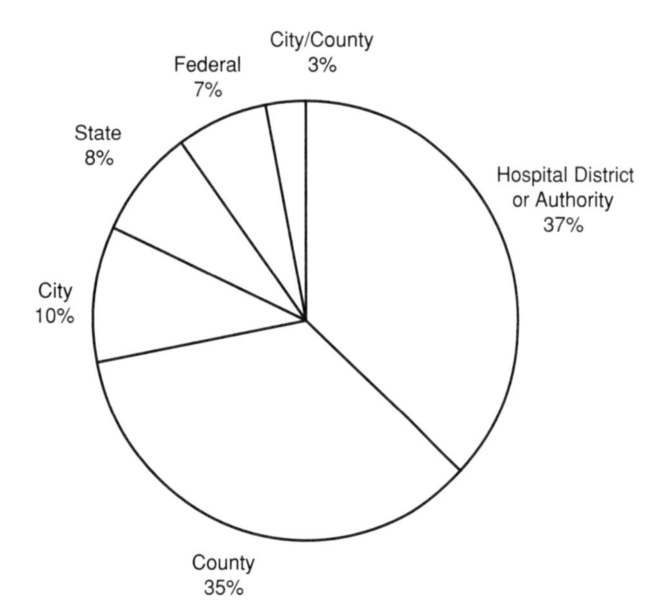

Figure 9.7. Type of control of public nonmetropolitan hospitals, 1996. Source: AHA, 1996.

through 1997, there were a total of 28 rural hospitals that closed, an average of seven a year. Rural hospitals, like their urban counterparts, began to adapt to new market realities, including the need for greater accountability under managed care and the need to more efficiently make use of available resources. Studies of the strategies rural hospitals used for survival showed the importance of local resources, especially income-generating characteristics of the community, including the relative wealth of the population, employment patterns, and state-level policies that supported the hospitals (Seavey, Berry, and Bogue 1992). It is clear from the analysis of hospital survival that the conditions that confront the smallest rural hospitals are fundamentally different from what other hospitals experience. This is reflected in the recent development of policy to support alternative hospital structures and designs including the Medical Assistance Facility (MAF), the Rural Primary Care Hospital (RPCH), and the Critical Access Hospital (CAH). Management strategies for survival have varied and there are no clear models for administrators (Mick et al., 1993); however, there are abundant models of successful integration into networks (Moscovice et al., 1995), innovation, and partnering (Bogue and Hall, 1997).

There are many examples of communities banding together to save their small, rural hospital; but to save hospitals, many of them had to change. The options for change were once limited because of strict license and payment rules from Medicare and state Medicaid agencies. Since the mid-1980s, those options have expanded, both for vehicles to finance hospitals beyond the traditional corporate, nonprofit foundation, and authority structures, as well as in the forms that hospitals can take as they adapt. The organizational forms that are possible can be described in a matrix that scales the operational autonomy against the range of services offered at the facility (Fig. 9.9).

The options included in Figure 9.9 include affiliations that may expand or reduce the number of services offered at the facility while it remains a general, acute care hospital. Rural hospitals are flexible and can expand and

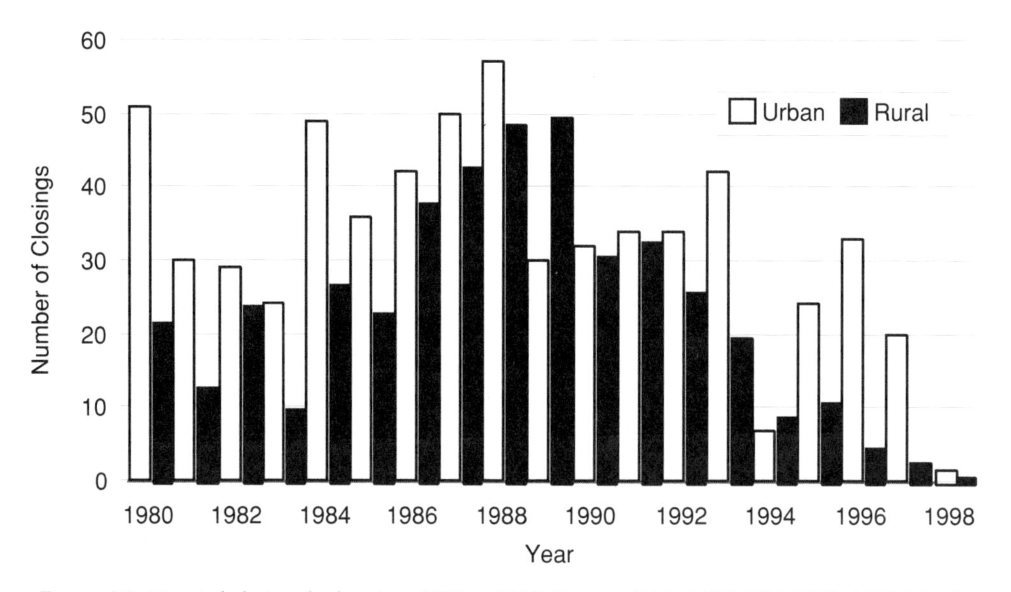

Figure 9.8. Hospital closings by location, 1980 to 1998. Source: AHA, 1997; US DHHS, 1997; North Carolina Rural Research Program, 1998.

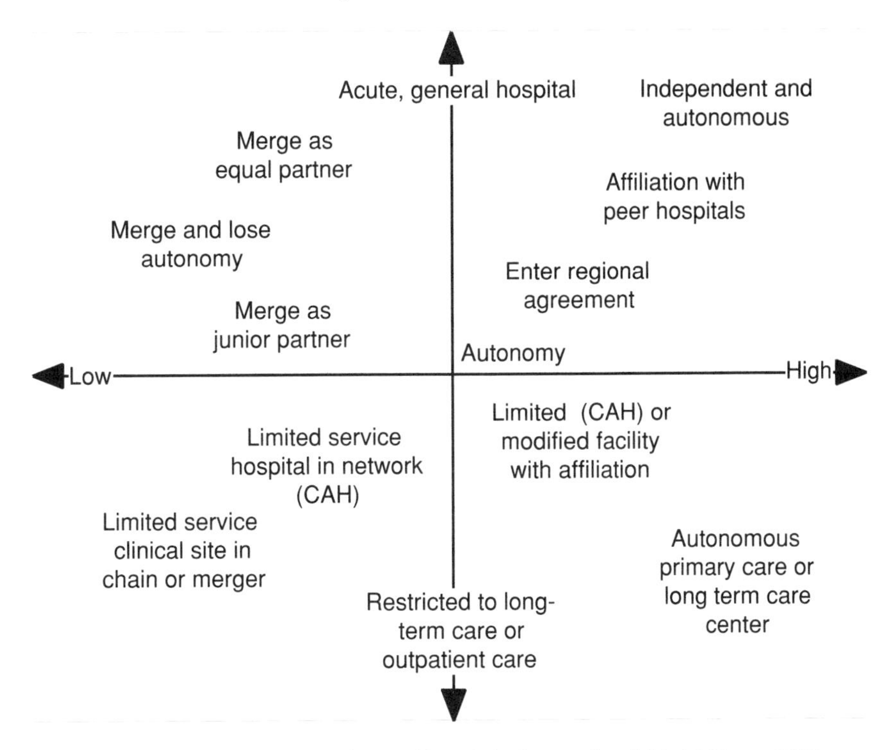

Figure 9.9. Strategic options for rural hospitals. Source: Rural Health News, 1997.

diversify their service offerings to meet local needs for long-term care and specialized services (Fig. 9.10).

Options for conversion include modifying the facility to the point where is ceases to be a hospital and becomes a primary care center or an outpatient facility that specializes in surgery or diagnostic and evaluation activities. Many rural hospitals have been converted into long-term care facilities because the existing physical structure allows for this modification. Conversion is one option that can keep the organization running and the community presence alive (Alexander, D'Aunno, and Succi, 1996). However, the loss of emergency or obstetric services, core components of a "real hospital," may force people to travel outside the community for certain health care services.

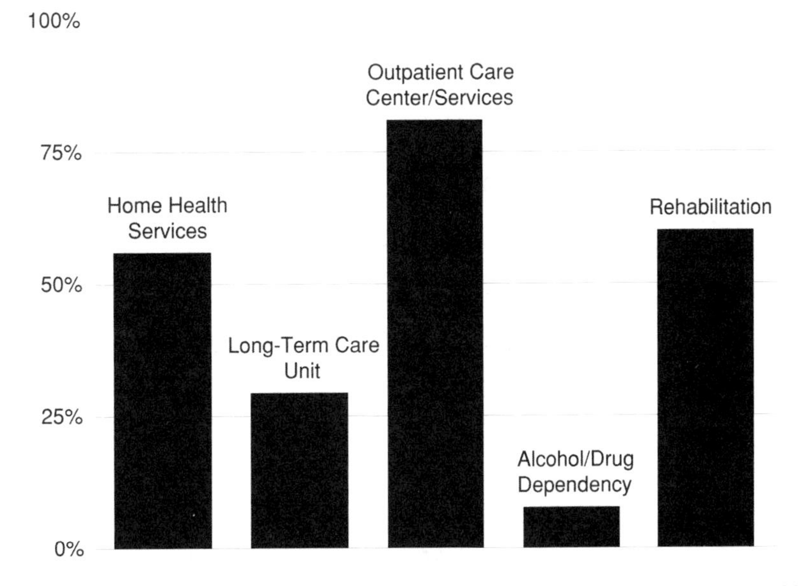

Figure 9.10. Nonmetropolitan hospitals with diversified services, 1996. Source: AHA, 1997.

Diversity: The Approach in Prairie du Chien, Wisconsin

Prairie du Chien Memorial Hospital, located in a community of 6,000 in Wisconsin, presents a case of an innovative hospital whose success can be attributed to its ability to do just about everything. This Crawford County hospital has a $6.5 million surplus and 15% operating margin. The hospital has 44 beds, of which 22 are long-term-care beds, and offers not only emergency, acute, and skilled nursing care but also respite care, home health, durable medical equipment, home oxygen, and rehabilitation services. It has even expanded beyond providing just hospital-related services and now delivers meals to home-bound elderly people, operates a senior meal site in its cafeteria, manages an assisted-living complex for seniors, operates a day-care center, and contracts with the local prison to provide linen service and meals. "With all of these services, many of which are private pay, we can spread our overhead and be very efficient," says CEO Harold Brown, "[And] except for the assisted living, none of this takes a lot of capital." The multiple programs have created spin-off effects.; the older people who come for lunch at the cafeteria will visit inpatients and the drivers who deliver meals to people at home check on them and report problems. Such an arrangement demonstrates the success of a diversification scheme that not only provides more services but also brings together community citizens.

Source: "Ready or Not: Rural Hospitals are Changing." Rural Health News 4(1): Spring 1997.

Rural hospitals have been able to reconfigure their structures to provide a broader or more appropriate mix of services; some have converted many or all of their beds to long-term care while others emphasize outpatient care. Networks have been created among rural hospitals or affiliations have been established with larger hospitals, physician groups, or other health care providers. In each case, the ultimate goal is to meet market needs and ensure institutional survival.

POLICY ISSUES AFFECTING RURAL HOSPITALS

The advent of Medicare and Medicaid was important for the survival of rural hospitals. These programs reimbursed the costs of patients who were previously more liable to need charity to pay for their care—the elderly and the poor. Medicare has been a more important source of revenue for rural hospitals than urban ones because rural communities have a higher proportion of the elderly (Table 9.2).

Medicare underwent an important change in the way it paid for hospital care in the 1980s. In 1982, the Prospective Payment System (PPS) was introduced. The PPS system paid a fixed fee for a specific diagnosis related group (DRG) allowing variations only for very serious cases that might require additional care and resources. The PPS system was meant to be based on the costs of inputs to the hospitals and the formula that calculated those inputs weighted labor costs very heavily. The labor cost estimates were based on prevailing labor rates for the areas in which the hospitals were located, and general labor costs were much lower in rural places than urban. Rural hospitals were paid, on average, less than urban hospitals for the same types of patients with the same diagnoses. These payment differentials created differences in the net payments over (or under) actual costs, also called the "margin," within the Medicare program. Rural hospitals lagged behind urban hospitals in their margins, then fell below the break-even level in 1987 (Fig. 9.11). These payment differentials prompted Congress, in 1990, to redesign the payment policies to reduce geographic difference in rates. The urban-rural gap in PPS margins narrowed in 1991 and 1992 but has widened again since 1993.

Utilization of hospitals has also changed significantly over recent years, with steady drops in use of hospitals since prospective payments and managed care became an important aspect of the market in health care. Between 1991 and 1995 in all nonmetropolitan hospitals, inpatient admissions fell by 1.6%, inpatient days by 5.8%, and lengths of stay by 4.3%; these changes were comparable to drops in overall hospital utilization. These

Table 9.2 Proportion of Nonmetropolitan Hospital Revenue from Medicare, Medicaid, Private Payer, and Uncompensated Care as Percent of Expenses 1986, 1991, 1995, as Percentage of Total Revenue

	1986	*1991*	*1995*
Payer	41.9	37.3	42.1
Medicare	8.7	9.2	11.0
Medicaid	1.0	0.9	1.2
Other Government	48.4	52.4	45.7
Non-Government	48.4	52.4	45.7
Uncompensated[a] Care as			
Percent of Hospital Expenses	Not available	5.3	5.7

[a]Uncompensated care includes both bad debt and charity care.
Source: AHA Profile of Nonmetropolitan Hospitals, Chicago, 1997.

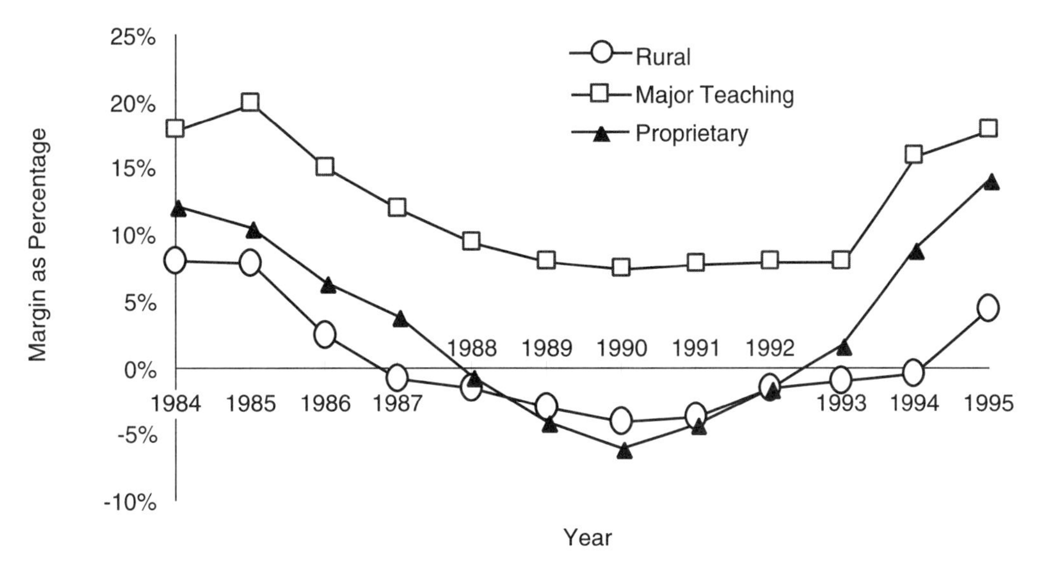

Figure 9.11. Aggregate PPS inpatient margins for selected hospital groups. Source: MEDPAC, 1998.

changes were not consistent across hospitals—interestingly, the smallest rural hospitals showed increases in admissions and bed days during the period. This may have been the result of the closing of low-performing hospitals or small hospitals or a reaction to increased need for services in these communities (Table 9.3).

The ability of a hospital to cover its expenses depends on the proportion of patients who are Medicare beneficiaries. The aggregate margin (excess of revenue over costs) for Medicare inpatients in urban hospitals is 7% in facilities where Medicare accounted for more than 75% of the caseload but only 1.1% where fewer than 60% of patients were enrollees. For rural hospitals, the aggregate Medicare inpatient margin was 6.3% in the

Table 9.3 Inpatient Use of Nonmetropolitan Hospitals by Bed Size, 1991–1995

Bed Size	*Year* *1991*	*1995*	*1991–1995 Percent Change*
ADMISSIONS			
6–49 beds	718,683	788,254	9.7%
50–99 beds	1,367,625	1,266,814	−7.4%
100+ beds	3,028,290	2,975,511	−1.7%
Total	5,144,598	5,030,579	−1.6%
INPATIENT DAYS			
6–49 beds	4,415,517	4,523,637	2.4%
50–99 beds	10,804,255	9,610,185	−11.1%
100+ beds	24,764,305	23,518,656	−5.0%
Total	39,984,077	23,518,656	−41%
LENGTH OF STAY, IN DAYS			
6–49 beds	6.1	5.7	-6.6%
50–99 beds	7.9	7.6	−3.8%
100+ beds	8.2	7.9	−3.7%
Total	7.8	7.5	−3.8%

Source: AHA Annual Survey of Hospitals, 1996. AHA, Profile of Nonmetropolitan Hospitals, Chicago, 1997.

greater-than-75% category and 2.9% in hospitals where fewer than 60% of patients were enrollees.

THE BALANCED BUDGET ACT OF 1997

Reinstatement of the Medicare Dependent Hospital Programs

Congress and the Health Care Financing Administration have developed through legislation a number of special rural hospital payment mechanisms. These systems define sole community hospitals, rural referral hospitals, and Medicare-dependent hospitals. The payments on behalf of Medicare beneficiaries to these hospitals are higher than normal payments to rural hospitals (Table 9.4).

The provision for Medicare-dependent small rural hospitals was originally established in the Omnibus Reconciliation Act of 1989 (OBRA, 1989). The original law provided special payments to small rural hospitals that had a high portion of their revenue derived from the Medicare program and, in effect, had limited ability to make up for any shortfalls in Medicare payments. Rural hospitals that had 100 or fewer beds, had at least 60% of their inpatient days or discharges attributable to Medicare beneficiaries, and were not classified as a sole community hospital could qualify as a Medicare-dependent hospital and receive funds until the provision expired in 1993. With the Balanced Budget Act of 1997, this program was reinstated until 2001 and the target amount for inpatient costs was updated. The provision also states that hospitals may decline geographic reclassification for the purposes of qualifying for this designation.

Rural Referral Centers

A rural referral center (RRC) may request reclassification if its average hourly wage is comparable to hourly wages of hospitals in the area in which the RRC is located. Any hospital classified as a RRC in 1991 was permanently classified as such beginning in 1998.

Geographic Classification for Purposes of Disproportionate Share

Disproportionate share adjustment was added in 1986 to provide additional funds to hospitals that treat a high proportion of low-income persons. The current provision allows all rural hospitals to seek geographic reclassification for the purposes of receiving increased disproportionate share payments (DSH payments).

Medicare Rural Hospital Flexibility Program

This new legislation replaces the current, seven-state EACH/RPCH program (and the Medical Assistance Facility demonstration in Montana) with a new Medicare Rural Hospital Flexibility Program (MRHFP) under which limited-service hospitals known as Critical Access Hospitals (CAHs) would be designated. The program is generally similar to the EACH/RPCH program, with all states eligible for participation. States wishing to have hospitals designated as CAHs must create a Rural Health Plan that describes how a rural hospital network would be created, the criteria for designation of CAHs, and how the development of the networks would enhance rural access. Hospitals 35 miles from the next nearest hospitals are automatically eligible (15 miles in mountainous areas) with states able to waive the distance criteria based on other reasonable standards.

The bed-size limit for CAHs is 15 beds, and the maximum length of stay is 96 hours, unless a longer period is required because of inclement weather or other emergency conditions, or a Professional Review Organization or other equivalent entity, on request, waives the 96-hour restriction. An exception to the bed-size require-

Table 9.4 Median Total Margins by Urban/Rural Location and Rural Type for Fiscal Years

	1990	*1991*	*1992*	*1993*	*1994*	*1995*
All Urban	2.2	2.4	2.3	2.3	2.5	2.9
All Rural	2.2	2.5	2.7	2.8	2.7	3.3
Rural, sole community	2.0	2.3	2.5	3.2	2.9	3.4
Rural, rural referral	3.9	3.9	4.3	3.6	4.3	4.5
Rural, other referral	2.0	2.4	2.4	2.4	2.3	2.9

Source: Mohr, PE et al. 1998. The Financial Dependence of Rural Hospitals on Outpatient Revenue. Bethesda, MD: The Project HOPE Walsh Center for Rural Health Analysis.

ment is made for swing-bed facilities, which may have up to 25 inpatient beds that can be used interchangeably for acute or skilled nursing facility (SNF)-level care, provided that not more than 15 beds are used at any one time for acute care. Current payment provisions for inpatient and outpatient RPCH services are repealed by the provision, and CAHs are to be paid for their reasonable costs of providing the services to Medicare beneficiaries who are, on average, almost half of the users of small, rural hospitals.

Critical Access Hospitals must be part of a rural network; in the seven-state demonstration, this involved an Essential Access Community Hospital (EACH). Now, a rural health network is defined as an organization consisting of at least one CAH and at least one full-service hospital, the members of which have entered into certain agreements regarding patient referral and transfer, communications, and patient transportation. Rural hospitals designated as EACHs under previous law would continue to be paid as sole community hospitals. All prior approved MAFs and RPCHs are automatically approved as CAHs under the new provisions once their state rural health plan has been approved by HCFA.

QUALITY OF CARE

The quality of care provided in rural hospitals has generally been accepted as equal to that provided in urban institutions with some exceptions. A controversial article by a team of RAND investigators (Park et al., 1990) brought the issue of quality in small rural hospitals to the attention of a wider group of researchers. The U.S. Agency for Health Care Policy and Research (AHCPR) contracted for a careful review of the evidence of effects on quality of care and health outcomes for patients who were admitted to smaller, rural hospitals to examine the effects of low volumes and other hospital characteristics. The results of that study, reported in the *Journal of Rural Health* (Schlenker et al., 1996), found that there was strong evidence of a volume-outcome effect, with low volumes associated with poorer outcomes for a certain set of conditions and procedures. However, most procedures for which a volume-outcome relationship has been demonstrated are not typically performed in small, rural hospitals. The strongest relationships between volume and outcomes have been found for coronary artery bypass graft/open heart surgery; total hip replacement, intra-abdominal artery operation/resection; cardiacatheterization and angiography; and transurethral prostatectomy. All but the last procedure were unlikely to be carried out in small, rural hospitals. The analysis highlights that many procedures and conditions commonly treated in rural and urban hospitals have not been studied for a volume-outcome effect and that all hospitals need to improve their assessment of their patient care quality.

Assessing quality of care, health outcomes, and provider performance is a growing area of health care. Some would say that it is becoming a common part of the health care system as reports of hospital and health plan performance are more commonly published and disseminated. The increasing interest in quality comes when many are concerned that managed care may negatively affect quality because of its focus on controlling costs. Although there is very little research evidence to support this belief, it has become a motivating reason to move away from a health care system based almost completely on price. Some hospitals have adopted continuous quality techniques as a means to improve care; many others with small staffs and limited resources have found it difficult to support a full-time quality assurance program. In spite of these limitations, many rural hospitals are addressing the needs of the community and finding opportunities to improve quality of care. In 1996, 78% of rural hospitals reported that they had worked in concert to conduct a health status assessment of the community; only 65% said that they use health status indi-

Table 9.5 Rural Hospital Focus on Quality and Community Health Needs

	Percent of Total		
	1993	*1996*	*Percent Change*
WORK IN CONCERT TO CONDUCT A HEALTH STATUS ASSESSMENT OF THE COMMUNITY			
Nonmetro	53.0	78.0	25.1
Metro	61.4	83.6	22.1
USED ASSESSMENT TO IDENTIFY UNMET HEALTH NEEDS, EXCESS CAPACITY, OR DUPLICATIVE SERVICES			
Nonmetro	56.4	61.7	5.3
Metro	64.8	74.0	9.2
USED HEALTH STATUS INDICATORS TO DESIGN OR MODIFY SERVICES			
Nonmetro	47.8	65.2	17.3
Metro	67.2	82.2	15.1
SHARE CLINICAL AND HEALTH INFORMATION WITH COOPERATING ORGANIZATIONS			
Nonmetro	47.2	61.8	14.7
Metro	65.5	78.6	13.1
DISSEMINATE COST AND QUALITY TO THE COMMUNITY			
Nonmetro	40.7	48.1	7.4
Metro	48.6	64.5	16.0

Source: AHA Annual Survey of Hospitals, 1997.

Clinical Care Program Improves Provider Coordination and Patient Care

Rutland Regional Medical Center is a 188-bed hospital that serves a six-county region in rural Vermont. In 1993, personnel at the hospital decided to assemble a working group to focus on the on going problem of long lengths of stay. After looking at the multiple factors that affect patient outcomes and utilization—patient, nursing, physician, organization, and environmental characteristics—the team decided to focus on improving the clinical coordination of care. Their solution was to establish a Clinical Care Coordinator Program headed by "super nurses." The goal of the program was to facilitate patient care, increase the efficiency and communication of medical teams, and implement the continuous quality improvement process. At the end of one year, it was determined not only that length of stay had decreased significantly but also that the medical staff was able to conduct rounds more smoothly; and patients and family members liked the access to a specific person who would listen and answer questions. Positive effects of the program include enhanced problem identification, improved communication, and patient satisfaction. The success of the program has not only improved the quality of care at Rutland Regional Medical Center but has led to its replication in the orthopedics service and community cancer center.

Source: Winstead-Fry P, Bormolini S, Keech RR. 1995. Clinical care coordination program—a working partnership. Journal of Nursing Administration 25(7/8): 46–51.

cators to design or modify services. The overall trend is toward an increased focus on quality and community needs, yet rural hospitals lag behind their urban counterparts (Table 9.5).

REFERENCES

Alexander JA, D'Aunno TA, Succi MJ. 1996. Determinants of rural hospital conversion. Medical Care 34(1): 29–43.

Bindman AB, Keane D, Lurie N. 1990. A public hospital closes: impact on patient's access to care and health status. JAMA 264: 2899–2904.

Bogue R, Hall CH Jr, eds. 1997. Health Network Innovations: How 20 Communities are Improving Their Systems Through Collaboration. Chicago: American Hospital Publishing.

Christianson JB, Faulkner L. 1981. The Contribution of Rural Hospitals to Local Economies. Inquiry 18(1): 46–60.

Doeksen GA, Altobelli JG. 1990. The Economic Impact of Rural Hospital Closure: A Community Simulation. Grand Forks, ND: University of North Dakota Rural Health Research Center.

Doeksen GA, Loewen RA, Strawn DA. 1990. A rural hospital's impact on a community's economic health. Journal of Rural Health 6(1): 53–64.

General Accounting Office. 1991. Rural Hospitals: Federal Efforts Should Target Areas Where Closures Would Threaten Access to Care. Washington, DC: HRD 91–41.

Hadley J, Nair K. 1991. The impact of rural hospital closure on Medicare beneficiaries' access to hospital care. Washington, DC: Georgetown University Center for Health Policy Studies. Prepared under Health care Financing Administration Cooperative Agreement Number 17-C-99499.

Kronick R, Goodman DC, Wennberg J, Wagner E. 1993. The marketplace for health reform: the demographic limitations of managed competition. New England Journal of Medicine 328(2): 148–152.

Lillie-Blanton MS, Felt S, Redmon P, Renn S, Machlin S, Wenmar E. 1992. Rural and urban hospital closures, 1985–1988: operating and environmental characteristics that affect risk. Inquiry 29(3): 89–102.

McDermott RE, Cornia GC, Parsons RJ. 1991. The economic impact of hospitals in rural communities. Journal of Rural Health 7(2): 117–132.

Mick SS, Morlock LL, Salkever D, de Lissovoy G, Malitz FE, Wise CG, Jones A. 1993. Rural hospital administrators and strategic management activities. Hospital and Health Services Administration 38 (3): 329–352.

Moscovice I, Wellever A, Christianson J, Kralewski J, Manning W. 1995. Building Rural Hospital Networks. Ann Arbor, Mich: Health Administration Press.

Mullner RM, Rydman RJ, Whiteis D. 1990. Rural hospital survival: An analysis of facilities and services correlated with risk of closure. Hospital & Health Services Administration 35(1): 121–137.

Park RE, Brook RH, Kosecoff J, Keesey J, Rubenstein E, Keeler E, Kahn KL, Rogers WH, Chassin MR. 1990. Explaining variations in hospital death rates: randomness, severity of illness, quality of care. JAMA 264(4): 484–490.

Rosenbach ML, Dayhoff DA. 1995. Access to care in rural America: impact of hospital closures. Health Care Financing Review 17(1): 15–37.

Rural Policy Research Institute. 1994a. Anticipated Impacts of the Health Secutiry Act (HR 3600) On the Rural Health Delivery System. Columbia, Mo: University of Missouri.

Rural Policy Research Institute. 1994b. The Rural Perspective on National Health Reform Legislation. Columbia, Mo: University of Missouri.

Schlenker RE, Hittle DF, Hrincevish CA, Kachny MM. 1996. Volume/outcome relationships in small rural hospitals. Journal of Rural Health 12 (5):395–409.

Seavey JW, Berry DE, Bogue RJ, eds. 1992. The Strategies and Environments of America's Small, Rural Hospitals. Chicago: Hospital Research and Educational Trust.

Succi MJ, Lee SYD, Alexander JA. 1997. Effects of market position and competition on rural hospital closures. Health Services Research (6):679–699.

10

Rural Managed Care

MICHELLE M. CASEY

This chapter provides a brief historical perspective on managed care in rural areas and presents national data on health maintenance organizations (HMO), rural service areas, and rural enrollment in commercial HMOs. Future prospects for the growth of managed care in rural areas are discussed, including the implications of changes in the Medicare and Medicaid programs authorized by the Balanced Budget Act of 1997 (PL 105–33).

There are many forms of managed care; however, this chapter will focus on rural enrollment in HMOs. Although other types of managed care plans such as preferred provider organizations (PPOs) serve rural areas, national data on rural enrollment in non-HMO plans are not available.

HISTORICAL PERSPECTIVE ON MANAGED CARE IN RURAL AREAS

Although prepaid health plans were established in rural areas of the United States in the 1920s and 1930s, most of the HMO development since the federal Health Maintenance Act of 1973 has occurred in urban areas. The limited presence of HMOs in rural areas has been attributed to several factors, including smaller populations, the relatively low number of large employers in many rural areas, resistance of some rural physicians to participation in HMOs, lack of available capital for HMO development, and low Medicare adjusted average per capita cost (AAPCC) payment rates (Christianson et al., 1986; Christianson, 1989; Office of Technology Assessment, 1990; Serrato, Brown and Bergeron, 1995; Wellever et al., 1996; Casey, 1998; Christianson et al., 1997).

HMOs AND RURAL SERVICE AREAS

For the purpose of this chapter, the term "rural" describes counties located outside a metropolitan statistical area. Service areas are commonly reported by county, and the definition of rural used by all studies cited for county-level data is metropolitan/nonmetropolitan. The many variations in rural-urban definition are examined in depth in Chapter 1, Populations and Places in Rural America.

The number of rural counties in HMO service areas and the number of HMOs serving rural areas have been used as measures of potential access to HMOs (Christianson et al., 1986; Serrato, Brown, and Bergeron, 1995; Ricketts, Slifkin, and Johnson-Webb, 1995). The number of rural counties in HMO service areas decreased from 1989 to 1991 but then increased substantially between 1991 and 1995 (Table 10.1). Growth was especially rapid between 1994 and 1995, when the percentage of rural counties in the service area of at least one HMO increased from 60% to 82%.

Rural counties located in HMO service areas differ significantly from those that are not in HMO service areas on several socioeconomic and health system characteristics (Table 10.2). Rural counties in HMO service areas have almost twice the average population and more than twice the average population density of rural counties that are not in HMO service areas. They also have a

Table 10.1 Percent of Rural Counties in Service Area of at Least One HMO by Year

Year	*Percentage*
1988	52.6
1989	53.2
1990	47.7
1991	43.0
1992	48.1
1993	53.8
1994	59.6
1995	82.3

Source: University of Minnesota Rural Health Research Center, *Rural Managed Care: Patterns and Prospects,* 1997, analysis of data from the InterStudy National HMO Census, 1988–1995.

Table 10.3 HMOs by Number of Rural Counties in Service Area, 1995 (n = 585 HMOs)

Number of Rural Counties	*Number of HMOs*	*Percentage*
0	162	28%
1–5	193	33%
6–10	82	14%
11–20	66	11%
21 or more	82	14%

Source: University of Minnesota Rural Health Research Center, *Rural Managed Care: Patterns and Prospects,* 1997, analysis of data from InterStudy National HMO Census, 1995.

significantly higher percentage of the population employed in manufacturing, and a lower percentage employed in agriculture.

Almost three fourths of all HMOs included at least one rural county in their service area (Table 10.3). In 1995, 193 HMOs served one to five rural counties and 229 HMOs served more than five rural counties. On average, HMOs with rural counties in their service areas have larger total enrollment than HMOs that serve only urban areas.

The most common HMO model in rural areas is the independent practice association (IPA) model, which accounts for 58% of the HMOs serving rural areas (Table

Table 10.2 Characteristics of Rural Counties in and not in HMO Service Areas, 1995 (n = 49 states)[a]

County Characteristics	*Counties in an HMO Service Area (n = 1702)*	*Counties not in an HMO Service Area (n = 553)*
Population, 1994	25,765[e]	14,102
Population density, 1994 (per square mile)	42.5[e]	20.6
Unemployment rate, 1992 (number unemployed/number in civilian labor force)	8.2[e]	6.3
College-educated, 1990 (percent of population 25 years of age and older)	15.9[e]	16.8
Income per capita, 1993 (1,000s of 1993 dollars)	15.5[e]	17.0
Percent of population 65 years of age and older, 1994	15.5[e]	17.0
Standardized AAPCC rate, aged Part A (FY 1996)	233.3	230.7
Standardized AAPCC rate, aged Part B (FY 1996)	124.8[e]	121.9
Community hospital beds, 1993 (per 1,000 residents)	3.6[e]	5.0
Hospital occupancy rates, 1993[b] (community hospital beds)	0.51[e]	0.47
Physicians per capita, 1994[c] (per 1,000 residents)	0.83[e]	0.72
Percent of population in agriculture, 1990	9.1[e]	16.2
Percent of population in construction, 1990	7.0[e]	6.2
Percent of population in health services, 1990	7.5[d]	7.2
Percent of population in white collar jobs, 1990	42.3[e]	40.5
Percent of population in manufacturing, 1990	20.0[e]	13.3

Source: University of Minnesota Rural Health Research Center, *Rural Managed Care: Patterns and Prospects,* 1997, analysis of data from InterStudy National HMO Census, 1995; Area Resource File, 1996; HCFA (AAPCC rates), 1996.

[a]Alaska is excluded because Area Resource file data on Alaska are available only on the state level.

[b]Counties without hospitals are not included.

[c]Includes MDs and DOs.

[d]Indicates a significant difference in mean values at the .05 level.

[e]Indicates a significant difference in mean values at the .01 level.

Table 10.4. Model Types of HMOs Serving Rural Counties and Percentages, 1995

Staff model	HMO delivers health services through a physician group that is employed by the HMO.	3%
Group model	HMO contracts with one independent group practice to provide health services.	7%
Network model	HMO contracts with two or more independent group practices, possibly including a staff group, to provide health services; it may contain a few solo practices, but is predominantly organized around groups.	10%
Mixed model	Any HMO that uses a combination of the other model types.	22%
IPA model	HMO contracts directly with physicians in independent practices, and/or contracts with one or more associations of physicians in independent practice, and/or contracts with one or more multi-specialty group practices.	58%

Source: University of Minnesota Rural Health Research Center, *Rural Managed Care: Patterns and Prospects*, 1997, analysis of data from InterStudy HMO Census 1995; HMO model definitions: InterStudy, 1996.

10.4). Mixed-model HMOs represent 22% of the HMOs serving rural areas. Only 14 HMOs (2.4% of all HMOs) are headquartered in rural areas (Table 10.5). The percentage of rural-based HMOs has declined over time, suggesting that expansion of urban-based HMOs into rural areas is likely to dominate the pattern of HMO development in rural areas.

RURAL COMMERCIAL HMO ENROLLMENT

Although the service areas of many HMOs now include rural counties, actual rural HMO enrollment rates are low. Only eight states report county-level commercial HMO data (Table 10.6). Two of these states, Pennsylvania and Wisconsin, have more than 10% of their rural population under age 65 enrolled in a commercial HMO as compared with the more than 30% enrollment in their urban counterparts. Five states (Florida, Missouri, Minnesota, North Carolina, and South Carolina) have between 4% and 7% rural HMO enrollment, and one state (Wyoming) has less than 1%.

The national rural HMO enrollment rate is unknown, but is likely to be lower than the 7.8% average of these eight states for two reasons. First, the two states with the highest rural enrollment rates, Pennsylvania and Wisconsin, have large rural-based HMOs, which are uncommon in other states. Second, most of the states with large rural populations (Alabama, Alaska, Arkansas, Georgia, Idaho, Indiana, Iowa, Kansas, Louisiana, Maine, Mississippi, Montana, Nebraska, North Carolina, Oklahoma, South Carolina, Tennessee, Texas, Virginia, West Virginia) have total HMO enrollment rates well below the national average, whereas four of these eight states have total HMO enrollment rates that are higher than the national average.

Urban residents in these eight states are more than three times as likely as rural residents to be enrolled in a commercial HMO. Rural HMO enrollment rates in the eight states vary by population density and adjacency to urban areas (Table 10.7). The highest rural HMO enrollment rates are found in counties that are adjacent to large metropolitan areas and contain a city of over 10,000 population.

MEDICAID MANAGED CARE

The role of Medicaid managed care in rural areas is described in detail in Chapter 8, Medicaid Managed Care in Rural Areas. With the exception of Arizona, which has operated a statewide Medicaid managed care system since 1982, nearly all of the early Medicaid managed care initiatives were in large urban areas. As a result, relatively little research has been done on Medicaid managed care programs in rural areas. As of 1995–96, over 700,000 rural Medicaid recipients, or about 10.5% of rural Medicaid recipients nationally, were enrolled in HMOs and prepaid health plans.* Recent changes in federal regulations, however, encourage states to implement Medicaid managed care programs, and therefore growth is expected in the coming years.

MEDICARE MANAGED CARE

Medicare managed care is discussed in Chapter 6, Medicare Program in Rural Areas. Historically, Medicare risk enrollment has been much lower in rural areas than in urban areas. As of September 1998, 2.6% of rural Medicare beneficiaries were enrolled in risk plans (RUPRI, 1999). The lower enrollment rate in rural areas

*This total includes enrollment in licensed HMOs and other prepaid health plans that contract on a risk basis with state Medicaid agencies, and excludes enrollees in Medicaid primary care case management programs, and dental and mental health managed care programs.

Table 10.5 HMOs Headquartered in Rural and Urban Areas: 1988–1995

	Location of HMO Headquarters			
	Rural		*Urban*	
Year	*Number*[a]	*Percent*	*Number*[a]	*Percent*
1988	28	4.7	568	95.3
1989	24	4.2	544	95.8
1990	19	3.5	518	96.5
1991	16	3.1	503	96.9
1992	15	2.9	499	97.1
1993	16	3.2	479	96.8
1994	12	2.4	497	97.6
1995	14	2.4	560	97.6

[a]HMOs that report financial data as a single entity are counted as one HMO.
Source: University of Minnesota Rural Health Research Center, *Rural Managed Care: Patterns and Prospects,* 1997, analysis of data from Interstudy National HMO Census, 1988–1995; Office of Management and Budget metropolitan statistical area designations, 1994–1995.

reflects a geographic discrepancy in the availability of Medicare risk plans. In 1996, 100% of Medicare beneficiaries residing in central urban areas and 68% of beneficiaries in other urban areas had at least one managed care option, while 92% of Medicare beneficiaries in rural nonadjacent areas and 79% of beneficiaries in rural adjacent areas had no managed care plans available (PPRC, 1997) Medicare risk enrollment was growing in both urban and rural areas during the 1990's. However, 43 HMOs decided not to renew their Medicare risk contracts and 53 plans reduced their service areas as of January 1999 (HCFA, 1998). Rural counties represent a disproportionate share of the counties affected and, in particular, of the counties with no other risk plans available to beneficiaries.

Table 10.6 Average Rural and Urban Commercial HMO Enrollment in 8 States, 1995

	Percent of Population under 65 Years of Age Enrolled in Commercial HMOs	
State	*Rural*	*Urban*
Florida	4.9	24.3
Minnesota	5.5	35.8
Missouri	6.3	26.2
North Carolina	4.2	13.6
Pennsylvania	12.0	30.8
South Carolina	4.6	9.7
Wisconsin	17.0	35.7
Wyoming	0.6	0.0
Total	7.8	25.7

Source: University of Minnesota Rural Health Research Center, *Rural Managed Care: Patterns and Prospects,* 1997.

SUMMARY AND CONCLUSIONS

Although rural HMO enrollment rates are very low and continue to be considerably below those of urban areas, significant increases in rural enrollment in commercial HMOs, Medicare risk plans, and Medicaid HMOs and prepaid health plans appear likely in the near future. Increased competition among HMOs for members in urban areas is providing HMOs with incentives to expand to rural areas. Both the number of HMOs with rural counties in their service areas and the number of rural counties in the service areas of HMOs have increased significantly over the past five years, indicating that HMOs have been expanding their capacity to serve rural commercial enrollees.

The 1997 BBA contains several provisions that should make it more attractive for HMOs and other managed care organizations to serve rural Medicare beneficiaries under risk plans. The legislation establishes a minimum AAPCC payment floor of $367 in 1998. It phases in a blending of national and local AAPCC rates over a 6-year period of time, with a goal of achieving a 50/50 blend by 2004. The legislation also creates three options for establishing Medicare payment areas within a state: statewide, all rural counties in a state, and groups of noncontiguous counties. Provider-sponsored organizations (PSOs) may contract with HCFA on a risk basis to serve Medicare beneficiaries, and a PSO may meet federal standards in lieu of state licensing requirements for up to 3 years.

An analysis by the Rural Policy Research Institute (RUPRI) indicated that rates in 30% of all rural counties and 44% of rural nonadjacent counties would be raised to the minimum AAPCC payment rate of $367 in 1998 (RUPRI, 1997). Blending of national and local AAPCC rates was expected to increase rates in many rural counties that were already above the minimum rate; however, the cost of the minimum payment floor and the 2% "hold harmless" increase left little money to blend national and local rates for 1998 (Reichard, 1997).

Many of the states that currently have the highest rural Medicaid HMO and prepaid health plan enrollment rates are those that have implemented statewide 1115 waivers. Several additional states recently implemented 1115 waivers, which may significantly increase rural Medicaid managed care enrollment over the next few years. In addition, the BBA eliminates the requirement

Table 10.7 Commercial HMO Enrollment in 8 States by Degree of Urbanicity, 1995

County Type	*Percent of Population under 65 Enrolled in Commercial HMOs*
Metropolitan	
Large—central and fringe counties of metro areas of 1 million or more population	33.3
Small—counties in metro areas of fewer than 1 million population	17.1
Non-metropolitan	
Adjacent to a large metro area with a city of 10,000 or more	13.7
Adjacent to a large metro area without a city of at least 10,000 population	10.6
Adjacent to a small metro area with a city of 10,000 or more population	9.5
Adjacent to a small metro area without a city of at least 10,000 population	8.9
Not adjacent to a metro area and with a city of 10,000 or more population	2.3
Not adjacent to a metro area and with a city of 2,500 to 9,999 population	4.3
Not adjacent to a metro area and with no city or a city with a population less than 2,500	3.9

Source: University of Minnesota Rural Health Research Center, *Rural Managed Care: Patterns and Prospects*, 1997.

that states obtain waivers to require mandatory enrollment of Medicaid beneficiaries in Medicaid managed care organizations and primary care case management programs. The legislation also allows states an option to require Medicaid managed care enrollment in rural areas with only one managed care entity, as long as an enrollee may receive care "through not less than two physicians or case managers" and obtain care from "any other provider in appropriate circumstances."

In order to monitor the impact of Medicare and Medicaid policy initiatives and changes in employer-provided health insurance on rural populations, it will be essential to analyze future changes in rural enrollment in Medicare risk plans, other Medicare managed care options, Medicaid HMOs/prepaid health plans, and commercial HMOs. Currently, county-level Medicare risk enrollment data are available from HCFA. However, only eight states report county-level data on commercial HMO enrollment, and Medicaid managed care definitions and reporting periods vary from state to state. Uniform collection of county-level Medicaid HMO and prepaid health plan and commercial HMO enrollment data at the state level would greatly improve researchers' abilities to analyze the impact of managed care on rural populations.

REFERENCES

Reichard J, ed. 1997. New Medicare HMO rates: one plan's ceiling is another plan's floor. Medicine and Health 51(36): 1.

Casey M. 1998. Serving rural Medicare risk enrollees: HMOs' decisions, experiences, and future plans. Health Care Financing Review 20(1): 73–81.

Christianson J, Shadle M, Hunter M, et al. 1986. The new environment for rural HMOs. Health Affairs 5: 105–121.

Christianson J. 1989. Alternative delivery systems in rural areas. Health Services Research 23: 6: 849–889.

Christianson JB, Wellever A, Hamer R, Knutson D. 1997. HMO financial arrangements with rural physicians. Journal of Rural Health 13(3): 240–252.

Health Care Financing Administration (HCFA). 1998. Status of Medicare non-renewals as of October 14, 1998. Internet. URL:http://www.hcfa.gov/Medicare/status.htm

Physician Payment Review Commission (PPRC). 1997. Annual Report to Congress. Washington, DC: PPRC.

Ricketts T, Slifkin R, Johnson-Webb K. 1995. Patterns of health maintenance organization service areas in rural counties. Health Care Financing Review 17(1): 99–113.

Rural Policy Research Institute (RUPRI). 1997. The Rural Implications of Medicare AAPCC Capitation Changes: Background Assessment and Simulation Results of Key Legislative Proposals. Columbia, MO: University of Missouri.

Rural Policy Research Institute. (RUPRI). 1999. Taking Medicare into the 21st Century: Realities of a Post-BBA World and Implications for Rural Health Care. Columbia, MO: University of Missouri.

Serrato C, Brown R, Bergeron J. 1995. Why do so few HMOs offer Medicare risk plans in rural areas? Health Care Financing Review 17: 85–97.

US Congress, Office of Technology Assessment. 1990. Health Care in Rural America.

Wellever A, Casey M, Krein S, Yawn B, Moscovice I. 1996. Rural Physicians and HMOs: An Uneasy Partnership. Rural Health Research Center Working Paper Series #17, University of Minnesota, Institute for Health Services Research.

11

Rural Health Care Networks

ANTHONY WELLEVER

Many rural health providers voluntarily collaborate with other health care providers to cope with the challenges of operating in a turbulent, rapidly changing health care delivery and financing environment. By coalescing into cooperatives, alliances, consortia, or networks, rural providers expect to reduce their costs, manage their scarce resources, and increase their bargaining position with other institutional actors, such as insurers and regulators (Zuckerman, Kaluzny, and Ricketts, 1995). The popularity of voluntary collaboration among rural providers may have accelerated in recent years in response to the Medicare prospective payment system and the anticipated expansion of managed care in rural areas, both of which caused rural hospitals and other providers to seek improvements in the management of their cost and utilization (Shortell, Gillies, and Devers, 1995; Shortell, Gillies, and Anderson, 1994).

This chapter will present a brief overview of rural health networks. The chapter begins with a discussion of conceptual issues concerning the definition of rural health networks. The types and characteristics of existing rural health networks are considered next. Descriptions of several recent state, federal, and private programs to support rural health network development and the results of formal evaluations of some of these programs are also presented.

RURAL HEALTH NETWORKS DEFINED

Defining rural health networks is not a clear-cut task. On the one hand, the term network is used to mean everything from casual contacts among rural providers to relations between commonly owned organizations. On the other hand, words such as alliances and consortia are used to describe arrangements that are, in essence, networking relationships. Bringing sense to the topic requires being fairly precise about what rural health networks are and what they are not. The following definition is intended to draw a bright line around what is and what is not a network. A rural health networks is:

> a formal organizational arrangement among rural health care providers (and possibly insurers and social service providers) that uses the resources of more than one existing organization and specifies the objectives and methods by which various collaborative functions will be achieved (Moscovice et al., 1996, p. 7).

This definition has four components:

1. *The organizational arrangement is formal.* Formal in this case means explicit and legal. Examples include memoranda of understanding, contracts, incorporation of a network in which the individual members are shareholders (if for-profit) or board members (if not-for-profit), and consolidation of functions by acquisition or merger up to consolidation into a single entity.
2. *The membership is specified.* Integrated rural health networks are composed of a variety of health care providers (i.e., they are not composed of only one type of provider, such as only hospitals or only community health centers). They may also include insurers and social service providers. Urban members may participate as network members, as

long as at least two rural providers also participate as members.

3. *Resources are committed by members.* Resources (e.g., money, time) are contributed to the network by its members (but not necessarily in the same proportion by all of its members). The network is composed of pre-existing organizations. New organizations created by the network (e.g., a mobile imaging service or a health maintenance organization) are not included.
4. *The network is purposeful.* A network is more than a mission statement; it must be productive. Networks perform functions and activities according to an explicit plan of action. Examples of collaborative functions range from sharing services to coordinating and integrating services provided by member organizations to the direct provision and financing of care (Moscovice et al., 1996).

Although a wide variety of rural health network types fall under this definition, a number of interorganizational arrangements are excluded by it (Table 11.1) Rural health networks, as defined above, occupy only the center band in this spectrum of inter-organizational arrangements. Informal networks are located on the left side of this spectrum. Like formal networks, informal networks are formed when rural providers join together voluntarily to achieve one or more objectives and each of the participants retains its autonomy. Informal networks differ from formal networks in that the roles and responsibilities of members and the purposes of the network itself are not set forth in a written agreement. Although informal networks may be quite effective at solving problems that arise from time to time, they are not created with the intention of serving as a forum for solving problems on a permanent basis. Formal networks, on the other hand, create a structure that is intended to last. Formal networks identify which issues they will pursue; who is in the network and who is not; and how authority is allocated among members. By committing the agreement to writing, the members are clear about the purpose of the network and the duties of membership. A written contract allows the members to be precise about the network's purposes and also provides a framework for modifying that purpose should it become desirable. By signing the agreement, members consent to its terms.

Health care systems are depicted on the other side of the spectrum shown in Table 11.1. In these arrangements, multiple providers work together, cooperatively integrating a variety of administrative and patient care functions. Unlike both informal and formal networks, participants in systems are not autonomous but are owned by a single entity. The roles, responsibilities, and relationships of participants to one another are spelled out in corporate documents such as articles of incorporation, bylaws, and policies and procedures. Theoretically, systems have a strategic advantage over networks in their ability to decide questions quickly and to compel their members to comply with corporate decisions. In reality, however, many systems—especially new ones—may be no more highly integrated than networks.

Organizational theorists suggest that as uncertainty in the environment grows, organizations tend to replace their reliance on markets for their needed resources with hierarchies. In other words, when recurring uncertainty about the outcome of transactions between organizations is prevalent, "the inefficiencies of bureaucratic organization will be preferred to the relatively greater costs of market transactions" (Powell, 1990). Although it is far too early to tell whether this theory will hold in regard to rural health networks, it is interesting to speculate that inter-organizational relations among rural health providers may become more hierarchical over time; that is, successful informal networks may become formal networks, and successful formal networks, under the right circumstances, might become integrated systems.

TYPES OF RURAL HEALTH NETWORKS

Several types of networks fall within the broad definition of rural health networks proposed above. These network types all satisfy the definition, but they differ from one another in terms of their purpose and membership. In this section, the similarities and differences of various

Table 11.1 Spectrum of Inter-organizational Arrangements

Type	*Informal Network*	*Formal Network*	*System*
Action	Joint action	Joint action	Joint action
Agreement	No written agreement	Written agreement	Written agreement
Level of Autonomy	Individual autonomy	Individual autonomy	Common ownership

Source: Moscovice et al., 1996.

Horizontal and Vertical Networks

Rural health networks are often described as either horizontal or vertical depending on the composition of their members. The term *horizontal network* has come to mean a network composed of all of the same types of members—for example, a rural health network composed only of hospitals. A *vertical network*, on the other hand, has come to mean a network composed of different types of members—for example, a network of doctors and hospitals or a network of community health clinics, hospitals, and public health agencies. Individual horizontal and vertical rural health networks will vary in their degree of integration from those that are highly integrated to those that are not integrated at all.

Horizontal rural health networks tend to be somewhat older than vertical networks. They typically are composed of members who do not compete actively with one another and who come together to share information and services of strategic value to them. Vertical rural health networks are a newer type of cooperation organization and are formed to reduce duplication across provides, improve continuity of care, and position providers to prosper in a managed care environment.

types of health care networks are noted. The network types are defined in the sidebar Rural Health Network Definitions.

Affiliations, Alliances, Consortia, and Cooperatives

The definitions of affiliations, alliances, consortia, and cooperatives in the sidebar—Rural Health Network Definitions—share the following attributes: (1) the method of linking members together is a formal agreement or a formal organization (which implies incorporation or some other form of defined structure); (2) the participants in these arrangements are independently owned; and (3) the members jointly participate in specific activities. Affiliation agreements are typically bilateral, with two entities forming a linkage between them. Frequently, one of the partners to the agreement is a larger facility located in either a rural or an urban setting. The larger partner provides a range of services to the smaller partner. The larger partner may charge for some services and provide others at no charge to the smaller facility. A larger facility may have a number of bilateral affiliation agreements with rural providers. This arrangements is often characterized as a "spoke-and-wheel" network, in which services, resources, and communications flow independently between the center (the large provider) and each of the nodes (the small providers) without the programmed exchange of services, resources, and communications between and among the various nodes.

In contrast to simple affiliations, alliances, consortia, and cooperatives encourage the exchange of services, resources, and communications among all of the members of the network. The agreement forming the network typically defines the nature of relationships among members. Because of the experience gained through the network participation, members may increase the number of informal transactions occurring among them. Some of these transaction may become formal over time.

Alliances, consortia, and cooperatives may have one or more large members that donate the majority of tangible resources to the network. Luke (1991) hypothesizes that the existence of a single large member stabilizes relationships within a network. The existence of a large, powerful member may be associated with better network performance, because a large member can finance new network enterprises and dedicate staff to network development. Moscovice and his colleagues (1995) found that 53% of 127 rural hospital networks had at least one urban (and presumably larger) member.

Although not true in every case—the vocabulary of networks is far from precise—alliances are often regional or national in scope and member attachment to the alliance is minimal. In many instances, the alliance serves as a vendor of services and products or as a conduit to vendors of services and products at reduced prices. Alliance membership in many cases is purely a group purchasing strategy. Consortia typically are composed of like members such as all hospitals or all community health clinics. Cooperatives may or may not be defined by law as a type of corporate entity.Cooperatives may be composed of all one type of member or various types of members and typically provide a range of services to consumers for agreed-on monthly fees (Casey, 1995; Kushner, 1991).

Independent Practice Associations (IPA)

A confusing term, IPA is used to describe both a Health Maintenance Organization (HMO) model type and an independent physician organization that contracts with an HMO. For the purpose of this chapter, an IPA is considered exclusively as a type of physician organization. An IPA is a rural health network if it is composed exclusively or primarily of rural physician practices. IPAs differ from other types of rural health networks in that they

Rural Health Network Definitions

Affiliation. An agreement (usually formal) between two or more otherwise independent entities or individuals that defines how they will relate to one another. Affiliation agreements between hospitals may specify procedures for referring or transferring patients from one facility to another, joint faculty and/or medical staff appointments, teaching relationships, sharing of records or services, or provision of consultation between programs (Alpha Center, 1998).

Alliance. A formal organization, usually owned by shareholder/members, that works on behalf of its individual members in the provision of services and products and in the promotion of activities and ventures. Examples of alliances: Voluntary Hospitals of America, Consolidated Catholic Health Care, and American HealthCare System (American Hospital Association, 1995).

Consortium. Two or more independently owned [like] entities [such as hospitals] having activities that are coordinated by a central management body (Provan, 1984, p. 495).

Cooperative. A formal organization working on behalf of its individual members for a specific purpose (e.g., sharing of services, development of staff education programs, legislative advocacy) (Office of Technology Assessment, 1990, p. 479).

Independent Practice Association (IPA). A health maintenance organization delivery model in which the HMO contracts with a physician organization [the IPA], which in turn, contracts with individual physicians. The IPA physicians practice in their own offices and continue to see fee-for-service patients. This type of system combines prepayment with the traditional means of delivering health care (Texas Medical Association, 1997).

Management Services Organization (MSO). A corporation owned by a hospital or hospital/physician joint venture that provides management services to one or more medical group practices. MSOs purchase the tangible assets of the practice and lease them back as part of a full-service management agreement. The MSO employs all nonphysician staff and provides all supplies and administrative systems for a fee (American Hospital Association, 1995).

Physician-Hospital Organization (PHO). A legal entity formed by a hospital and a group of physicians to further mutual interests and to achieve market objectives. A PHO generally combines physicians and a hospital into a single organization for the purposes of obtaining payer contracts. Doctors maintain ownership of their practices and agree to accept managed care patients according to the terms of a professional services agreement with the PHO. The PHO serves as a collective negotiating and contracting unit. It is typically owned and governed jointly by a hospital and shareholder physicians (Alpha Center, 1998).

Provider Sponsored Network (PSN)/Provider Service Organization (PSO). Formal affiliations of providers, organized and operated to provide an integrated network of health care providers with which third parties, such as insurance companies, HMOs, or other health plans, may contract for health care services to covered individuals. Some models of integrated include Physician Hospital Organizations (PHOs) and Management Service Organizations (MSOs) (Alpha Center, 1998).

have a specific function and their membership is limited to certain kinds of providers.

The primary purpose of an IPA is to contract with a managed care organization (MCO) on behalf of a group of individual physicians. The IPA contracts with an MCO as an independent organization and in turn contracts with individual physicians or physician practices to provide services. Using an IPA makes provider contracting easier for an MCO, because the MCO does not have to contract with each provider individually. Contracting through an IPA may be beneficial for physicians in small practices also: their overall bargaining power with MCOs may be increased because of the size of the IPA. IPAs frequently limit their activities to contracting with MCOs and individual providers, but some may perform other services as well. For example, an MCO may contract with an IPA to provide utilization and quality management services on behalf of the MCO. In these arrangements, the IPA may own or lease its own management information system, or it may use the systems of the MCO. In either case, physician members of the IPA are responsible for the utilization and quality management of the MCO's enrollees. In accepting this responsibility, the members of the IPA are typically at risk for poor performance. On the other hand, the physicians of the IPA are free to set the performance standards they prefer, thus maintaining a sizable portion of their clinical autonomy.

Some IPAs contract directly with self-insured firms to provide medical services to the firm's employees. Insurance commissioners and consumer advocates in some states have criticized this practice because they believe there are not adequate safeguards to protect consumers in the event of unexpectedly high costs or high utilization of services.

The membership criteria for an IPA is highly prescriptive. Membership is typically limited to individual physicians or group practices. Nonphysician providers, such as nurse practitioners or physician assistants, may also participate as members in some IPAs. Other institutional providers, however, such as hospitals and nursing homes, may not participate as members of IPAs.

Physician-Hospital Organizations (PHO) and Management Service Organizations (MSO)

Physician-Hospital Organizations (PHOs) perform many of the same functions as IPAs, except that PHOs perform these functions, as the name implies, for both physicians and hospitals. PHOs contract with MCOs and, in turn, the PHO pays the hospital and physicians for services provided to MCO enrollees according to the terms outlined by the PHO-provider contract. Like IPAs, PHOs may contract with MCOs only to provide services to the MCOs enrollees, or the PHO may agree to provide services and managed utilization and quality. PHOs may also contract directly with self-insured employers.

PHOs are composed of physicians and hospitals. The physicians may join the PHO as individuals, as practices, or as an IPA. In situations in which a PHO is composed of an IPA and a hospital, governance may be shared equally by the two entities. In these cases, the PHO typically will contract with an MCO on a capitation basis. The PHO may then contract with the IPA on a capitation or partial capitation basis, and the IPA may, in turn, pay physicians on a fee-for-service basis.

PHOs are usually local organizations formed by a single hospital and its medical staff. There is a variety of PHO, however, referred to as a "super-PHO" that combines several hospitals and their medical staffs into a single organization. Some of these super-PHOs, in essence, are networks of local PHOs. Although MCO contracts are negotiated for the super-PHO as a whole, payments to individual providers are determined by the local PHO.

Management services organizations (MSOs) were initially developed as a method of binding physicians to hospitals, thereby improving physician retention. By removing physicians from many of the business aspects of medical practice, MSOs allow physicians to concentrate more fully on patient care. Like PHOs, MSOs are composed of physicians and hospitals. Like PHOs, MSOs also engage in a limited number of functions. MSOs offer practice and real estate management services to physicians for a fee. MSOs may also negotiate managed care contracts on behalf of an integrated group of physicians. An MSO may be wholly owned by a hospital that contracts individually with physicians and practices, or it may be owned as a joint venture between a hospital and some or all of its medical staff that contracts individually with physicians and practices.

Provider Service Organizations (PSO)

Created by the Balanced Budget Act of 1997, Provider Service Organizations (PSOs) are networks of health care providers who deliver a "substantial portion" of the health care items and services required by Medicare beneficiaries directly through the network or an affiliated group of providers and that accept a "substantial amount" of financial risk in providing such items and services. In essence, PSOs function as both insurance companies and providers. The Health Care Financing Administration will contract with PSOs on a risk basis to cover care provided to Medicare beneficiaries under the Medicare + Choice program. PSOs may choose to be licensed by their states as HMOs or they may seek a 3-year federal waiver. Under the waiver, PSOs must fulfill federal solvency, financial planning, benefits design, quality assurance, and premiums and cost-sharing regulations (*Federal Register,* May 7, 1998). In some cases, the waiver regulations may be more onerous than state licensure as an HMO. At this time, the ultimate impact this provision of the Medicare statute will have on rural health networks that wish to contract with Medicare is not known. The ability and willingness of providers to comply with either state or federal waiver regulations is likely to create special problems for some rural providers that want to form networks to serve Medicare patients on a risk basis. To assure a critical mass of Medicare+ Choice enrollees and to obtain adequate start-up financing, successful rural PSOs will likely need to cover a broad geographic area. Other rural providers who wish to participate in Medicare risk ventures will likely have to join an urban-based, regional PSO. In some markets (e.g., small urban markets that rely heavily on rural referrals), these urban-based, regional PSOs may provide ample opportunities for rural providers to participate in PSO governance and management.

WHY DO RURAL HEALTH NETWORKS FORM?

Rural health networks form for a variety of personal and institutional reasons. These motivations can be grouped

Table 11.2 Reasons Why Rural Hospitals Joined Their Networks (n = 303)

	Level of Importance (%)				
Reason	*Not at All Important 1*	*2*	*3*	*4*	*Extremely Important 5*
Expand revenue base	29.3	26.9	22.6	13.5	7.7
Improve quality of service	9.0	10.0	25.8	33.4	21.8
Promote cost efficiency	4.0	8.3	14.0	24.3	49.3
Gain political power with federal/ state government	19.3	21.7	20.7	18.3	20.0
Improve balance of power with urban hospitals and physicians	17.7	19.7	28.4	19.4	14.8
Gain window into other hospitals	7.7	11.3	21.0	26.0	34.0
Gain operations help from network staff	11.0	11.4	25.4	26.4	25.8

Source: Moscovice et al., 1995.

broadly into three categories: resource acquisition, information needs, and political gains (Knoke, 1988). Using these categories as a framework, Moscovice and colleagues (1995) in 1992 asked 303 rural hospital members of networks to rate each of seven statements in terms of the potential gains they expected to obtain when they joined their respective networks (Table 11.2).

The primary motivation cited by rural hospital administrators for joining a network was promotion of cost efficiency. On a 5-point scale, with 5 representing "extremely important" and 1 representing "not at all important," 73% of respondents said that promotion of efficiency rated either a 4 or 5. The second major motivation was to gain a window into other organizations (i.e., improve information about services and operating practices). Two other motivations were cited by more than one half of the respondents as being important (i.e., the statement was rated either 4 or 5): improve the quality of service and gain operations help from network staff.

Well over one half of administrators said that expanding the revenue base was not important (those rating the statement either 1 or 2). The responses to the two statements in the political gains category, improve balance of power with urban providers and gain political power with state/federal government, were relatively evenly distributed across the five levels of importance. Much of the recent rural health network formation activity, however, appears to be directed at improving the competitive and bargaining positions of rural health providers in their relations with urban providers and health plans.

CHARACTERISTICS OF RURAL HEALTH NETWORKS

Current knowledge of rural health network characteristics is limited to those networks with at least one rural hospital member. Although rural health networks without rural hospital members exist, no studies have been conducted to date to identify them and report on their structural and operating characteristics.

Hospitals Participating in Rural Health Networks

Rural hospitals are among the primary participants in rural health networks. In 1995, the American Hospital Association (AHA) asked rural hospitals whether or not they participated in either a network* or alliance, PHO, MSO, IPA, or system (see definitions in sidebar Horizontal and Vertical Networks). Eighty-seven percent (87%) of rural hospitals (1,914 out of 2,204) responding to the survey answered all the questions conerning their participation in collaborative organizations. The results of the survey are displayed in Table 11.3. Not-for-profit, nongovernmental rural hospitals were significantly more likely to participate in alliances and

*AHA defines "network" as "a group of hospitals, physicians, and other providers, insurers, and/or community agencies that work together to coordinate and deliver a broad spectrum of services to the community (AHA, 1995). Because this definition is broader than the one proposed earlier, the responses to "networks" and "alliances" were combined. An affirmative response to either network or alliance participation or both was counted as a single case of membership in the alliance/network category.

Table 11.3 Percent of Rural Hospitals Participating in Various Collaborative Organizations by Hospital Characteristic (n=1914)

	Number	*Alliance/Network*	*PHO*	*MSO*	*IPA*	*System*
HOSPITAL TYPE						
Not-for-profit	965	45.1%	24.9%	10.8%	17.5%	38.1%
Government, non-federal	816	40.9%	17.2%	4.3%	14.6%	9.2%
For profit	133	33.1%	36.8%	23.3%	16.5%	79.0%
Total	1914	42.5%	22.4%	8.9%	16.2%	28.6%
BED SIZE (ACUTE CARE ONLY)						
25 or fewer beds	417	36.7%	12.5%	5.5%	15.4%	19.9%
26–50 beds	752	40.7%	16.8%	5.3%	15.2%	23.9%
51–100 beds	465	41.3%	28.6%	12.3%	15.5%	36.8%
101–200 beds	230	54.8%	40.0%	18.3%	21.7%	38.3%
201 or more beds	50	72.0%	52.0%	16.0%	20.0%	52.0%
OCCUPANCY RATE						
25% or less	408	35.8%	11.8%	4.2%	13.2%	19.6%
26%–50%	986	42.6%	22.9%	8.6%	16.0%	29.5%
51%–75%	477	49.1%	30.2%	13.2%	18.5%	33.3%
76%–100%	43	30.2%	25.6%	11.6%	23.3%	41.9%
AVERAGE DAILY CENSUS						
10 or fewer patients	372	43.6%	13.4%	3.8%	15.9%	16.9%
11–25 patients	480	37.9%	18.8%	7.9%	14.4%	25.2%
26–50 patients	438	40.4%	24.2%	10.7%	16.0%	34.9%
51–100 patients	390	42.1%	24.1%	8.0%	18.0%	32.1%
101 or more patients	234	54.7%	38.0%	17.1%	18.0%	36.8%
URBANICITY/ RURALITY						
Adjacent to a large metro area with a city of 10,000+	91	42.9%	37.4%	23.1%	20.9%	40.7%
Adjacent to a large metro area without a city of 10,000+	84	27.4%	16.7%	7.1%	14.3%	26.2%
Adjacent to a small metro area with a city of 10,000+	224	45.4%	32.6%	16.1%	17.9%	36.2%
Adjacent to a small metro area without a city of 10,000+	452	39.8%	19.5%	8.0%	15.3%	26.6%
Not adjacent with a city of 10,000+	279	52.7%	34.1%	12.9%	20.1%	33.7%
Not adjacent without a city of 10,000 or more but with a city of 2,500–9,999 residents	523	42.5%	19.1%	5.5%	14.9%	25.6%
Completely rural: no city with >2,500 residents	261	38.3%	9.6%	2.3%	13.8%	23.0%
REGION						
New England[a]	50	48.0%	30.0%	6.0%	12.0%	14.0%
Middle Atlantic[b]	71	38.0%	25.4%	11.3%	21.1%	25.4%
East North Central[c]	275	33.5%	23.6%	10.9%	12.7%	27.3%
West North Central[d]	480	49.0%	17.5%	5.6%	12.5%	28.8%
South Atlantic[e]	236	53.0%	25.0%	9.8%	16.5%	29.2%
East South Central[f]	219	39.7%	23.7%	9.6%	15.1%	40.6%
West South Central[g]	303	42.2%	25.7%	10.2%	15.5%	22.4%
Mountain[h]	186	32.8%	19.4%	7.5%	21.0%	26.3%
Pacific[I]	94	36.2%	23.4%	13.8%	38.3%	37.3%

[a]New England = ME, VT, MA, NH, CT, RI.
[b]Middle Atlantic = NY, NJ, PA.
[c]East North Central = OH, MI, IN, IL, WI.
[d]West North Central = MN, IA, MO, KS, NE, SD, ND.
[e]South Atlantic = DE, MD, VA, WV, NC, SC, GA, FL.
[f]East South Central = KY, TN, MS, AL.
[g]West South Central = AR, LA, TX, OK.
[h]Mountain = MT, WY, CO, NM, AZ.
[i]Pacific = WA, OR, CA, AK, HI.
Source: AHA, 1996; University of Minnesota, Rural Health Research Center, 1997.

networks than were government and for-profit rural hospitals. On the other hand, for-profit rural hospitals were much more likely to participate in a PHO, MSO, or system. Rural governmental hospitals (e.g., county, district, or municipal hospitals) were much less likely than the other two types of rural hospitals to participate in MSOs. This is possibly a reflection of the reluctance of local government officials to use public money to support ostensibly private, profit-making enterprises such as physician practices.

Larger rural hospitals, as measured by number of beds (bed size), were more likely to participate in all manner of collaborative organizations. Particularly striking is the level of their involvement in alliances and networks: 72% of rural hospitals with more than 201 beds participate in alliances/networks. These larger rural hospitals often serve a catalyst for bringing network members together and act as a chief source of funding for the network during the early stages of development (Moscovice et al., 1995).

Rural hospitals in New England, the East North Central, and South Atlantic census regions are significantly more likely to participate in alliances/networks than rural hospitals in other regions of the country. Fifty-three percent (53%) of the rural hospitals in the South Atlantic region participate in networks. Within this region, two states (Florida and West Virginia) have state-sponsored or state-coordinated rural health networking initiatives, and at least two other states in the region have active state offices of rural health that encourage networking (North Carolina and Georgia). The region of the country in which rural hospitals are least likely to participate in alliances/networks is the Mountain region, possibly because of the large distances between communities.

Rural hospitals in the Pacific region are two to three times more likely to participate in an IPA than rural hospitals in most of the other regions. This is no doubt a reflection of greater rural managed care penetration in California, Washington, and Oregon, and the small number of rural hospitals in the Alaska and Hawaii, which are less penetrated states. Rural hospitals in the East South Central region and the Mountain region are significantly more likely to belong to a hospital system than rural hospitals in other sections of the country. Tennessee and Kentucky, in the East South Central region, have a long history of for-profit and not-for-profit system development. The development of rural hospital participation in systems in the Pacific region is probably the result of the growing consolidation of the health care system on the West Coast and escalating competition among these health care giants.

Rural hospitals in counties with a city of at least 10,000 residents that are not adjacent to an urban county are significantly more likely to participate in a rural network than rural hospitals in other counties. Over one half of these hospitals said they were members of an alliance/network. Many of the hospitals in this group are larger and likely serve as the sponsor for rural health networks. Rural hospitals with a city of at least 10,000 residents that are adjacent to a large metropolitan area are significantly more likely to participate in PHOs and MSOs. Because these rural hospitals are close to metropolitan competitors, they may have attempted to establish linkages with and provide services to members of their medical staffs in an effort to bond the physicians to the hospital. These relationships are intended to improve physician retention, affect referral patterns, and improve bargaining strength with managed care organizations.

Rural Health Networks: A Recent Snapshot

In 1996, the University of Minnesota Rural Health Research Center identified and surveyed all 180 rural health networks distributed over 44 states with at least one rural hospital member (Plate 11.1). (Moscovice, Wellever, and Krein, 1997). The Midwest region had the highest proportion of rural health networks in the country (72 of 180). Five categories of network composition emerged from the survey responses. These networks were composed of

1. Rural hospitals only
2. Rural and urban hospitals only
3. Hospitals and physicians
4. Hospitals, physicians, and others
5. Hospitals and others (no physicians)

Among rural health networks with at least one hospital member, the most common networks are composed exclusively of hospitals (46.7%). However, approximately 60% of new networks (i.e., less than 2 years old) that include at least one hospital include a more diverse membership (Table 11.4). Widespread rural health network development is a relatively recent development. Although some rural health networks have existed for 20 years or more, approximately 70% are quite young—3 years old or less.

By definition, all rural health networks in this study have at least one rural hospital as a member. In these networks, physicians are the next most common member. However, fewer than one half of all rural health networks have physician members. Approximately one in four rural health networks in this study reported having urban hospital members. Participation of other health and social service providers or health care insurers is much less common (Table 11.5).

Table 11.4 Percent of Integrated Rural Health Networks, 1996

	Rural Hospitals Only	*Rural & Urban Hospitals Only*	*Hospitals & Physicians*	*Hospitals, Physicians & Others*	*Hospitals & Others (No Physicians)*
NETWORK AGE (IN YEARS)					
<2 (n = 49)	22.5	18.4	26.5	20.4	12.2
2–3 (n = 72)	23.6	15.3	29.2	22.2	9.7
>3 (n = 53)	43.4	20.8	11.3	11.3	13.2
NETWORK SIZE (IN NUMBER OF MEMBERS)					
<5 (n = 44)	41.9	11.3	35.5	6.5	4.8
5–10 (n = 41)	22.5	16.3	26.5	20.4	14.3
11–20 (n = 34)	29.6	18.2	11.4	27.2	13.6
21–30 (n = 27)	13.3	33.3	0	26.7	26.7
>30 (n = 34)	0	40.0	20.0	40.0	0

Source: Moscovice, Wellever, and Krein, 1997.

Eight of ten rural health networks are incorporated as either for-profit or not-for-profit corporations. Approximately 90% of incorporated rural health networks are not-for-profit organizations. Eleven percent (11%) of rural health networks are bound together by a written contract (e.g., affiliation agreement or memorandum of understanding) (Table 11.6). Over 90% of networks have a governing board that is responsible for the conduct of the network. Eighty percent (80%) of networks have developed written bylaws to outline the roles and responsibilities of the network and its members, officers, and managers. The level of structure implicit in incorporation and bylaw development may indicate the members' belief that the network is a "going concern" and not simply a forum for solving a transitory problem (Table 11.7).

Member dues are the primary source of income for networks in this study, with over one half of the respondents saying that they rely on dues to finance operations. More than 40% of networks depend on the sale of network services to members or others as a source of revenue. The third most common form of network funding is government grants, with approximately one third of the rural health networks in the study reporting that they receive grants from either the state or the federal government (Table 11.8). This survey was conducted before the 1997 development of the Federal Office of Rural Health Policy's (FORHP) Rural Network Development Grant Program. Presumably, the proportion of networks relying on government grants for a portion of their funding would be higher if the survey were conducted today.

Table 11.5 Rural Health Network Membership, 1996

Member Type	*Percent of Networks with This Type of Member*
Rural hospitals	100.0
Physicians	42.2
Urban hospitals	39.4
Mental health providers	10.6
Home health agencies	10.0
Public health agencies	10.0
Nursing homes	9.4
Ambulance services	6.1
Social service agencies	6.1
HMO/Insurance companies	5.0

Source: Moscovice, Wellever and Krein, 1997.

STATE, FEDERAL, AND PRIVATE PROGRAMS TO SUPPORT RURAL HEALTH NETWORK DEVELOPMENT

Over the past 10 years, a number of programs to support rural health network development have been created. Varying in sponsorship and purpose, each of these pro-

Table 11.6 Legal Status of Integrated Rural Health Networks, 1996

Legal Status	*Percent*
For-profit	9.4
Not-for-profit	70.0
Cooperative	6.1
Government	2.2
Contract	10.6
Other	1.7

Source: Moscovice, Wellever, and Krein, 1997.

Table 11.7 Rural Health Network Governing Board Attributes, 1996

Percent of networks with a governing board	90.6%
Average size of governing board	12.3 people
Percent of networks with community board members	35.6%
Average number of community board members	5.6 people
Percent of networks with written bylaws	80.6%

Source: Moscovice, Wellever, and Krein, 1997.

grams offered rural providers with grants to develop co-operative solutions to the problems of rural health care delivery.

New York State Rural Health Network Demonstration Program

In 1986, the New York legislature authorized the creation of the Rural Health Network Demonstration Program as "a pilot project program for the purpose of assisting local and regional health care providers, consumers and organizations in underserved rural areas to promote more effective health care delivery systems and to maintain essential community services through the development of contracts or joint or cooperative agreements among health care providers" (Chapter 624, Laws of 1986, New York State). The legislation called for funding projects that would result in the merger, integration, reorganization, or coordination of similar or different types of health care providers into unified health care delivery systems. It defined a network as any two providers entering a joint venture or cooperative agreement that resulted in improvements in resource sharing, access to services, or efficiency of delivery. Between 1986 and 1993, the New York demonstration program made awards totaling $1.8 million for rural health network development.

In 1994, rural health network development in New York state entered a new phase. Capitalizing on the lessons learned in the demonstration project, the state legislature institutionalized rural health network development by creating a program for networks within the state's rate-setting legislation, New York Prospective Hospital Reimbursement Methodology (NYPHRM V). Funds for rural health network development were tied to reimbursement legislation. Between 1994 and 1996, $1 million per year was made available to networks in the form of grants, and $3 million per year were made available as rate enhancements to providers participating in certain kinds of networking relationships. In the demonstration phase, any collaborative activity was viewed favorably. In the second phase of network development, emphasis focused on two types of networks: "vertically integrated" rural health networks and those established under the EACH Program (see below). Approximately 20 networks were funded during this period.

Rate enhancements were eliminated in 1996. Rural health network development in the state, however, did not suffer. The Health Care Reform Act of the State of New York made available $7 million per year for network development between 1997 and 1999. Thirty-four awards ranging from approximately $50,000 to $340,000 were made in 1997. In this, the third phase of rural health network development in New York, the emphasis shifted from planning and organizational development to implementation of specific action plans.

Over the course of the past decade, New York has pioneered rural health network development, moving in an orderly fashion from experimentation to integrated net-

Table 11.8 Sources of Network Funding and Reliance on Those Sources, 1996

Sources of Network Income	*Percent of Networks That Use This Source of Funding*	*Percent of Networks That Use Only This Source of Funding*
Government grants	31.4	10.0
Private foundation grants	10.7	1.4
Member dues	52.9	19.3
Sale of network services	43.6	10.7
Health insurance premiums	5.7	2.1
Loans from members	1.4	0.0
Contributions from members	15.0	6.4
Contributions from non-members	5.0	0.7

Source: Moscovice, Wellever, and Krein, 1997.

work infrastructure development to implementation. The first phase of the New York State Rural Health Demonstration Program was evaluated formally in 1994. For more information about rural health network development in New York State, call 518-474-5565.

Robert Wood Johnson Foundation Rural Hospital Network Program

Established in 1987, the Rural Hospital Network Program (RHNP) was designed not to demonstrate the efficacy of any one collaborative strategy for improving rural health care but instead to support the development of a range of strategies to improve the delivery of health care services in rural areas. The Robert Wood Johnson Foundation (RWJF) hoped that the successful demonstrations would serve as models to be replicated in other rural communities. The foundation provided grant support to networks of rural hospitals or networks including both rural hospitals and other providers. Four-year awards of up to $600,000 were made to each of the 13 networks selected to participate in the program. Grant funds were used to support personnel, consultants, travel, supplies and equipment, and startup and marketing expenses associated with new services. The variety of programs developed by RHNP participants included shared services, primary care and specialty clinics, and professional recruitment. Grant funds were also used for network development. The participating networks were also eligible to apply for up to $500,000 in low-interest loans. The Foundation arranged for faculty from the New York University Graduate School of Public Administration to provide technical assistance to RHNP grantees. For more information, call 609-452-8701.

Essential Access Community Hospital Program

The Essential Access Community Hospital (EACH) Program was the first attempt by the federal government to assure the availability of primary care, emergency services, and limited acute inpatient services in rural areas where it was no longer feasible to maintain a full-service hospital. Established by Congress as part of the Omnibus Budget Reconciliation Act (OBRA) of 1989, the Program created the Rural Primary Care Hospital (RPCH), a Medicare-certified limited-service hospital. RPCHs were required to establish network relationships with larger supporting hospitals designated as EACHs. The rural health network of the program was defined as an organization that included at least one RPCH and one other acute care hospital that had mutual agreements regarding patient referral and transfer, the development and use of communications systems, and the provision of emergency and nonemergency transportation among members.* The EACH Program awarded $21.7 million in grants to 59 RPCHs,† 37 EACHs, and seven state governments (Wright et al., 1995). Limited to only seven states, the EACH Program was superseded by the Medicare Rural Hospital Flexibility Program in 1997 (see below). For more information, call 410-786-6675.

Florida Rural Health Network Initiative

In 1993, the Florida legislature created the Rural Health Network Initiative, whose purpose was to establish rural health networks to promote the coordinated delivery of quality health care services in rural areas of the state. A rural health network was defined as a nonprofit legal entity consisting of rural and urban health care providers and others that is organized to plan and deliver health care services on a cooperative basis in a rural area except for some secondary and tertiary services (s.381.0406, Florida Statutes). A key feature of the legislation creating the initiative was the authorization of a grant program to develop four rural health "laboratories" in the state to test alternative methods for delivering health care services.

At present, Florida has certified nine integrated rural health networks. The network service areas contain approximately 988,265 residents living in 25 rural counties. The networks include 693 health care providers and 40 hospitals. Through the networks, local providers have established IPAs, PHOs, and Provider Service Networks (PSNs). Improvement of emergency medical services and the broader diffusion of telemedicine are explicit goals of the Florida networks. Three networks have negotiated with insurance companies to develop and market low-cost managed care plans targeted at small businesses and the uninsured, and three networks have contracted with the Florida Healthy Kids Program, an insurance program for children. Two networks received grants under the FORHP Network Development Program (see below). The networks have developed a variety of other services. A primary goal of each network is to prepare local medical communities for "integration into managed care systems." For more information, call 850-413-0113.

*An RPCH was not required to be linked with an EACH. The program required only linkage with "one other acute care hospital."

†All "RPCH grantees" did not covert to RPCH status, but all did establish a relationship with an EACH or other supporting hospital.

Table 11.9 Rural Networks Participating in the CCN Demonstration Program

Name	*City*	*State*
Northwest Georgia Healthcare Partnership	Dalton	Georgia
Southcentral Health Network	Twin Falls	Idaho
Franklin Community Partnership	Farmington	Maine
Itasca Partnership for Quality Health Care	Grand Rapids	Minnesota
Healthcare 1999	Pembroke	North Carolina
Sullivan County Community Health Network	Claremont	New Hampshire
Tioga County Partnership for Community Health	Wellsboro	Pennsylvania
Bamberg County Multi Disciplinary Committee	Denmark	South Carolina
Rural Health Outreach Program	Arlington	Virginia
Lincoln County Public Health Coalition	Odessa	Washington

West Virginia Rural Health Networking Project

The West Virginia Rural Health Networking Project was a 3-year program sponsored by the Claude Worthington Benedum Foundation of Pittsburgh to plan for and establish integrated health networks in rural areas of West Virginia. Beginning in 1994, the program was administered by the West Virginia Office of Community and Rural Health Services, which received a grant of $144,500 from RWJF for the purpose of planning and administering the project. Two types of grants were offered: Type A grants of up to $15,000 for one year, available to providers who would use the funds to support network planning and development; and Type B grants of up $150,000 over 3 years to assist established networks in implementing network plans. Three networks were funded under this project, which was administered cooperatively with the West Virginia EACH Program and the Agency for Health Care Policy and Research Rural Managed Care Centers Program (see below). For more information, call 304-558–0580.

Community Care Network Demonstration Program

The Community Care Network (CCN) Demonstration Program involves 25 networks of health care and health promotion, which are testing the AHA's vision for locally reformed health care delivery and financing (Table 11.9). That vision has four elements that CCN must incorporate: community health focus, management within fixed resources, seamless continuum of care, and community accountability. The network members include health care, business, government, and community organizations serving a wide range of rural, suburban, and inner-city communities. In addition to 25 sites participating in the program, 24 finalists from a pool of 283 applicants share information about their success in pursuing the CCN vision.

The program is a collaborative effort of the Health Research and Education Trust (formerly the Hospital Research and Education Trust), the AHA, Catholic Health Association of the United States, and Voluntary Hospitals of America (VHA, Inc.). The W. K. Kellogg Foundation and The Duke Endowment provided $7 million to start the program in 1995. In 1996, the program's scope of activity was expanded to include an evaluation component to look at the long-term potential for the CCN model with $1.2 million in grants from the Robert Wood Johnson Foundation, W. K. Kellogg Foundation, the California Wellness Foundation, and the U.S. Public Health Service. Another grant of $750,000 was awarded by the W. K. Kellogg Foundation to examine the networks' ability to sustain their efforts over time as well as governance issues within each of the CCNs.* For more information, call 312-422–2600.

AHCPR Rural Managed Care Centers Program

In October 1994, AHCPR awarded cooperative agreements to five university-based groups to promote the "establishment of managed care institutions and the development of rural health networks." This program was created by Congress at a time when many policy makers believed that national health care reform would be based on managed competition and that many rural areas lacked the necessary infrastructure to implement managed care systems. AHCPR made awards to investigators at the Universities of Arizona, Oklahoma, Southern Maine,

*A mid-term evaluation of the Community Care Network Demonstration is Health Network Innovations: How 20 Communities Are Improving Their Systems Through Collaboration. Richard Bogue and Claude H. Hall, eds. 1997. Chicago: American Hospital Publishing.

West Virginia, and a partnership between the Universities of Nebraska and Iowa. Intended as a 5-year program, AHCPR project officers have adhered to the original intent of the initiative despite the demise of federal health care reform. Primarily a demonstration program rather than AHCPR's traditional focus on research, the awards were intended to foster "innovations in delivery of health care services," with an emphasis on the development of rural health networks. The activities undertaken by the demonstration sites vary, but include provider and community education about managed care, network development, health care information system development, communication systems development, and managed care contracting support. For more information, contact: Arizona, 520-626–7946; Maine, 207-780–4430; Nebraska/Iowa, 402-559–5260; Oklahoma, 405-271–3230; and West Virginia, 304-293–6753.

Federal Office of Rural Health Policy Rural Network Development Grant Program

At the direction of Congress in 1997, FORHP offered grants of up to $200,000 per network per year to "vertically integrated" rural health networks to support planning, development, and evaluation. The goals of these networks were to (1) expand access to care in rural areas, (2) coordinate care in rural areas, (3) restrain the cost of health care, and (4) improve the quality of care in rural areas. From over 130 applications, 34 awards were made in September 1997. For more information, call 301-443–0835.

Medicare Rural Hospital Flexibility Program

The successor program to the EACH Program, the Medicare Rural Hospital Flexibility Program features a limited-service rural hospital model named the Critical Access Hospital, which functions in a network relationship with a larger rural or urban acute care hospital. Unlike the EACH Program, which was open to only seven states, the Medicare Rural Hospital Flexibility Program is open to all states, upon application to HCFA. A "rural health network" is defined by the legislation as an organization consisting of at least one critical access hospital and one other hospital. Agreements among the members of the network must address referral and patient transfer, development of communication (including telemetry and electronic sharing of patient data where feasible), emergency and nonemergency transportation, and medical staff credentialing and quality assurance. Grants of $25 million per year for five years were authorized in the 1997 legislation creating the program, and appropriated in 1998 to be awarded in 1999. The grants are to be used for developing state rural health plans and for certifying critical access hospitals and rural health networks. For more information, call 202-232–6200.

Evaluating Rural Health Network Programs

The effectiveness of rural health networks at achieving their goals is still unknown. The youth of most networks and the difficulties inherent in measuring rural health network performance have produced few evaluations of rural health networks or of the programs that support their development* (see Christianson, Moscovice, and Wellever, 1995). The results from the evaluations that have been conducted are far from conclusive. Major findings from three rural health network evaluations are outlined in this section. The section concludes with a list of outstanding evaluation issues.

Robert Wood Johnson Foundation Rural Hospital Network Program

The evaluators of the Rural Hospital Network Program highlighted six major findings (Moscovice et al., 1995):

1. Joining a network is a popular strategic response for rural hospitals in an uncertain environment. Although almost one half of all rural hospitals in the country participated in a rural hospital network during 1985–1990, the evaluators found few examples of integrated networks whose members shared decision making, contributed significant resources to the network, or sacrificed individual autonomy. Simply joining a network does not assure improvement in a rural hospital's condition.
2. Rural hospital networks are a relatively unstable organizational form. The evaluators found that in a 3-year period (1988–1991), approximately one third of rural hospital networks in the country ceased to exist and a majority of the remaining networks added or deleted members.
3. Joining a network can be a low-cost strategy for rural hospitals, both in terms of financial commitment and in terms of the degree of authority relinquished to the group. The evaluators found that the majority of rural hospital networks did not pay dues and that hospital executives exercised influence over network decisions.

*Evaluations of the AHCPR's Rural Managed Care Centers Program and FORHP Rural Network Development Grant Program are currently in progress.

4. Rural hospitals join networks primarily to improve cost efficiency, but, on average, hospitals do not appear to realize short-term economic benefits from network membership. The evaluators stressed, however, that their findings did not indicate that specific hospitals did not benefit financially from network participation, nor that specific network activities were not effective.
5. Mutual resource dependence and formalization of governance structure signify transition of networks from temporary to more permanent organizations. The evaluators found that rural hospital network survival was positively related to mutual resource dependence of its members (measured by participation in a shared activity) and the presence of a formalized management structure (measured by the presence of a paid director and a governing board). "Networks may form primarily as defense mechanisms for rural hospitals to adapt to an uncertain health care environment," the evaluators said, "but to survive over time those networks must add value to their member institutions" (p. 210).
6. Some of the benefits of rural hospital networks may be realized outside of the communities in which rural hospitals are located. Many rural hospital networks included urban and large rural hospital members, who may benefit from their association with rural hospitals by establishing or improving referral relationships.

New York State Rural Health Network Demonstration Program

In 1994, New York conducted an evaluation of 14 networks funded during its 1988–1992 rural health network demonstration program (HMS Associates, 1994). The evaluators made several observations about network development, including:

- A distinction exists between networking—an ad hoc collaborative behavior—and network development, which concentrates on the creation of permanent, formal structures for providing services and developing systems of care.
- Network development is a time-consuming process: future policy initiatives should recognize both the time consumed by and the value of the process and take measures to accommodate it.
- Networks that concentrate on fewer activities often are able to achieve successes sooner. However, networks with too narrow a focus may be unable to expand into other areas of need.

In sum, the evaluators noted that "successful networks were grounded in compelling need, local leadership committed to compromise, clear cut benefits to participants, and highly focused objectives" (HMS Associates, 1994, p. v). Additionally, they pointed out the key roles played by outside consultants (technical assistance and disinterested third-party) and the role of external funding (in this case, state funding) to facilitate development that would not have occurred otherwise. The evaluators point out that New York could improve its network development program by "clarifying program objectives, encouraging self-evaluation, providing levels of fiscal support, establishing a technical assistance program, and acting more as facilitator than regulator" (HMS Associates, 1994).

Essential Access Community Hospital Program

A primary goal of the Essential Access Community Hospital Program was to encourage the development of rural health networks in order to reduce fragmentation in rural health services, eliminate redundant services, and better support limited-service rural hospitals (Wright et al., 1995). Accordingly, the rural health networks developed under the EACH Program were a key component of the EACH Program evaluation sponsored by HCFA. The evaluators found:

- Only 37% of EACH Program grantees formed active formal networks
- The moderate increase in the number of linkages between EACHs and RPCHs seems to indicate that informal or formal relationships existed between EACHs and RPCHs before the networks were formed
- Although the number of transfers and the amount of communication between EACHs and RPCHs increased during the program, it was not clear that the increased transactions were the result of the establishment of the rural health network or the effect of the service limitation
- Fewer than 50% of rural health network participants reported "positive changes" as a result of network participation [Note: The majority of these networks were 2 years old or newer at the time of the evaluation]
- Participation in a rural health network was not related to the "success" of an RPCH.

In conclusion, the evaluators noted: "The program-wide data and case studies may jointly suggest that expectations for network-building should be toned down. Our initial expectation—that EACH-RPCH networks could provide critical and wide-ranging support for all or most of the small struggling hospitals seems misplaced, given our findings over the program period" (Wright et al., 1995, p.59).

Evaluation Issues

The evaluations of rural health networks have left many questions unanswered. The most fundamental question—whether rural health networks benefit either their members or the rural residents they serve—has not been answered convincingly. The evaluations conducted to date have concentrated on networks formed through grant programs intended to create rural health networks. Whether these networks are representative of networks formed without grant funding is not known. Certainly, these evaluations suffer from their short time-horizon. Most of the networks evaluated were in formative stages of their development when studied. Benefits to members and residents not readily apparent at the time of the evaluation may have become more evident as the networks matured. That time is needed to cement relationships within a network and to begin meaningful, collaborative work has been noted by several researchers (Moscovice et al., 1996; HMS Associates, 1994).

Chief among the unresolved evaluation questions are the following (Christianson et al., 1995):

- Do rural health networks improve the health and well-being of rural residents?
- If networks do generate benefits for rural residents, what types of networks accomplish this for the smallest expenditure of resources?
- How does network structure affect the types of services undertaken by networks?
- How does network structure affect network performance?
- What groups receive the greatest benefits from network development?
- Do networks change their organizational structure and activities over time? If so, how does this affect their economic efficiency?
- What are the organizational and environmental characteristics that predict successful network performance?

REFERENCES

Alpha Center. 1998. Glossary of Terms Commonly Used in Health Care, Washington, D.C.: Alpha Center. URL: http://www.alphacenter.com

American Hospital Association (AHA). 1995. 1995 Annual Survey, Chicago: American Hospital Association.

Casey M. 1997. Integrated networks and health care provider cooperatives: new models for health care delivery and financing. Health Care Management Review 22: 41–48.

Christianson J, Moscovice I, Wellever A. 1995. The structure of strategic alliances: evidence from rural hospital networks. In: Kaluzney A, Zuckerman H, Ricketts T eds., Partners for the Dance: Forming Strategic Alliances in Health Care. Ann Arbor, MI: Health Administration Press.

Federal Register. May 7, 1998. 63(88): 25359–25379.

HMS Associates. 1994. Rural Health Care Networks in New York State: Impacts and Recommendations. Getzville, NY: Healthcare Management Services Associates.

Knoke D. 1988. Incentive in collective action organizations. American Sociological Review 53: 311–329.

Kushner C. 1991. The Feasibility of Health Care Cooperatives in Rural America: Learning From the Past to Prepare for the Future. Chapel Hill, NC: North Carolina Foundation for Alternative Health Programs, Inc., North Carolina Rural Health Research Program.

Luke R. 1991. Spatial competition and cooperation in local hospital markets. Medical Care Review 48: 207–237.

Moscovice I, Christianson J, Johnson J, Kralewski J, Manning W. 1995. Building Rural Hospital Networks. Ann Arbor, MI: Health Administration Press.

Moscovice I, Wellever A, Christianson J, Casey M, Yawn B, Hartley D. 1996. Rural Health Networks: Concepts, Cases and Public Policy. Minneapolis: University of Minnesota, Rural Health Research Center.

Moscovice I, Wellever A, Krein S. 1997. Rural Health Networks: Forms & Functions. Minneapolis: University of Minnesota, Rural Health Research Center.

Office of Technology Assessment (Congress of the United States) 1990. Health Care in Rural America. Washington, DC: U.S. Government Printing Office.

Powell W. 1990. Neither Market Nor Hierachy: Network Forms of Organization. In Skaw B, Cummings L, eds. Research in Organization Behavior. Greenwich, CT: JAI Press, vol. 12, 295–336.

Provan K. 1984. Interorganizational cooperation and decision making autonomy in a consortium multihospital system. Academy of Management Review 9: 494–504.

Shortell S, Gillies R, Anderson D. 1994. The new world of managed care: creating organized delivery systems. Health Affairs 13: 46–64.

Shortell S, Gillies R, Devers K. 1995. Reinventing the American Hospital. The Milbank Quarterly 73(2): 131–159.

Texas Medical Association. 1997. Managed Care Glossary. URL:http://gateway.texmed.org/tmamss/library/tma_002/ tma_002.htm.

Wright G, Felt S, Wellever A, Lake T, Sweetland S. 1995. Limited-Service Hospital Pioneers: Challenges and Successes of the Essential Access Community Hospital/ Rural Primary Care Hospital (EACH-RPCH) program and Medical Assistance Facility (MAF) Demonstration, HCFA Contract No. 500–87–0028. Washington, D.C.: Mathematica Policy Research, Inc.

Zuckerman H, Kaluzny A, Ricketts T. 1995. Strategic alliances: a worldwide phenomenon comes to health care. In: Kaluzney A, Zuckerman H, Ricketts T. eds., Partners for the Dance: Forming Strategic Alliances in Health Care, Ann Arbor, MI: Health Administration Press.

12

Rural Maternal and Perinatal Health

DENISE M. LISHNER, ERIC H. LARSON, ROGER A. ROSENBLATT, AND SARAH J. CLARK

Maternal and newborn care is a critical component of rural health services and integral to the health of the rural community (Council on Graduate Medical Education, 1997; Gavin and Leong, 1989). A high-quality system provides prenatal, obstetric, and neonatal services locally and, at the same time, an efficient system for linking higher-risk women and infants with nonlocal services when required. In the 1960s and 1970s, many rural areas lagged behind urban ones in terms of sentinel health outcomes such as infant mortality and rates of low birthweight (Sherman, 1992). Research on rural birth outcomes and the organization of maternal and neonatal services revealed that obtaining optimal birth outcomes required an accessible and efficiently used constellation of local and nonlocal services (Gortmaker et al., 1987; Hein and Lathrop, 1986). Efforts to build such regionalized systems of care substantially decreased the most glaring of rural/urban differentials in infant mortality. Questions remain, however, about the magnitude and importance of remaining rural/urban differences in access to perinatal care, birth outcomes, and the long-term stability of the systems of care that have been so successful in reducing infant mortality among rural residents of the United States.

While rates of infant mortality have decreased among rural residents overall, access to maternal and perinatal care has diminished in some rural areas and remains a pressing public policy issue. Some rural areas are losing their capacity to provide basic maternal and infant services (Nesbitt and Baldwin, 1993; Office of Technology Assessment, 1990; Rosenblatt, 1989). The loss of local care is not simply an inconvenience for women; the absence of local care creates barriers that may limit access to other parts of the maternal and perinatal care system. Importantly, lack of local care has been shown to be independently associated with poorer perinatal outcomes and higher costs (Nesbitt et al., 1990; Nesbitt et al., 1997).

This chapter describes major issues surrounding maternal and perinatal health care in rural areas of the United States. It presents a profile of rural maternal and perinatal health in the 1990s, describing rural birth rates by maternal characteristics and geographic location; the utilization of prenatal care services; birth outcomes including low birthweight and fetal, neonatal, and postneonatal mortality rates; ingredients of a cohesive maternal and perinatal health care system; obstacles impeding access to these systems of care in rural areas; effects of insufficient local services on access, quality, and outcomes of care; issues surrounding the provision of reproductive health services; and implications for the future. The chapter uses recent national data as well as findings from regional and national outcome studies to describe the current situation, suggest recent trends, and inform policy decisions concerning maternal and perinatal health care in rural America.

Space limitations do not allow the consideration of many additional and important women's health services such as health promotion and disease prevention, especially cancer screening and treatment, and care for elderly women. Care for children is described in Chapter 13, Rural Children's Health.

BIRTH AND ITS CONTEXT IN RURAL AREAS

Although the United States has the world's most advanced perinatal technology, it fails in making these marvels equally available to the entire populace. Neonatal intensive care units have become increasingly accessible to most very low birthweight infants, but for some populations, routine care is not always within reach. Although these inequalities and inequities are present throughout the country, rural areas bear additional burdens because of their remoteness and low population densities, burdens that translate into some of the demographic disparities between rural and urban areas that are explored in this chapter.

RURAL BIRTHS AND BIRTH RATES BY MATERNAL CHARACTERISTICS AND GEOGRAPHIC LOCATION

Over four million infants were born in the United States in 1992, with about 20% born to rural mothers. About 60% of pregnancies in the United States are unintended, with potentially serious risks and consequences such as late or no prenatal care, low birthweight, neonatal mortality, economic hardship, and interference with educational and career goals (Brown and Eisenberg, 1995). A disproportionate share of women bearing unintended children are unmarried or at either end of the reproductive age span (Brown and Eisenberg, 1995).

The age distribution of live births in rural and urban areas is presented in Table 12.1. Overall, greater proportions of rural compared to urban mothers were teenagers or in their 20s. This pattern is consistent when stratified by race, but more pronounced among blacks; over 25% of rural black infants were born to teenage mothers, compared to 15% of rural white infants.

Trends over time in distribution of live births by mother's age are presented in Table 12.2. Since 1980, the percentage of births to girls younger than 15 years has remained constant in both rural and urban areas. The percentage of births to older teens decreased in both rural and urban locations from 1980 to 1988, and then increased slightly in 1990 and has remained stable to date. The percentage of births to mothers aged 30–39 years and over 40 years has increased consistently in both rural and urban areas since 1980, coinciding with the decision of many women to pursue a career and postpone child rearing.

Table 12.3 presents more comprehensive information about fertility among women aged 22 to 44 years. Rural women were more likely than urban or suburban women to have had three or more children, and were less likely to have no pregnancies and to have borne no children.

INSURANCE

The percentage of uninsured people in the United States rose from 11.8% in 1980 to 17.3% in 1995 (Council on Graduate Medical Education, 1997), presenting a major barrier to medical care. Insurance status among women in their childbearing years differs substantially among rural, urban, and suburban populations (Table 12.4). Rural women are less likely than either urban or subur-

Table 12.1 Live Births by Age of Mother, 1992

	Total		*<15 Years of Age*		*15–19 Years of Age*		*20–29 Years of Age*		*30–39 Years of Age*		*40+ Years of Age*	
	Number	*Percent*	*Number*	*Percent*	*Number*	*Percent*	*Number*	*Percent*	*Number*	*Percent*	*Number*	*Percent*
All—Total	4065014	100	12220	.03	505415	12.4	2249754	55.3	1239915	30.5	57710	1.4
Metro	3263248	100	9788	.03	380983	11.7	1771276	54.2	1051779	32.2	49422	1.5
Nonmetro	801766	100	2432	.03	124432	15.5	478478	59.7	188136	23.5	8288	1.0
White—Total	3201678	100	5367	.02	342739	10.7	1779008	55.6	1028127	32.1	46437	1.5
Metro	2528179	100	4230	.02	248685	9.8	1372897	54.3	863048	34.1	39319	1.6
Nonmetro	673499	100	1137	.02	94054	14.0	406111	60.3	165079	24.5	7118	1.1
Black—Total	673633	100	6448	1.0	146800	21.8	374017	55.5	139728	20.7	6640	1.0
Metro	576964	100	5260	.09	121802	21.1	319569	55.3	124418	21.6	5915	1.0
Nonmetro	966669	100	1188	1.2	24998	25.9	54448	56.3	15310	15.8	725	.07

Source: Vital Statistics of the United States, 1992. Volume I—Natality. National Center for Health Statistics, 1996.

Table 12.2 Percent Distribution of Births by Maternal Age, 1980–1992

	<15 Years of Age	*15–19 Years of Age*	*20–29 Years of Age*	*30–39 Years of Age*	*40+ Years of Age*
1980					
Metro	0.3	14.4	64.3	20.3	0.7
Nonmetro	0.3	17.8	65.5	15.7	0.7
1985					
Metro	0.3	11.7	61.6	25.6	0.8
Nonmetro	0.3	14.9	64.6	19.5	0.7
1988					
Metro	0.3	11.6	58.1	29.0	1.0
Nonmetro	0.3	14.7	62.2	22.0	0.8
1990					
Metro	0.3	11.8	56.1	30.5	1.3
Nonmetro	0.3	15.5	60.7	22.5	0.9
1992					
Metro	0.3	11.7	54.2	32.2	1.5
Nonmetro	0.3	15.5	59.7	23.5	1.0

Source: Vital Statistics of the United States.

ban women to be covered under health insurance sponsored by their own employers. Rural married women are more likely than their urban or suburban counterparts to purchase their own insurance or to be enrolled in Medicaid; rural unmarried women are less likely than urban women, but more likely than suburban women, to be enrolled in Medicaid. More unmarried rural women are covered under a parent's health insurance policy, compared with unmarried urban and suburban women. In rural areas, 10% of married women and 16.6% of unmarried women lack health insurance. While this is less of a problem for rural than urban women, it suggests that financial factors may impede access to appropriate health care for substantial numbers of childbearing women.

Similar patterns are observed when examining payment sources for women's most recent labor and delivery charges (Table 12.5). A small proportion of rural women had full coverage for obstetric care under their insurance. Rural women were slightly more likely than urban or suburban women to pay out-of-pocket expenses (in part or in whole) for costs associated with labor and delivery; they are less likely than urban but more likely than suburban women to have labor and delivery charges covered under Medicaid.

Table 12.3 Characteristics of Current and Potential Mothers Aged 22–44, 1995

	Metro, Central City	*Metro, Noncentral City*	*Nonmetro*
Total number (thousands)	18,550	29,303	12,347
Number of pregnancies			
0	35.0%	33.2%	31.5%
1	16.9%	16.3%	15.9%
2	18.4%	20.4%	22.5%
3 or more	29.7%	30.0%	29.9%
Number of children born			
0	44.7%	41.7%	38.2%
1	18.2%	17.6%	17.6%
2	20.0%	24.0%	25.3%
3 or more	17.0%	16.6%	18.9%

Source: 1995 National Survey of Family Growth.

Table 12.4 Source of Insurance Coverage for Women Aged 15–44 Years, 1995 (expressed as percent of all women)[a]

	Metro, Central City	*Metro, Noncentral City*	*Nonmetro*
MARRIED WOMEN			
Uninsured	11.4	7.8	10.0
Woman's employer	39.9	39.2	34.6
Husband's employer	39.6	49.8	46.6
Medicaid	11.0	6.2	11.5
Champus	3.8	3.0	2.2
Self-purchased	4.5	5.3	7.2
UNMARRIED WOMEN			
Uninsured	14.2	12.9	16.6
Woman's employer	33.3	37.6	26.1
Parent's employer	19.1	28.5	29.2
Medicaid	29.7	16.2	24.5
Champus	1.9	1.9	1.8
Self-purchased	4.0	3.6	2.8
Other	3.5	5.2	4.2

[a]Because categories overlap, percentages will total more than 100.
Source: 1995 National Survey of Family Growth.

UTILIZATION OF PRENATAL CARE

Inadequate prenatal care is associated with high incidence of low birthweight, preterm delivery, and infant mortality (Health Resources and Services Administration, 1992). Prenatal care is regarded as a major factor in positive pregnancy outcome; however, the percentage of births to women with late or no prenatal care increased in the 1980s and early 1990s (Moore, 1992). Prenatal care, which should begin early in pregnancy, provides an opportunity to encourage healthy behaviors, treat chronic conditions, intervene with mothers who use tobacco and other drugs, screen for birth defects, and manage problems associated with pregnancy and delivery such as gestational diabetes and pregnancy-induced hypertension. Table 12.6 indicates that for rural women, rates of early initiation of prenatal care were lower than that for suburban women but higher than the rate for urban women. More rural than suburban women had delayed initiation of prenatal care (fifth month of pregnancy or later) and urban mothers had the highest proportion of late initiation of prenatal care.

FETAL DEATH, INFANT MORTALITY AND LOW BIRTHWEIGHT

Among the most sensitive markers of the general health of a population are rates of fetal death, infant morta-

Table 12.5 Payment Source for Labor and Delivery Charges, 1995 (as percent of all deliveries)

Payment Source for Most Recent Delivery	*Metro, Central City*	*Metro, Noncentral City*	*Nonmetro*
Own income only	7.2	6.9	6.1
Insurance only	32.7	44.2	28.4
Own income plus insurance	14.5	23.6	26.0
Medicaid	44.5	24.2	38.5
Other sources	1.1	1.1	1.0

Source: 1995 National Survey of Family Growth.

Table 12.6 Percentage of Current and Potential Mothers 22–44 Years of Age Receiving Prenatal Care, 1995

	Metro, Central City	*Metro, Noncentral City*	*Nonmetro*
Total (in thousands)	18,550	29,303	12,347
<3 months pregnant	86.1%	89.7%	87.4%
3–4 months	5.5%	5.0%	6.0%
5 months or more	8.4%	5.4%	6.5%

Source: 1995 National Survey of Family Growth.

lity, and low birthweight (weight less than 2,500 grams at birth). The prevention of these poor outcomes has been a focus of maternal and child health policy in the United States for over a century (Meckel, 1990; Miller, 1988; Schmidt and Wallace, 1988). In the 1960s and 1970s, rates of rural infant mortality compared unfavorably to rates for urban residents. Infant mortality review, training in neonatal stabilization skills, and regionalization of care for high-risk women all contributed to a dramatic drop in the rural/urban gap in infant mortality during the 1980s (Gortmaker et al., 1987; Hein and Lathrop, 1986; Larson, Hart, and Rosenblatt, 1992; Rosenblatt, Reinkin, and Shoemack, 1985). The successful regionalization of perinatal care in the 1980s is one of the great success stories in rural health care. At the same time, however, some important perinatal outcome differences remain, especially in postneonatal mortality (death between the ages of 28 and 364 days). In this section, the perinatal outcomes experienced in rural populations are described and compared to urban ones.

The fetal death ratio is a measure of the number of late fetal deaths (after 20 weeks gestation) per 1000 live births during a year. Table 12.7 shows that in 1992, fetal death ratios were higher in the nonmetropolitan population overall (7.6 compared to 7.3 in the metropolitan population) and in various racial subpopulations. The fetal death ratio among African Americans was approximately twice that of whites (13.3 versus 6.2). Since 1980, however, the nonmetropolitan fetal death ratio has dropped steadily (from 9.9 in 1980 to 7.6 in 1992) and the metro/nonmetro gap has steadily narrowed since 1980 as well. In 1980 the nonmetro rate was 10% higher than the metro ratio of 9.0. In 1992, it was only about 4% higher than the metro ratio of 7.3.

The infant mortality rate is generally divided into two component rates, the neonatal death rate and the postneonatal death rate (Plate 12.1). Neonatal mortality occurs before the 28th day of life and postneonatal deaths occur between the 28th and 364th day. The distinction is made because the dominant causes of death in the neonatal period are quite distinct from the those in the later period. In general, deaths occurring in the neonatal period are more commonly associated with prematurity, congenital anomalies, or complications of pregnancy and delivery. Deaths in the postneonatal period are associated more often with non-pregnancy-related causes such as infectious disease and injuries.

Analysis of mortality data from the 1991 Linked Birth Death Data Set (National Center for Health Statistics, 1995), indicates that, in general, rural and urban rates of neonatal mortality are not very different (Table 12.8). Within racial subpopulations some rural-urban differences are found. Among rural American Indians, for example, the neonatal mortality rate is somewhat lower than the metropolitan rate (4.77 vs. 6.38); for whites, the rural rate is somewhat higher than the urban rate (4.64

Table 12.7 Fetal Deaths, 1992

	U.S. Total		*Metro*		*Nonmetro*	
Fetal Deaths	*Total*	*Rate/1000*	*Total*	*Rate/1000*	*Total*	*Rate/1000*
Total	30256	7.4	24085	7.3	6171	7.6
White	20131	6.2	15573	6.1	4558	6.7
Nonwhite	10125	11.6	8512	11.4	1613	12.4
Black[a]	9055	13.3	7669	13.1	1386	14.1

[a]Black is a subset of nonwhite.
Source: Vital Statistics of the United States, 1992. Volume II—Mortality. Part B.

Table 12.8 Poor Birth Outcome in the United States by Metro/Nonmetro Residence and Race, 1991

	Total births	*Percent of total births*	*Percent Low Birthweight (<2500 g)*	*Neonatal death rate*	*Postneonatal death rate*
U.S.	4,111,059	100.0	7.1	5.44	3.20
Metro	3,369,023	72.0	7.2	5.47	3.13
Nonmetro[a]	742,036	18.0	6.8[b]	5.31	3.52[b]
WHITE					
U.S.	3,241,355	100.0	5.8	4.41	2.65
Metro	2,618,256	80.8	5.8	4.36	2.53
Nonmetro[a]	623,099	19.2	6.0[b]	4.64[b]	3.12[b]
AFRICAN AMERICAN					
U.S.	682,669	100.0	13.6	10.72	5.92
Metro	593,930	87.0	13.6	10.79	5.96
Nonmetro[a]	88,739	13.0	13.0[b]	10.25[b]	5.63[b]
AMERICAN INDIAN					
U.S.	38,843	100.0	6.2	5.48	5.87
Metro	17,081	44.0	6.4	6.38	4.77
Nonmetro[a]	21,762	56.0	5.9[c]	4.77[c]	6.74[b]
OTHER					
U.S.	148,192	100.0	6.5	3.57	2.22
Metro	139,756	94.3	6.5	3.55	2.21
Nonmetro[a]	8,436	5.7	6.6	3.91	2.61

[a]Statistical comparisons are to residents of metropolitan counties.
[b]Significant at .01.
[c]Significant at .05.
Source: National Center for Health Statistics, 1995.

vs. 4.36). In contrast, rural/urban differences are pronounced in postneonatal mortality. Overall, and among white and American Indian infants, nonmetropolitan rates were significantly higher than metropolitan rates. Rural American Indians in particular experience very high rates of postneonatal mortality (6.74 per thousand live births) despite relatively low rates of low birthweight (5.9%).

About 7% of the infants born in 1991 weighed less than 2,500 grams at birth. Most of those infants were born at gestational ages of less than 37 weeks. Low-birthweight infants are of special concern because they are 40 times more likely to die during the neonatal period, and five times more likely to die during the postneonatal period than normal birthweight infants (McCormick and Richardson, 1995). If they survive, they are much more likely to experience mild to severe morbidity and developmental difficulties. The most common cause of death among low-birthweight infants is respiratory distress related to pulmonary immaturity. The higher rates of low birthweight among black infants account for much of the neonatal mortality differentials observed among black infants compared to white ones. As with neonatal mortality, there were some differences in urban versus rural rates of low birthweight outcome. In 1991, overall rural and urban rates were 6.8 and 7.2, respectively. Plate 12.2 shows the distribution of low-birthweight rates from 1991 through 1993 for nonmetropolitan counties. Often, observed rural/urban differences in the rates of poor birth outcome reflect underlying differences in the demography of rural and urban populations (Clarke and Coward, 1991). However, a recent study by Larson, Hart, and Rosenblatt (1997) attempted to adjust for such differences in a national-level analysis of rural and urban rates of poor birth outcome. It was shown that rural residence was not an independent risk factor for low birthweight or neonatal mortality at the national level or in most states after correcting for demographic and biological risk factors (Larson et al., 1997). At the same time, rural residence was found to be a significant independent risk factor for postneonatal mortality nationally and in many states. Rural residence was also shown to be an independent risk factor for a greater chance of receiving late or no prenatal care. Although the regionalization movement eliminated drastic differences in rural versus urban rates of neonatal mortality, rural infants continue to experience a higher risk of death in the postneonatal period compared to urban infants.

ACCESS TO MATERNAL AND PERINATAL HEALTH CARE IN RURAL AREAS

Some improvements in rural birth outcomes have occurred over time, yet persistent differences favoring urban and white women suggest that inequities in availability of, and access to, maternal and perinatal care still prevail among rural and disadvantaged populations.

Local availability of obstetric care is a prerequisite for ensuring the health and welfare of mother and baby. Access to care for rural residents is predicated on the availability of local providers, facilities, services, transportation, and health insurance/ability to pay. When any of these are not available locally, access to care is compromised, with potentially detrimental health consequences. Regionalized perinatal care systems that refer those at high risk to centralized systems of technologically intensive services are also critical for providing quality and accessible care, and optimizing birth outcomes. Unfortunately, a variety of factors have converged to limit the availability of essential maternal and perinatal services in many rural communities.

Nonavailability of Local Providers

About 20% of the U.S. population live in rural areas, yet only 9% of the nation's physicians practice in rural communities (Council on Graduate Medical Education, 1997). Obstetricians provide 84% of obstetric care, family physicians provide 13%, and nurse practitioners provide 3% nationally, but many states have counties with no obstetricians at all (Health Resources and Services Administration, 1992). The capacity of rural health care systems to provide adequate perinatal care was disrupted in the past decade by provider shortages, the decision by many providers to discontinue obstetrics, rural hospital closures, and obstetric malpractice liability concerns (Health Resources and Services Administration, 1992). There was a 20% decrease in the number of rural obstetric providers in the United States between 1984 and 1989 (Office of Technology Assessment, 1990), and the proportion of rural family physicians providing obstetric care fell from 43% in 1988 to only 37% in 1992 (Schmittling, 1993). A survey of family physicians who moved to rural areas nationwide from 1987 through 1990 showed that fewer family physicians practice maternity care than a decade ago. Family physicians were more likely to provide maternity care if they owned their practice and were not solo practitioners, or if they practiced in counties that were less populated, had fewer obstetricians, and had more family physicians (Pathman and Tropman, 1995).

Data describing trends in the supply of primary care physicians are provided in Chapter 3, Physicians and Rural America. Obstetricians are heavily concentrated in urban areas, with fewer than three obstetrician/gynecologists per 100,000 residents in rural counties with largest city populations of fewer than 10,000. The more highly specialized the physician, the less likely that the physician will settle in a rural area, because specialists require a large population base, sophisticated hospitals and laboratories, and specialty colleagues (Council on Graduate Medical Education, 1997). This creates a reliance on family physicians and general practitioners, as well as mid-level providers (e.g., nurse midwives) for obstetric care of rural mothers. Although rural generalist providers offer excellent obstetric care, they require the ready availability of obstetric consultation and the ability to refer patients to their consulting physicians (Council on Graduate Medical Education, 1997).

Nonavailability of Facilities

Obstetrics is an integral part of the rural health care system and is instrumental in maintaining the health care community in rural areas as well as the viability of the local hospital. However, rural areas often have difficulty maintaining viable obstetrical units (Rosenblatt et al., 1994). The past decade has witnessed a dramatic loss of rural hospitals and hospital-based obstetric care, although smaller hospitals (fewer than 300 beds) in rural areas are more likely to offer delivery services than are comparable urban hospitals (Office of Technology Assessment, 1990). Furthermore, sophisticated resources are not always available in small rural hospitals. Closures of rural hospitals or their obstetrical units and the perception that local facilities are inferior in quality may result in bypassing of local hospitals for care (Nesbitt et al., 1990).

Rural hospitals perform relatively few deliveries and are often far from tertiary care centers where high-risk neonates are best cared for (Gortmaker et al., 1985). Assuring optimal outcomes for high-risk rural infants requires effective regionalized systems of perinatal care in rural areas (Rosenblatt et al., 1985). Major efforts in the 1980s to regionalize systems of perinatal care for high-risk rural infants and their mothers resulted from the recognition that the survival of rural infants born at low birthweight or with other medical risks did not compare favorably with the survival of high-risk urban infants (Gortmaker et al., 1985; Hein, 1980; Hein and Lathrop, 1986; Rosenblatt et al., 1985).

In a regionalized perinatal care system, women at high risk are referred to more technologically intensive facilities better equipped to meet the medical requirements of neonates, thereby minimizing differences in outcomes attributable to geographic location (Hein and Lathrop, 1986). Local obstetric care providers serve as the entry point to regionalized systems of perinatal care (Nesbitt et al., 1997). Evidence has shown that outcomes can be improved by early identification of high-risk pregnancies and referral to tertiary perinatal centers before delivery (McCormick and Richardson, 1995). Birthweight-specific survival of high-risk rural infants born in regionalized centers has improved dramatically (Gortmaker et al., 1987; Larson et al., 1992; Larson et al., 1997).

Adverse effects of regionalization include initial separation of the newborn and its family, costs of prolonged neonatal hospital stays, disruption of established patient-physician relationships and continuity of care, and loss of local medical services (McCormick and Richardson, 1995). Changes in the health care environment have resulted in a reversal of the trend toward regionalization, with a deterioration in perinatal regionalization, replacement of cooperation by competition, and the blurring of traditional levels of care as all facilities escalated the level of care provided (McCormick and Richardson, 1995). Powell and colleagues (1995) suggest that the penetration of managed care into rural areas and technological sophistication of small hospital nurseries could decrease referrals and promote retention of high-risk neonates at level I and II hospitals.

Nonavailability of Services

Perinatal services are important factors in reducing neonatal and infant mortality rates. For most perinatal services, the proportion of hospitals offering such care is higher in urban than rural areas (Table 12.9). However, much progress has been made in rural areas to narrow this gap. Rosenblatt and colleagues (1994) found that although smaller and more rural hospitals in the state of Washington refer most premature and low-birthweight infants to regional referral centers, sophisticated prenatal and intrapartum technologies are available in the majority of rural units, even the smallest and most remote. The most striking rural/urban difference in perinatal technology levels are found in the nursery. Rural hospitals generally do not have the resources, trained personnel, or patient volume to sustain the highest levels of neonatal intensive care.

Table 12.9 Percentage of Hospitals Providing Select Perinatal Services, 1995

	Metro	*Nonmetro*
INPATIENT SERVICES		
Obstetric care	63	68
Neonatal intensive care	36	7
Neonatal intermediate care	27	8
OUTPATIENT SERVICES		
Reproductive health	32	11

Source: 1995 Annual Survey of Hospitals, American Hospital Association.

Pathman and Tropman (1995) observe that hospitals providing routine obstetrical services must maintain staff with the ability to perform cesarean sections; many small rural hospitals have no obstetricians on staff, so family physicians are often relied upon to perform this procedure. A survey of rural hospitals in Washington State showed that 75% provided obstetric services, and of these, 60% had no obstetrician on staff. Family physicians performed the majority of cesarean sections in all but eight of the largest rural hospitals, where they did 28% of the cesarean sections (Norris et al., 1996), suggesting that most rural hospitals have the capacity to offer this important service.

Financial Barriers

Financial barriers may also limit access to health care for rural residents. These include lack of transportation, the inability to pay or lack of insurance coverage, and the reluctance of some rural providers to accept Medicaid patients (Office of Technology Assessment, 1990). Klerman and Scholle (1992) note that rural women may have difficulty obtaining maternity care because they are more likely than their urban counterparts to be poor and uninsured and less likely to have Medicaid coverage. Rosenblatt and colleagues (1991) found that family physicians, obstetrician/gynecologists, and certified nurse midwives in four northwestern states were reluctant to provide care to Medicaid patients and limited the amount of care they provided to this population.

A series of federal laws mandating coverage of pregnant women at 133% of Federal Poverty Level have decreased financial barriers to prenatal care for many women, and state outreach programs and other interventions have improved provider participation by increasing reimbursement in some states (Baldwin and Curry, 1992). Policy makers have also sought to address the social service needs of Medicaid-enrolled pregnant women by offering state matching funds for services to enhance prenatal care; by the early 1990s, over 80% of states were offering such services to this population. Examples include Washington State's First Steps Program, which provides maternity support services and targeted maternity case management in addition to expanding and streamlining Medicaid eligibility and increasing reimbursement (Baldwin et al., 1998), and a North Carolina program that provides bonuses to physicians who offer obstetric care to poor rural women in conjunction with the local health department (Taylor and Ricketts, 1993).

Although these programs enhance prenatal care initiation and Medicaid enrollment, there is no evidence that they have lowered rates of low birthweight in a targeted population (Ray, 1997). However, there has been some progress in reducing inequities in care caused by financial barriers. A recent study demonstrated that Medicaid status had no meaningful association with prenatal, intrapartum, or overall resource use, with similar care and resources expanded on Medicaid-insured patients compared with privately insured women (Dobie et al., 1997).

Minority Status

Low-income and minority women are more likely to have poor obstetric outcomes, despite efforts to expand Medicaid eligibility and to improve access to prenatal care (Wilcox and Skjoerven, 1992). While 22% of all U.S. births are to women living in rural areas, 62.5% of Native American births are to rural women (Larson et al., 1997). Grossman and colleagues (1994) report that Native American women have higher prenatal risk profiles than white women, with a higher proportion of births to teenagers, unmarried women, smokers, and alcohol users. They found that rural Native American mothers were more likely to receive early and adequate prenatal care and were less likely to deliver a low birthweight infant than their urban counterparts, yet the neonatal and postneonatal mortality rates of infants born to rural Native American mothers were not lower, raising questions about access to newborn and infant health services.

Effect of the Malpractice/Liability Crisis on the Provision of Obstetrics

Despite state legislative reforms, the number of obstetric-related malpractice claims and insurance premium rates continued to rise, causing many obstetric providers to reduce or eliminate the obstetric portion of their practices or to refuse care of high-risk patients (Office of Technology Assessment, 1990). A review of national and state studies showed significant attrition of obstetric providers and reductions in their participation in obstetric practice; the specialty most affected was family practice, and the patients affected most were rural residents and the poor and uninsured (Health Resources and Services Administration, 1992).

Declines in the proportion of physicians offering obstetric services were reported in a study of four northwestern states, largely because of rising medical malpractice premiums. The study found that the majority of general practitioners and family physicians in these states no longer provide obstetrical care, whereas 80% of obstetrician/gynecologists do. However, although only a minority of family physicians continue to practice obstetrics, most rural family physicians in all four states still deliver babies (Rosenblatt et al., 1991). Similar trends have been observed for rural physicians in other studies (Office of Technology Assessment, 1990). Over 50% of rural family physicians in the Midwest and almost 50% of rural family physicians in the Pacific region provide routine obstetric care, whereas their urban counterparts are much less likely to perform obstetrics in all regions (American Academy of Family Physicians, 1991). There is some evidence that the tendency of physicians to discontinue the provision of obstetrics has decelerated (Rosenblatt et al., 1990).

Concerns have been raised that physicians may be altering their practice patterns and performing more tests and cesarean deliveries in response to the litigious environment. However, Baldwin and colleagues (1995) found that after controlling for patient, physician, and sociodemographic characteristics, there was no difference in prenatal resource use or cesarean delivery rate for low-risk patients between Washington State obstetric providers with more or less exposure to malpractice claims. Managed care and community clinics are changing the nature of the obstetric insurance penalty; as these organizational forms replace solo and small group practice modes, the prohibitive effect of malpractice insurance may be mitigated.

IMPLICATIONS OF INSUFFICIENT LOCAL SERVICES ON ACCESS, QUALITY, AND OUTCOMES

A comprehensive report produced by the Office of Technology Assessment (1990) concluded that fetal, infant, and maternal mortality rates were somewhat higher and late prenatal care more of a problem in rural as compared with urban areas. Mothers in rural areas are more at risk for receiving inadequate prenatal care than those in more urban areas and are more likely to emigrate from the home towns for delivery; and their infants die in their first year of life at a rate greater than the standards of infant mortality set by the Surgeon General (Health Resources and Services Administration, 1992). A number of studies have investigated health outcomes in light of the problems emanating from lower availability of, and access to, certain providers and services in rural versus urban areas, lower volumes of deliveries, and related problems that could have an impact on the health of mother and children. Larson and colleagues (1997) observe that results of state-based studies comparing rural and urban birth outcomes vary widely, in part because of methodological differences. Findings from recent regional and national birth outcome studies are presented below.

Baker and Kotelchuck (1989) found interstate differences in birthweight-specific mortality when comparing South Carolina and Massachusetts, and partially attributed this to rural and urban differences in the two populations. In Alabama, Hale and Drushell (1989) noted a significantly increased risk of postneonatal mortality among normal-birthweight infants in rural areas and showed that the association between African-American race and increased risk of postneonatal mortality was greater among residents of rural than urban areas. In a study based in Florida, Clarke and Coward (1991) found that rural residence was not associated with increased risk of infant death after other social factors related to rurality were accounted for.

Larson and colleagues (1992) demonstrated that rural residence in Washington State was not associated with increased risk of death or low-birthweight outcomes but was associated with significantly higher rates of inadequate prenatal care. Nonwhites living in rural areas were at much higher risk for low-birthweight infants, infant death, and inadequate prenatal care than whites. In Washington State, rural residence did not seem to be a risk factor for low birthweight or infant mortality despite barriers to access to prenatal care in rural areas.

Larimore and Davis (1995) reported that 47 counties in rural Florida were lacking in maternity care services, and 45 of these had family physicians who practiced in the county but did not provide maternity services. They found a negative correlation between availability of these services and infant mortality and concluded that increasing infant death rates can be predicted by decreasing physician availability. Deprez and colleagues (1996) documented prenatal care utilization and provider participation in the Maine Medicaid program for 1985–89 and found that women from rural areas experienced lower physician availability and greater outmigration for care with no detrimental effect on adequacy of prenatal care.

Nesbitt and colleagues (1990) reported that women living in rural areas where most of their obstetric care was obtained outside their local community were more likely to experience adverse perinatal outcomes such as complicated deliveries and higher rates of prematurity than were women from communities where most patients delivered in the local community hospital. Costs for neonatal care for patients in "high outflow areas," where the majority of women deliver outside their home community, were significantly higher among those covered by Medicaid. Nesbitt and colleagues (1997) showed that women in Washington State from high outflow areas were less likely to have a normal neonate; this was true for both Medicaid and privately insured patients. Births to privately insured women were more likely to result in higher charges and longer hospital lengths of stay.

A national study of over 11 million births in the United States between 1985 and 1987 (Larson et al., 1997) revealed that residence in a nonmetropolitan county was not associated with increased risk of low birthweight or neonatal mortality at the national level or in most states, after controlling for demographic and biological risk factors. Rural residence was associated with a greater risk of postneonatal mortality at the national level, and strongly associated with late initiation of prenatal care at the national level and in a majority of states. Although rural residence does not appear to be associated with a higher risk of low birthweight or neonatal mortality, higher levels of late prenatal care among rural residents suggest a persistent problem of access to routine care that may be associated with higher levels of postneonatal mortality and childhood morbidity.

These studies generally indicate that the large rural/urban differences in neonatal mortality that characterized the 1970s and 1980s have diminished somewhat, likely because of perinatal care regionalization. However, important rural/urban differences in postneonatal mortality across populations and regions may reflect differences in rates of inadequate prenatal care as well as problems accessing maternal, postneonatal, and pediatric care in rural communities. It should be emphasized that this is not a homogeneous trend: there are many intrarural as well as intraurban differences. Reasons for differences in birth outcomes may vary by region and population and may be governed by income and racial/ethnic demographics as well as by health care access and utilization trends.

OTHER REPRODUCTIVE HEALTH SERVICES

Despite the fact that family planning services are an important part of the continuum of services related to ma-

Table 12.10 Number and Distribution of Family Planning Clinics, 1994

	Percent Distribution		*Total Numbers*	
Type of Provider	*Metro*	*Nonmetro*	*Metro*	*Nonmetro*
Health Department	34.2	54.9	1294	1830
Hospital	16.1	5.2	610	174
Community Health Center	17.8	16.3	676	543
Independent	14.1	15.7	534	524
Planned Parenthood	17.8	7.9	675	262

Source: Frost JJ. 1996. Family planning clinic services in the United States, 1994. Family Planning Perspectives 28(3):92–100.

ternal and child health, and critical to the ability of women to control their fertility, these services are not widely available to all who need them. Brown and Eisenberg (1995) claim that Americans have major gaps in knowledge about contraception and the risks and benefits of various birth control methods. Quality instruction in schools is not uniformly available, access to contraception is limited, and too few providers address the problems of contraception and unintended pregnancy. They add that the group at greatest risk of unintended pregnancy is that aged 18 to 29, and that among females aged 13 to 19, a higher proportion of teens from families in poverty are at risk. It is estimated that 70% of young women aged 18 and 19 are at risk of unintended pregnancy (Henshaw and Forrest, 1993), despite recent efforts to reduce teen pregnancy.

As shown in Table 12.10, the overall number of family planning clinics is roughly equal in metropolitan and nonmetropolitan areas. In nonmetropolitan areas, the predominant providers of family planning services are health departments and community/migrant health centers, whereas hospitals and Planned Parenthood affiliates are more common in metropolitan areas.

The distribution of family planning clients parallels the distribution of facilities (Table 12.11). In nonmetropolitan areas, over half the clients are served at health departments; hospitals and Planned Parenthood affiliates serve over half of all metropolitan clients.

Through June 1997, a cumulative total of 612,078 AIDS cases were reported in the United States: 15% of these cases were among women (CDC, 1997). Between 1990 and 1995, the overall incidence of AIDS increased through the United States (Table 12.12), with substantially lower rates in rural than urban areas. However, the gap between urban and rural narrowed substantially over this period, indicated by the steady decline in the rate ratio. In fact, the rate in rural areas is increasing at a proportionally higher rate. This pattern is evident for AIDS cases among women aged 13 to 34 years.

The increasing incidence of AIDS among women is an area of great concern because over 90% of new cases of pediatric AIDS since 1990 were transmitted from mother to infant (CDC, 1997). Awareness of maternal HIV status is critical to enable obstetric and neonatal care to focus on the prevention of perinatal HIV transmission. According to 1995 data, utilization of HIV testing differs among rural and urban women in their childbearing years (Table 12.13).

Table 12.11 Number and Distribution of Clients Served at Family Planning Clinics, 1994

	Percent Distribution		*Total number served (in 1000s)*	
Type of Provider	*Metro*	*Nonmetro*	*Metro*	*Nonmetro*
Health department	21.4	55.4	1193	933
Hospital	19.8	4.0	967	68
Community health center	0.5	8.1	465	136
Independent clinic	12.2	16.1	596	271
Planned parenthood	34.1	16.4	1667	276

Source: Unpublished tabulations, Alan Guttmacher Institute, 1994.

Table 12.12 Trends in AIDS Cases, 1990–1995 (rates per 100,000 population)

	1990	1993	1995
ALL AIDS CASES			
Metro	21.91	26.43	27.25
Nonmetro	4.65	6.26	7.29
(rate ratio)	(4.72)	(4.22)	(3.74)
WOMEN 13–34 YEARS OF AGE[a]			
Metro	7.80	12.06	13.81
Nonmetro	1.85	3.52	4.57
(rate ratio)	(4.21)	(3.43)	(3.02)

[a]Age at initial diagnosis of AIDS.
Source: Unpublished data from the Centers for Disease Control and Prevention.

Among younger women (aged 15 to 29 years), education about HIV, other sexually transmitted diseases, and birth control differed by residence. Although more rural than urban women had received instruction in "safe sex" to prevent HIV transmission, slightly more rural women reported receiving no formal sex education at all. Rates of instruction about birth control methods, other sexually transmitted disease, and "saying no to sex" were similar for rural and urban young women (Table 12.14).

Unintended pregnancies lead to approximately 1.5 million abortions annually in the United States, yet abortion remains a highly controversial issue (Brown and Eisenberg, 1995). Declines in abortion rates are largely the result of the lack of providers willing to perform this procedure. Henshaw and Van Vort (1994) report that 94% of nonmetropolitan counties in the United States have no legal medical provider willing to provide abortion services. A study in rural Idaho showed that while most physicians provided a wide range of reproductive health services, only 3.6% performed abortions, necessitating that women travel long distances for this procedure (Rosenblatt et al., 1995). A majority (65%) of residents of family medicine programs responding to a 1995 survey stated that they certainly would not perform abortions, although most agreed that first-trimester training should be optional within family practice residency programs (Steinauer et al., 1997).

Although abortion rates are not available, there appears to be a greater discrepancy between total number of pregnancies and total number of births among urban than rural women, suggesting that either urban women miscarry at a higher rate than rural women or that abortions are less common among rural women. The latter interpretation may reflect poorer access to family planning and abortion services among some rural women.

THE FUTURE OF MATERNAL AND PERINATAL HEALTH CARE IN RURAL AMERICA

The provision of safe and adequate maternal and perinatal care in rural areas is predicated on the forging of strong linkages with urban providers, facilities, and institutions. A prime example is perinatal care regionalization through which high-risk pregnant women and neonates are transported to centralized facilities in more urban locations to ensure that they receive timely and appropriate health care. The threats of deregionalization discussed earlier could have adverse consequences in

Table 12.13 HIV Testing among Women 22–44 Years of Age, 1995

	Metro, Central City	*Metro, Noncentral City*	*Nonmetro*
Total population	18,550	29,303	12,347
HISTORY OF HIV TESTING (%)			
Never tested	48.7	52.3	56.8
Tested in previous 12 months	21.3	16.1	14.6
Tested prior to 12 months ago	30.0	31.6	28.6
REASON FOR TESTING (%)			
Hospitalization/surgery	6.0	7.0	7.9
Applying for insurance	6.8	8.5	6.6
Prenatal care	22.2	22.4	25.5
Finding out if infected	44.6	37.9	36.5
Doctor's referral	8.1	6.5	6.4
As part of blood donation	14.5	17.8	16.5

Source: 1995 National Survey of Family Growth.

Table 12.14 Sex Education among Women 15–29 Years of Age as Percentages, 1995

Received Instruction in	*Metro, Central City*	*Metro, Noncentral City*	*Nonmetro*
Birth control methods	63.3	61.4	61.5
STDs	63.8	62.4	62.0
Safe sex to prevent HIV	51.0	50.5	57.0
How to say no to sex	56.9	53.8	55.0
Received no formal sex education	26.5	27.0	29.0

Source: 1995 National Survey of Family Growth.

terms of the survival rates of babies born to rural women with complicated pregnancies.

Rural areas also depend on training institutions, many located in large urban centers, for the education of health care professionals and their deployment to rural locations. There has been increasing emphasis on preparing providers for rural practice by increasing their exposure to small town medicine and lifestyles. Training institutions that include students from rural backgrounds, and that offer rural-oriented curricula, rural rotations and residencies, and basic training in perinatal care are essential in preparing providers for rural practice.

A number of policies have been advocated to address the issue of geographic maldistribution of physicians (Council on Graduate Medical Education, 1997), many of which are also pertinent for ensuring an adequate supply of obstetric providers in rural communities. These include continued support for federal and state programs that increase the number of physicians choosing generalist careers; sustained federal support for undergraduate and residency training of family physicians; support for medical education and health care delivery programs that increase the flow of physicians to rural areas; development of primary care residencies that prepare and deploy graduates for rural practice; exploration of strategies that enhance the likelihood that female physicians will locate in rural areas; and promotion of rural practice opportunities for nonphysician providers as a complement to rural physicians.

New Patterns of Health Care Provision—Midwives and Other Mid-Level Providers

Most family practice residents do not deliver babies after they finish their training and enter practice, underscoring the need for alternative providers of obstetric care. Certified nurse midwives (CNMs) are a potential source of care in small towns with a dearth of obstetric providers (Rooks, 1997). Nesbitt (1996) advocates collaborative practice between CNMs and family physicians to extend access to high-quality maternal care in rural communities. Recent studies show that CNMs are highly capable of handling normal, uncomplicated deliveries and that women benefit from avoiding unnecessary interventions (Harvey et al., 1996; Rooks, 1997). Rosenblatt and colleagues (1997) found that midwives were less likely than family physicians or obstetricians to intervene in the course of labor, and their patients had lower cesarean section and episiotomy rates. However, obstacles to the wider utilization of CNMs, such as resistance from physicians, limitations on prescriptive privileges and restrictive hospital admitting privileges, need to be addressed if CNMs are to play a more prominent role in rural obstetric care (Rooks, 1997).

Physician assistants (PAs) are another source of obstetric care for rural women. Fifteen percent (15%) of PAs practice in rural areas, and although only about 4% specialize in obstetrics and gynecology, one third of those in family practice provide care to pregnant women (Rooks, 1997). The roles of NPs and PAs in rural areas are further described in Chapter 4, Nonphysician Professionals and Rural America.

Family Planning, Immunization, and Basic Prenatal Care

One indicator of a nation's effectiveness in addressing health needs is its infant mortality rate, yet the United States falls below other industrialized countries in this regard (Stoto et al., 1990). This highlights the need for social and medical programs targeted at improving maternal and perinatal public health measures (Shiono and Behrman, 1995). Objectives of the 1990 Healthy People

2000 report (Stoto et al., 1990) include an emphasis on adequate prenatal care, reduction of risk factors in pregnant women, and reductions in the proportion of low-birthweight babies and in infant mortality. These important public health goals can only be achieved if basic maternal and perinatal care services, as well as other essential services such as family planning and immunization, are made available nationwide and within local communities.

Continued efforts directed at expanding Medicaid and health insurance coverage so that rural and economically disadvantaged women have increased access to basic prenatal and obstetrical care are also critical for reducing high infant mortality and morbidity in rural communities, and in the nation as a whole.

The Impact of Managed Care

Managed care is beginning to affect rural areas of the nation, with over 90% of all rural counties in the service area of at least one HMO by the end of 1995 (Council on Graduate Medical Education, 1997). Rural counties with low population density and predominantly agricultural economies are less likely to be included in an HMO service area (University of Minnesota Rural Health Research Center, 1997). The recent ascendancy of managed care organizations that emphasize the gatekeeper role of the family physician has resulted in an increased number of residents choosing family practice careers (Rooks, 1997), which may in turn mitigate the effects of physician maldistribution in rural areas. In addition, managed care networks can provide the organizational vehicles to hire and deploy physicians to rural and underserved areas (Council on Graduate Medical Education, 1997). Moreover, the move to managed care and accompanying organizational arrangements may reduce provider apprehensions about malpractice insurance premiums and liability and obviate any inclination to discontinue obstetrics based on these concerns.

Possible negative effects of managed care include the loss of local control of health care systems and the reluctance of privately managed care systems to care for the uninsured (Council on Graduate Medical Education, 1997). Rook (1997) observes that managed care is having serious effects on services provided to low-income pregnant women whose care is paid for by Medicaid, and restricts their use of programs designed to meet their special needs. Another major concern is that managed care organizations will direct all obstetric care into lower-level hospitals because of their lower operating costs (McCormick and Richardson, 1995). As managed care is just beginning to penetrate remote rural areas, the impact of such changes can only be anticipated. The potential cost-saving priorities of managed care organizations should not limit the basic services provided to rural women and children, whose rights to access and quality care must be protected.

CONCLUSIONS

The organization and provision of health care changed rapidly in the 1990s. On a positive note, there are many indications that maternal and perinatal care for rural and other underserved populations has improved over the past decade—with consequent improvements in health outcomes. These include an increase in the number of students choosing primary care careers with the potential for offsetting provider shortages in rural areas; a slowing down or reversal of the tendency for providers to eliminate the obstetric portions of their practices arising from malpractice insurance costs and liability concerns; the implementation of regionalized perinatal care systems that have enhanced the survival chances of high-risk rural infants; greater local availability of a range of obstetric services and sophisticated technologies; efforts to reduce financial barriers to health care by expanding Medicaid and other services needed by poor and underserved pregnant women; and evidence that rural pregnant women and their babies are receiving care comparable to that obtained by their urban counterparts.

Simultaneously, a number of trends have emerged or persisted over the past decade that are cause for concern. These include continued low rates of early prenatal care among rural women, especially those from certain minority groups; high rates of childbearing among rural teenagers and limited access to family planning services; marked disparities in postneonatal death rates among rural as compared to urban residents; signs that regionalized perinatal care systems may be unraveling; and evidence that economically disadvantaged rural women continue to experience significant barriers to obstetric care.

The solid gains achieved in rural obstetric care in recent years must be carefully preserved, and vigorous efforts must be marshaled toward eliminating persistent geographic and demographic inequities in health care and disparities in birth outcomes. These efforts should involve a synergistic package of educational, social, medical, and economic interventions supported by state and federal policies. Only then can our nation be assured that early and continuous access to a full spectrum of maternal and perinatal care will become the birthright of the community and each of its inhabitants.

REFERENCES

American Academy of Family Physicians. 1991. Facts About Family Practice. Kansas City, Mo: AAFP.

Baker SL, Kotelchuck M. 1989. Birthweight-specific mortality: important inequalities remain. Journal of Rural Health 5: 155–70.

Baldwin L-M, Curry MA. 1992. Chapter 3: Designing programs. In: Moore ML, Paul NW, eds. Improving Access to Prenatal Care: Innovative Responses to a National Dilemma. March of Dimes Birth Defects Foundation; 6–17.

Baldwin L-M, Hart LG, Lloyd M, Fordyce M, Rosenblatt RA. 1995. Defensive medicine and obstetrics. JAMA 274: 1606–1610.

Baldwin L-M, Larson EH, Connell FA, Nordlund D, Kain KC, Cawthon ML, Byrns P, Rosenblatt RA. 1998. The effect of expanding Medicaid prenatal services: does it improve birth outcomes? American Journal of Public Health. 88(11): 1623–1629.

Brown SS, Eisenberg L. 1995. The Best Intentions: Unintended Pregnancy and the Well-Being of Children and Families. Washington, DC: Institute of Medicine, National Academy Press.

Centers for Disease Control and Prevention. 1997. Unpublished data from AIDS/HIV Surveillance System. Atlanta, GA.

Clarke LL, Coward RT. 1991. A multivariate assessment of the effects of residence on infant mortality. Journal of Rural Health 7: 246–65.

Council on Graduate Medical Education. 1997. Ninth Report: Graduate Medical Education Consortia: Changing the Governance of Graduate Medical Education to Achieve Physician Workforce Objectives. Washington (DC): Government Printing Office.

Deprez RD, Agger MS, McQuinn LB. 1996. Access to physicians, obstetric care use, and adequacy of prenatal care for Medicaid patients in Maine: 1985–1989. Obstetrics and Gynecology 88(3): 443.

Dobie S, Hart LG, Fordyce M, Andrilla H, Rosenblatt RA. 1997. Obstetrical care and payment source: do Medicaid women get less care? American Journal of Public Health 10(4): 272–279.

Gavin K, Leong D. 1989. Maternity care as an essential public service: a proposed role for state government. Journal of Rural Health 5(4): 404–412.

Gortmaker S, Sobol A, Clark C, Walker DK, Geronimus A. 1985. The survival of very low-birth weight infants by level of hospital of birth: a population study of perinatal systems in four states. American Journal of Obstetrics and Gynecology 152: 517–524.

Gortmaker SL, Clark CJG, Graven SN, Sobol AM, Geronimus A. 1987. Reducing infant mortality in rural America: evaluation of the Rural Infant Care Program. Health Services Research 22(1): 91–116.

Grossman DC, Krieger JW, Sugarman JR, Forquera RA. 1994. Health status of urban American Indians and Alaska Natives: a population-based study. JAMA 271(11): 845–850.

Hale CB, Druschel CM. 1989. Infant mortality among moderately low birthweight infants in Alabama, 1980 to 1983. Pediatrics 84: 285–289.

Harvey S, Jarrell J, Brant R, Stainton C, Rach D. 1996. A randomized, controlled trial of nurse-midwifery care. Birth 23(3): 128–35.

Health Resources and Services Administration, Bureau of Health Professions. 1992. Study of Models to Meet Rural Health Care Needs through Mobilization of Health Professions Education and Services Resources. Vol. 1. Rockville, MD: National Rural Health Association.

Hein HA. 1980. Evaluation of rural perinatal care system. Pediatrics 66: 540–546.

Hein HA, Lathrop SS. 1986. The changing pattern of neonatal mortality in a regionalized system of perinatal care. American Journal of Diseases of Children 140: 989–993.

Henshaw SK, Forrest JD. 1993. Women at Risk of Unintended Pregnancy, 1990 Estimates: The Need for Family Planning Services, Each State and County. New York: Alan Guttmacher Institute.

Henshaw SK, Van Vort J. 1994. United States abortion services in 1991 and 1992. Fam Plann Perspect 26: 100–12.

Klerman LV, Scholle SH. 1992. Issues in the provision of maternity care. In: Kotch JB, et al., eds. A Pound of Prevention: The Case of Universal Maternity Care in the U.S. Washington, DC: APHA.

Larimore WL, Davis A. 1995. Relation of infant mortality to the availability of maternity care in rural Florida. Journal of the American Board of Family Practice 8(5): 392–399.

Larson EH, Hart LG, Rosenblatt RA. 1992. Rural residence and poor birth outcome in Washington State. Journal of Rural Health 8: 162–70.

Larson EH, Hart LG, Rosenblatt RA. 1997. Is rural residence a risk factor for poor birth outcome? A national study. Social Science and Medicine 45(2): 171–188.

McCormick MC, Richardson DK. 1995. Access to neonatal intensive care. The Future of Children: Low Birth Weight 5(1): 162–175.

Meckel RA. 1990. Save the Babies: American Public Health Reform and the Prevention of Infant Motality, 1850–1929. Baltimore, MD: Johns Hopkins University Press.

Miller CA. 1988. Development of MCH services and policy in the Unites States. In: Wallace HM, Ryan G, Oglesby AC, eds. Maternal and Child Health Practice. Oakland, CA: Third Party Press.

Moore ML. 1992. Introduction. In: Moore ML, Paul NW, eds. Improving Access to Prenatal Care: Innovative Responses to a National Dilemma. March of Dimes Birth Defects Foundation.

National Center for Health Statistics. 1995. Public Use Data File Documentation: Linked Birth/Infant Death Data Set: 1991 Birth Cohort. Hyattsville, MD: NCHS.

Nesbitt T, Connell F, Hart LG, Rosenblatt RA. 1990. Access to obstetrical care in rural areas: effects on birth outcomes. American Journal of Public Health 80: 814–818.

Nesbitt TS. 1996. Rural maternity care: new models of access. Birth 23: 161–165.

Nesbitt TS, Baldwin L-M. 1993. Access to obstetric care. Primary Care 20(3): 509–522.

Nesbitt TS, Larson EH, Rosenblatt RA, Hart LG. 1997. Neonatal outcomes and resource utilization in rural areas: effect of access to maternity care. American Journal of Public Health 87(1): 85–90.

Norris TE, Reese JW, Pirani MJ, Rosenblatt RA. 1996. Are rural family physicians comfortable performing cesarean sections? Journal of Family Practice 43(5): 455–460.

Office of Technology Assessment. 1990. Health Care in Rural America. OTA Publication No. OTA-H-434. Washington, DC: U.S. Government Printing Office.

Pathman D, Tropman S. 1995. Obstetrical practice among new rural family physicians. Journal of Family Practice 40(5): 457–464.

Powell SL, Holt VL, et al. 1995. Recent changes in delivery site of low-birth-weight infants in Washington: impact on birth weight-specific mortality. American Journal of Obstetrics and Gynecology 173(5): 1585–1592.

Ray WA, et al. 1997. Effect of Medicaid expansion on preterm birth. American Journal of Preventive Medicine 13: 292–297.

Rooks J. 1997. Midwifery and Childbirth in America. Philadelphia, PA: Temple University Press.

Rosenblatt RA. 1989. A lack of will: the perinatal care crisis in rural America. Journal of Rural Health 5: 293–298.

Rosenblatt RA, Bovbjerg RR, Whelan A, Baldwin L-M, Hart LG, Long C. 1991. Tort reform and the obstetric access crisis: the case of the WAMI states. Western Journal of Medicine 154: 693–699.

Rosenblatt RA, Dobie SA, Hart LG, et al. 1997. Interspecialty differences in obstetric care. American Journal of Public Health 87: 344–351.

Rosenblatt RA, Mattis R, Hart LG. 1995. Access to legal abortions in rural America: a study of rural physicians in Idaho. American Journal of Public Health 85(10): 1423–5.

Rosenblatt RA, Reinken J, Shoemack P. 1985. Is obstetrics safe in small hospitals?—evidence from New Zealand's regionalised perinatal system. Lancet 149: 98–102.

Rosenblatt RA, Sanders GR, Tressler CJ, Larson EH, Nesbitt TS, Hart LG. 1994. The diffusion of obstetric technology into rural U.S. hospitals. International Journal of Technology Assessment in Health Care 10(3): 479–489.

Rosenblatt RA, Whelan A, Hart LG. 1990. Obstetric practice patterns in Washington State after tort reform: has the access problem been solved? Obstetrics and Gynecology 76: 1105–1110.

Schmidt WM, Wallace HM. 1988. The development of health services for mothers and children in the United States. In: Wallace HM, Ryan G, Oglesby AC, eds. Maternal and Child Health Practices. Oakland, CA: Third Party Publishing Company.

Schmittling G. 1993. Facts about Family Practice, 1993. Kansas City, MO: American Academy of Family Physicians.

Sherman A. 1992. Falling by the Wayside: Children in Rural America. Washington, DC: Children's Defense Fund.

Shiono PH, Behrman RE. 1995. Low birth weight: analysis and recommendations. The Future of Children: Low Birth Weight 5(1): 4–17.

Steinauer JE, DePineres T, Robert AM, Westfall J, Darney P. 1997. Training family practice residents in abortion and other reproductive health care: a nationwide survey. Family Planning Perspectives 29: 222–227.

Stoto MA, Behrens R, Rosemont, C. 1990. Healthy People 2000: Citizens Chart the Course. Washington, DC: National Academy Press.

Taylor DH, Ricketts TC III. 1993. Increasing obstetrical care access to the rural poor. Journal of Health Care for the Poor and Underserved 4(1): 9–20.

University of Minnesota Rural Health Research Center. 1997. Rural Managed Care: Patterns and Prospects. Minneapolis, MN: University of Minnesota.

Wilcox AJ, Skjoerven R. 1992. Birthweight and perinatal mortality: the effect of gestational age. American Journal of Public Health 82(3): 378–82.

13

Rural Children's Health

SARAH J. CLARK, LUCY A. SAVITZ, AND RANDY K. RANDOLPH

This chapter presents a profile of rural children's health in the 1990s, describing demographic changes, mortality patterns, health status indicators, health insurance, and the availability of health care providers and institutions. It utilizes recent, national data only; findings from small-area or single-state studies and from research conducted prior to 1990 are not included in statistical comparisons, although they are referenced occasionally to support or clarify statements about related issues. The purpose is to describe the current situation, suggest recent trends, and inform policy decisions concerning child and adolescent health in rural America.

The following analyses of rural child health use the best available data sets to frame the discussion, including the National Health Interview Survey, the United States (U.S.) Census, the National Survey of Family Growth, the Area Resource File (ARF), the National Crime Survey, and the American Hospital Association's (AHA) Annual Survey of Hospitals. Unpublished data were provided by individual staff at the Centers for Disease Control and Prevention (CDC) and the National Center for Health Statistics (NCHS).

The data sets used for this chapter generally classify children based on their residence in a metropolitan or nonmetropolitan county. For some variables, metropolitan residency is further stratified as either central city or noncentral city. For ease of reading, the more familiar terms *urban, suburban,* and *rural* are used throughout this chapter; however, they are not intended to represent more precise classifications of "rural" or "urban" (Ricketts and Johnson-Webb, 1997). Chapter 1—Populations and Places in Rural America—discusses these differences in detail.

DEMOGRAPHICS

As of 1996, 16 million children (under 21 years of age) resided in nonmetropolitan areas (Table 13.1)—a significant decrease from the 1984–85 estimate of 21 million (McManus and Newacheck, 1989). Rural children account for 21% of all U.S. children and represent 31% of the total nonmetropolitan population.

Rural children continue to reside predominantly in the South and Midwest. In contrast, the Northeast and West regions comprise very small rural populations, and their proportions have decreased considerably over the past decade.

Several important demographic differences exist between rural and urban populations. A greater proportion of rural children are white, compared with the urban population. Black children and children of Asian and Hispanic descent constitute a greater proportion of the urban child population; the rural population includes a larger proportion of Native American children. Rural children are more likely to live in larger families with married parents, whereas a greater proportion of urban children live in families headed by a single mother. Rural preschool-aged children are more likely to have both or their only parent working.

Rural families are, on the whole, poorer than urban families. Overall, 23.2% of rural children under the age of 18 live in poverty, compared with 21.0% of urban children. This difference is consistent across all categories of age, gender, and family status (Table 13.2).

Several housing characteristics pertain directly to

Table 13.1 Demographic Characteristics of U.S. Children, 1996

	Percent Distribution		*Population (in 1000s)*	
	Metro	*Nonmetro*	*Metro*	*Nonmetro*
AGE (IN YEARS)				
Under 1	1.5	1.3	3,246	656
1 to 5	7.8	7.4	16,639	3,780
6 to 17	17.4	18.9	36,986	9,680
18 to 20	4.1	4.1	8,605	2,127
>20 (adults)	69.2	68.3	146,876	35,093
Total Population	100	100	212,352	51,336
GENDER[a]				
Male	51.1	51.4	29,080	7,249
Female	48.9	48.6	27,791	6,866
RACE[a]				
White	77.1	83.9	43,875	11,845
Black	17.2	12.0	9,809	1,691
Native American	0.9	2.4	521	337
Asian	4.7	1.7	2,667	242
HISPANIC ORIGIN[a]	17.8	7.8	10,115	1,107
RESIDENCE BY REGION[a]				
Northeast	20.5	10.0	11,685	1,414
Midwest	21.9	31.4	12,429	4,430
South	32.2	42.5	18,326	6,001
West	25.4	16.1	14,431	2,271
FAMILY SIZE[b]				
Four or fewer	79.3	73.3	23,877	5,358
Five or more	20.7	26.7	6,221	1,949
FAMILY COMPOSITION[b]				
Married parents	72.5	73.8	19,189	4,742
Single, female-headed	22.8	20.9	6,044	1,342
Single, male-headed	4.7	5.4	1,236	344
PARENTAL EMPLOYMENT[c]				
Married, both working	53.3	58.5	7,062	1,738
Single, female-headed, mother working	46.9	53.8	1,638	415
Single, male-headed, father working	76.7	78.3	503	106

[a]Children younger than 18 years only.
[b]Families with children younger than 18 years.
[c]Families with children younger than 6 years.
Source: 1996 Current Population Survey.

health issues in the daily lives of children (Table 13.3). Rural families are less likely to obtain water for residential use from a public system or private company, and much more likely to use well water or another source. This may place rural children at a disadvantage in terms of the need for fluoride supplementation, the availability of safe water for mixing infant formula, and the potential for bacterial contamination of drinking water. Rural families are also significantly more likely to use a septic tank or other sewage source, rather than a public system, and to have incomplete plumbing facilities; again, this may have a direct impact on health related to the transmission of bacteria and water-borne diseases.

Table 13.2 Percent of U.S. Children Under 18 Living in Poverty, 1996

	Metro	*Nonmetro*
AGE (IN YEARS)		
Under 1	23.8	29.7
1 to 5	24.1	27.3
6 to 17	19.4	21.2
GENDER		
Male <18 years	20.5	23.1
Female <18 years	21.5	23.4
FAMILY STATUS		
Married parents	9.5	12.2
Single, female-headed	49.1	52.7
Single, male-headed	30.2	33.9

Source: 1996 Current Population Survey.

HEALTH INSURANCE

Insurance status is a strong predictor of the adequacy of children's health care. Research has demonstrated that uninsured children experience problems with access to medical care, delays in necessary treatment and inadequate immunization (Holl et al., 1995; Newacheck, Hughes, and Stoddard, 1996; Himmelstein and Woolhandler, 1995). Being uninsured is more prevalent among rural (15%) than urban (13.6%) children (Table 13.4). Urban children were somewhat more likely than rural children to have private insurance coverage (65% versus 63%). Of those privately insured, a greater proportion of rural than urban children were on a self-purchased policy; more urban children were covered under an employer-sponsored group plan. The proportions of Medicaid-enrolled children were roughly equal, even though a higher proportion of rural children live in poverty.

Over the past two decades, the most prominent change in the area of health insurance has been the dramatic increase in managed care organizations. Although more than 80% of rural counties are currently included in the service area of at least one commercial health maintenance organization (HMO), actual enrollment rates are very low (University of Minnesota, 1997).

An important component of managed care is its emphasis on prevention, including immunizations and well-child visits. However, rural children may be less likely than urban children to receive these preventive services, because they are not generally covered in a traditional fee-for-service environment. Managed care in rural areas is addressed in more detail in Chapter 10, Rural Managed Care.

AVAILABILITY OF HEALTH CARE PROVIDERS AND SERVICES

The presence of primary care providers (PCPs) in a community is an important marker for availability of health care for children. PCPs deliver basic preventive and acute care for most U.S. children. The trends in PCP supply are

Table 13.3 Health-Related Characteristics of Family Dwellings, 1990

	Percent Distribution		*Population (in 1000s)*	
	Metro	*Nonmetro*	*Metro*	*Nonmetro*
WATER SOURCE				
Public/private	89.5	64.4	72,076	13,993
Drilled well	9.0	28.6	7,244	6,224
Dug well	1.0	3.9	813	852
Other	0.5	3.1	387	676
SEWAGE SOURCE				
Public system	81.8	48.6	65,891	10,564
Septic tank/cesspool	17.5	48.5	14,121	10,550
Other	0.6	2.9	506	631
PLUMBING				
Complete	99.5	98.5	57,766	13,174
Incomplete	0.5	1.5	317	205

Source: 1990 Census of Population and Housing, Standard Tape File 3c.

Table 13.4 Health Insurance Status of Children 0 to 18 Years of Age, 1996

	Metro		*Nonmetro*	
	Number	*Percent*	*Number*	*Percent*
Private, employer-sponsored	33,800,920	59.4	7,769,107	55.1
Private, self-purchased	3,234,503	5.7	1,128,542	8.0
Medicaid	11,123,131	19.6	2,859,262	20.3
Champus	945,860	1.7	218,035	1.5
Medicare	41,868	0.1	17,223	0.1
No health insurance	7,724,784	13.6	2,123,727	15.0

Source: 1996 Current Population Survey.

discussed in Chapter 3, Physicians in Rural America, and Chapter 4, Nonphysician Providers in Rural America. Although the percentage of physicians practicing in rural areas decreased from 1985 to 1995 in almost every specialty, the overall number of PCP physicians practicing in rural areas increased from 43,099 to 50,166. Family physicians and general practitioners continue to provide care for many rural children; over 20% of these physicians practice in rural areas, but pediatricians are predominantly concentrated in metropolitan areas. This likely creates a reliance on family physicians and general practitioners, as well as mid-level providers (e.g., physician assistants and licensed nurse practitioners), for pediatric care of rural children.

Health services for children and adolescents—inpatient and outpatient hospital-based care—are considered specialty services, and as such are less available in rural versus urban areas (Table 13.5). However, it is encouraging to note that half of all rural hospitals are providing inpatient surgical services for general pediatric cases. Increases in outpatient child wellness and teen outreach services in both rural and urban areas are an important expansion of the continuum of health care delivery offered in hospital-based settings.

Table 13.5 Percentage of Hospitals Providing Child and Adolescent Services, 1995

	Metro	*Nonmetro*
INPATIENT SERVICES		
Pediatric general medical surgery	63	50
Pediatric intensive care	23	6
Child/adolescent psychiatry	45	18
OUTPATIENT SERVICES		
Child wellness	24	11
Teen outreach	22	7

Source: 1995 Annual Survey of Hospitals, American Hospital Association.

CHILDREN'S HEALTH STATUS AND SOURCE OF CARE

Children are, in general, very healthy. It is difficult to detect differences in health status or health outcomes according to certain characteristics, especially measures of function typically used with adults. Furthermore, the primary focus of children's health care is prevention: immunization, growth monitoring, vision and hearing screening, lead screening, developmental assessment, and counseling for parents. These components of preventive care usually are provided during the course of well-child visits, recommended at scheduled intervals during the first years of a child's life* (American Academy of Pediatrics, 1988).

Because many aspects of preventive care are not routinely or uniformly recorded in the medical record or collected in national or state data sets, immunization rates have historically served as a proxy for the overall delivery of children's well-child care. CDC data from 1994 for the primary immunization series† found that 66% of rural children received appropriate vaccinations, compared with 71% of suburban children and 62% of urban children (CDC, 1993). National immunization rates for the primary series have risen considerably over the past 5 years, but recent data published by the CDC have not included national rural-urban trends. The sampling frames used to generate immunization rates have been altered to allow for stable estimates by state and for select urban areas, but the ability to analyze trends in rural areas is limited. Furthermore, computerized immunization registry systems that can generate small-area immunization

*Well-child visits are recommended at 1–2 weeks, 2 months, 4 months, 6 months, 9 months, 12 months, 15 months, 18 months, 24 months, and every year thereafter.

†Primary immunization series consists of four doses of diptheria-teatanus-pertussis (DTP) vaccine, three doses of polio vaccine, one dose of measles-mumps-rubella (MMR) vaccine, and three doses of *H. influenzae* type b (Hib) vaccine.

Table 13.6 Percent of U.S. Children with Unmet Medical Needs, 0 to 17 Years of Age, 1993

	Metro, central city	*Metro, noncentral city*	*Nonmetro*
Any unmet need	10.3	9.8	13.4
Needed but not able to get care	2.2	1.8	1.8
Delayed care due to cost	3.8	3.7	5.4
Needed dental care	6.1	5.3	8.4
Needed prescription	1.5	1.3	1.2
Needed glasses	1.4	1.2	1.6
Needed mental health care	0.4	0.5	0.3

Source: Vital Statistics of the United States, 1993. Access to Health Care Part 1: Children.

rates (and enable providers to determine which children are behind on immunizations) are being developed almost exclusively in urban areas.

Another indicator of the adequacy of children's health care pertains to ability to obtain needed medical care. Rural children are at increased risk for unmet medical need (Table 13.6). Overall, rural children were more likely to need but not receive dental care, and were more likely to delay care because of cost.

Having a regular source of medical care—often referred to as a "medical home"—enhances the likelihood that children receive recommended well-child care and appropriate follow-up for acute and chronic conditions (National Center for Health Statistics—NCHS, 1997). In 1993, 6% of U.S. children (4.2 million) had no regular source of care. Overall, poor and black and Hispanic children were at increased risk for having no source of care. Most children with insurance have a regular source of medical care; fewer uninsured children have a regular source of care (Table 13.7). However, when compared, rural children are as likely as urban children to have a regular source of care. In fact, among children who are uninsured or enrolled in Medicaid, rural children have a greater likelihood of having a regular source of care, compared with urban and suburban children. Nationally, the most common reasons for having no source of care were not being able to afford care (34%), not needing a physician (31%), and care being unavailable or not convenient (17%) (NCHS, 1997).

Regarding the setting of the regular source of care (private physician, public clinic, or emergency room) for children with different types of insurance, rural children, particularly those who are uninsured or enrolled in Medicaid, are substantially more likely than urban children to name a private practice as their regular source of care (Table 13.8). Margolis and colleagues (1992) found that rural physicians are more likely to accept patients of varying insurance status, possibly because they must retain a high proportion of the available patient pool in order to remain financially viable, whereas urban practices

Table 13.7 Percentage of Children with Regular Source of Medical Care by Insurance Status, 0 to 17 Years of Age, 1993

	Metro, central city	*Metro, noncentral city*	*Nonmetro*
HAD REGULAR SOURCE OF CARE			
All	92.3	94.4	94.1
Private health insurance	96.9	97.1	96.0
Public health insurance	94.4	92.5	95.6
No health insurance	73.3	79.8	85.3
NO REGULAR SOURCE OF CARE			
All	7.7	5.6	5.9
Private health insurance	3.1	2.9	4.0
Public health insurance	5.6	7.5	4.4
No health insurance	26.7	20.2	14.7

Source: Vital Statistics of the United States, 1993. Access to Health Care Part 1: Children.

Table 13.8 Type of Regular Source of Care by Child's Insurance Status by Percentages of Children, 1993

	Metro, central city	*Metro, noncentral city*	*Nonmetro*
PRIVATE INSURANCE			
Private MD	90.9	95.1	93.8
Public clinic	7.1	3.3	4.7
Emergency room	1.0	0.1	0.7
PUBLIC INSURANCE			
Private MD	49.1	69.8	85.2
Public clinic	42.3	24.7	6.6
Emergency room	5.5	4.2	2.8
NO INSURANCE			
Private MD	62.7	76.6	84.0
Public clinic	28.1	20.8	9.7
Emergency room	3.4	1.0	4.1

Source: Vital Statistics of the United States, 1993. Access to Health Care Part 1: Children.

"self-select" their patient population by limiting numbers of Medicaid or uninsured children.

An interesting contrast to the discussion of regular sources of care for rural children is that although rural physicians are more likely to accept a broad patient base, they are less likely to offer immunizations (Hueston, Mainous, and Farrell, 1994). Those who do provide immunization services are more likely to refer uninsured and Medicaid-enrolled children to the health department for immunizations (Ruch-Ross and O'Connor, 1994). Such referrals may be attributed to the high cost of vaccines or to the fact that rural physicians do not see enough children to warrant offering costly immunization services (Bordley et al., 1994; Szilagyi et al., 1994).

Generally, any disruption of the medical home is thought to create additional barriers to care related to increased waiting time, problems with transportation, and parental loss of work. However, an analysis of public health department immunization data from 11 states found that health departments in rural areas are highly effective in providing timely immunizations, often more so than urban health departments and private practices (Slifkin et al., 1997).

Additionally, the federal Vaccines for Children program (VFC) and several state programs aim specifically to reduce the referral of children for immunizations only by decreasing patient charges for vaccines. There is some evidence that such programs are effective for this purpose (Hueston, Mainous, and Ferrell, 1994; Freed et al., 1997; Zimmermann et al., 1997).

DEATH AND INJURY AMONG CHILDREN

Mortality rates among children over one year of age reflect both the quality of children's health care and societal problems such as violence and substance abuse. In 1992, over 84,000 children under the age of 25 died (Table 13.9). Twenty-three percent (23%) of deaths were among rural children. Infant mortality, defined as the death of a child under one year of age, is discussed in Chapter 12, Rural Maternal and Perinatal Health. For children over one year of age, mortality is associated primarily with injury: motor vehicle crashes, firearm injuries, drowning, burning, suffocation, and poisoning. Data from the National Vital Statistics System demonstrate that in 1992, fatal injuries were 44% higher among rural children aged 1 to 19 years compared with their urban counterparts. Among children aged 1 to 14 years, death rates for all races were at least 20% higher in rural than urban areas. Among children 15 to 19 years, mortality among urban blacks was 50% higher than among rural blacks; for all other ethnicities, mortality rates were higher in rural areas. Homicide rates were four times higher among urban males 15 to 19 years, whereas suicide rates were higher among rural males 15 to 19 years old. In all age groups, mortality from motor vehicle crashes is higher in rural areas, reflecting the increased travel time and distance required of rural populations. Finally, over the period of 1985 to 1992, rural injury mortality rates remained consistently higher than urban rates with one exception: the mortality rate for rural and urban males aged 15 to 19 years is equal (Fingerhut and Gunderson, 1995).

HIV/AIDS

Through June 1997, a cumulative total of 612,078 AIDS cases were reported in the United States: nearly 1% of these cases occurred in among children under the age of 13 (CDC, 1997). Between 1990 and 1995, the incidence of pediatric AIDS cases decreased 19% despite an increase of 30% in the overall incidence of AIDS nationwide (Table 13.10). However, while the incidence of pediatric AIDS cases declined 24% in metro areas, the incidence in rural areas increased 5%.

CRIME AND VIOLENCE

Detailed data on victims of criminal activity are collected through the National Crime Survey (NCS). Over the

Table 13.9 Deaths among Persons under 25 Years of Age, 1992

	Total <25 years		*<1 year*		*1–4 years*		*5–14 years*		*15–24 years*	
	Number	*Percent*	*Number*	*Percent*	*Number*	*Percent*	*Number*	*Percent*	*Number*	*Percent*
US—Total	84,133	100	34,628	41.2	6,764	8.0	8,193	9.7	34,548	41.1
Metro	64,898	100	27,701	42.7	5,171	8.0	5871	9.0	26,155	40.3
Nonmetro	19,235	100	6,927	36.0	1,593	8.3	2,322	12.1	8393	43.6
White—Total	57,179	100	22,164	38.8	4,685	8.2	5,989	10.5	24,341	42.6
Metro	42,276	100	17,048	40.3	3,498	8.3	4,112	9.7	14,618	41.7
Nonmetro	14,903	100	5,116	34.3	1,187	8.0	1,877	12.6	6723	45.1
Nonwhite—Total	26,954	100	12,464	46.2	2,079	7.7	2,204	8.2	10,207	37.9
Metro	22,622	100	10,653	47.1	1,673	7.4	1,759	7.8	8,537	37.7
Nonmetro	4,332	100	1,811	41.8	406	9.4	445	10.3	1,670	38.6
Black[a]—Total	24,005	100	11,348	47.3	1,799	7.5	1,876	7.8	8,982	37.4
Metro	20,588	100	9,854	47.9	1,492	7.2	1,541	7.5	7,701	37.4
Nonmetro	3,417	100	1,494	43.7	307	9.0	335	9.8	1,281	37.5
Male—Total	54,641	100	19,545	35.8	3,809	7.0	5,080	9.3	26,207	48.0
Metro	42,046	100	15,569	37.0	2,879	6.8	3,634	8.6	19,964	47.5
Nonmetro	12,595	100	3,976	31.6	930	7.4	1,446	11.5	6,243	49.6

[a]Black is a subset of nonwhite.
Source: Vital Statistics of the United States, 1992. Volume II—Mortality. Part B.

past 20 years, victimization of rural residents to violent crime has increased, while crimes of theft and household crimes have decreased (Table 13.11). Overall victimization rates are lowest in rural areas and highest in urban areas. However, in all areas, rates have substantially increased among youths 12 to 19 years. In each of the three criminal categories, the victimization rate for rural youths is higher than the rate for the overall urban population. Further, the urban-rural rate ratio is 1.9 for all categories of the total population; among youths, that gap narrows, with a rate ratio of 1.4 for crimes of theft and 1.2 for household crimes.

Table 13.10 Trends in AIDS Cases, 1990–1995 (rates per 100,000 population)

	1990	*1993*	*1995*
ALL AIDS CASES	26.56	32.69	34.54
Metro	21.91	26.43	27.25
Nonmetro	4.65	6.26	7.29
(rate ratio)	(4.72)	(4.22)	(3.74)
CHILDREN <13 YEARS[a]	2.42	2.68	1.95
Metro	2.04	2.13	1.55
Nonmetro	0.38	0.55	0.40
(rate ratio)	(5.30)	(3.86)	(3.82)

[a]Age at initial diagnosis of AIDS.
Source: Unpublished data from the Centers for Disease Control and Prevention.

In 1989, a special supplement to the NCS contained questions on youths' victimization experiences at school, their opinions about crime, the availability of drugs, and awareness of gangs (Table 13.12). Only a narrow difference existed in crime experiences among students in rural versus urban locations—a stark contrast to the larger rural-urban differences found in the regular NCS data.

Gang activity in school was cited three times more fre-

Table 13.11 Victims of Violent Crimes, Theft, and Household Crimes, 1991 (victimizations per 1000 households or persons)

	Metro, central city	*Metro, noncentral city*	*Nonmetro*
CRIMES OF VIOLENCE			
Total population	40.6	26.0	21.1
Age 12–19 years	86.2	63.0	47.9
CRIMES OF THEFT			
Total population	86.0	70.1	45.1
Age 12–19 years	128.2	115.5	93.1
HOUSEHOLD CRIMES			
Total population	232.1	152.7	120.4
Age 12–19 years	410.5	382.4	356.0

Source: Donnermeyer JF. 1995. Crime and violence in rural communities. In: Blaser SM, Blaser J, Pantoja K, eds. Perspectives on Violence and Substance Use in Rural America. North Central Regional Educational Laboratory, Midwest Regional Center for Drug-Free Schools and Communities.

Table 13.12 Crime in the School Setting, 1989 (percent reporting various criminal activities)

Activity Reporting	*Metro, Central City*	*Metro, Noncentral City*	*Nonmetro*
Being a victim of property crime	8	7	7
Being a victim of violent crime	2	2	1
Drugs available at their school	66	67	71
Have attended drug education classes	40	35	44
Gangs active in their school	25	14	8
Avoiding certain places at school	8	5	6
Fear of being attacked at school	24	20	20
Fear of being attacked going to/from school	19	12	13

Source: Bastian LD, Taylor BM. 1991. School Crime: A National Crime Victimization Survey Report. Washington, DC: Office of Justice Programs, Bureau of Justice Statistics. NCJ-131645.

quently among urban than rural youths. However, a substantial number of rural students exhibited fear about violence at school. These results indicate that rural youth are experiencing crime at a level and in ways similar to youth from the cities and suburbs.

SUBSTANCE ABUSE

Criminal activity is often linked to drug use, particularly among children. A 1992–1993 survey of rural and urban 8th and 12th graders demonstrated that rural-urban differences in drug use have decreased nationwide (Table 13.13). More rural students reported that drugs were readily available at their school, and rural students were more likely to have attended drug education classes. Of the observed trends, most surprising was that inhalants were more common than marijuana among 8th graders. It appears that during the 1990s inhalants, which are inexpensive and easily accessible, have replaced marijuana as the "gateway" drug (Edwards, 1993). For all other drugs, lifetime prevalence among 12th graders was higher than for 8th graders. With respect to rural-urban differences, urban youths are more likely to have used marijuana, cocaine, and

Table 13.13 Lifetime Prevalence of Drug Use Among 8th Graders and 12th Graders, 1993 (percent reporting any use)

	8th Graders		*12th Graders*	
	Metro	*Nonmetro*	*Metro*	*Nonmetro*
Marijuana	12.7	11.2	40.3	30.3
Cocaine	2.6	2.3	6.8	5.7
Crack	2.4	2.0	2.3	2.7
Inhalants	15.3	14.7	11.9	11.5
LSD	3.9	3.4	12.4	7.7
Stimulants	5.2	5.5	21.5	18.5
Smokeless Tobacco	19.0	25.1	32.5	39.7
Alcohol—any	71.3	70.3	90.2	90.2
Alcohol—got drunk	25.7	27.3	69.6	69.6
Cigarettes	46.5	45.7	63.0	63.1

Source: Edwards RW. 1995. Alcohol, tobacco, and other drug use by youth in rural communities. In: Blaser SM, Blaser J, Pantoja K, eds. Perspectives on Violence and Substance Use in Rural American. North Central Regional Educational Laboratory, Midwest Regional Center for Drug-Free Schools and Communities.

Table 13.14 Intensity of Drug Use Among 8th Graders and 12th Graders, 1993 (percent classified in each category)

	8th Graders		*12th Graders*	
	Metro	*Nonmetro*	*Metro*	*Nonmetro*
High drug involvement[a]	3.6	3.5	16.1	14.3
Moderate involvement[b]	12.6	11.9	18.4	13.4
Drug experimenters	11.1	10.7	14.4	14.1
Light alcohol users	13.8	13.0	20.3	24.7
Negligible or no use	58.9	60.9	30.8	33.5

[a]Defined as multidrug user, stimulant user, heavy marijuana user, and/or heavy alcohol user.

[b]Defined as occasional drug user or light marijuana user.

Source: Edwards RW. 1995. Alcohol, tobacco, and other drug use by youth in rural communities. In: Blaser SM, Blaser J, Pantoja K, eds. Perspectives on Violence and Substance Use in Rural American. North Central Regional Educational Laboratory, Midwest Regional Center for Drug-Free Schools and Communities.

LSD and rural youths are more likely to have used smokeless tobacco. Use of alcohol and cigarettes is high in both groups.

Patterns of the intensity of drug use among youths are helpful in evaluating the effectiveness of school or community drug education efforts, which are targeted toward youths who are moderately involved in drug use or who abstain from use. These data also assist in determining the need for drug treatment programs for youth who are heavily involved with drugs. Among 8th graders, urban youth have slightly greater involvement in drugs (Table 13.14); the same pattern holds true for 12th graders, with the exception of slight alcohol use, which is more common among rural youth. Furthermore, rural 12th graders are more likely to report using alcohol while "driving around," which greatly contributes to the higher rates of motor vehicle fatalities among rural youth (Edwards, 1995).

SUMMARY

Overall, the profile of rural children in the United States in the 1990s has changed very little from that in the 1980s (McManus and Newacheck, 1989). Demographic changes include a decrease in the total number of rural children, a decrease in the proportion of rural children who live in the Northeast or West, and a slight increase in the proportion of rural residents who are white. Changes in many aspects of children's health status cannot be determined, largely because of inadequacies in available data. However, the health of rural children appears to be deteriorating with regard to crime, substance abuse, and AIDS, and fatal injuries continue to affect a disproportionate number of rural children.

In contrast, rural areas appear to be experiencing an increase in the availability of health care services and health care providers. A provision in the 1997 Balanced Budget Act that allocates funds to states for offering coverage to uninsured children holds great potential. However, as eligibility and implementation will vary from state to state, the national effects of this policy—both from the urban and rural perspectives—are unclear and remain to be seen.

REFERENCES

American Academy of Pediatrics Committee on Psychosocial Aspects of Child and Family Health. 1988. Guidelines for Health Supervision II. Elk Grove Village, IL: American Academy of Pediatrics.

Bordley WC, Freed GL, Garrett JM, Byrd CA, Meriwether R. 1994. Factors responsible for immunization referrals to health departments in North Carolina. Pediatrics 94: 376–380.

Centers for Disease Control and Prevention. 1994. Vaccination coverage of 2-year-old children—United States, 1993. Morbidity and Mortality Weekly Report 43: 705–709.

Centers for Disease Control and Prevention. 1997. HIV/AIDS Surveillance report. 9: 3–37.

Edwards RW. 1993. Drug use among 8th graders is increasing. International Journal of Addictions 28: 1621–1623.

Edwards RW. 1995. Alcohol, tobacco, and other drug use by youth in rural communities. In: Blaser SM, Blaser J, Pantoja K (eds). Perspectives on Violence and Substance Use in Rural America. Oak Brook, IL: North Central Regional Educational Laboratory, Midwest Regional Center for Drug-Free Schools and Communities.

Fingerhut LA, Gunderson P. 1995. Rural children and injury: lessons from the data. Presented at: Child and Adolescent Rural Injury Control. Madison, WI.

Freed GL, Clark SJ, Pathman DE, Konrad TR, Biddle AK, Schectman RM. 1997. Impact of a new universal purchase vaccine program in North Carolina. Archives of Pediatric and Adolescent Medicine 151: 1117–1124.

Himmelstein DU, Woolhandler S. 1995. Care denied: US residents who are unable to obtain needed medical services. American Journal of Public Health 85: 341–344.

Holl JL, Szilagyi PG, Rodewald LE, Byrd RS, Weitzman ML. 1995. Profile of uninsured children in the United States. Archives of Pediatric and Adolescent Medicine 149: 398–406.

Hueston WJ, Mainous AG III, Farrell B. 1994. Childhood immunization availability in primary care practices. Archives of Family Medicine 3: 605–609.

McManus MA, Newacheck PW. 1989. Rural maternal, child, and adolescent health. Health Services Research 23: 807–848.

Margolis PA, Cook RL, Earp JA, Lannon CM, Keyes LL, Klein JD. 1992. Factors associated with pediatricians' participation in Medicaid in North Carolina. JAMA 267: 1942–1946.

National Center for Health Statistics. 1997. Vital Statistics of the United States, 1993. Access to Health Care Part 1: Children.

Newacheck PW, Hughes DC, Stoddard JJ. 1996. Children's access to primary care: differences by race, income, and insurance status. Pediatrics 97: 26–32.

Ricketts TC, Johnson-Webb KD. 1997. What is "rural" and how to measure "rurality": a focus on health care delivery and health policy. Working Paper of the Rural Health Research Center, University of North Carolina at Chapel Hill.

Ruch-Ross HS, O'Connor KG. 1994. Immunization referral practices of pediatricians in the United States. Pediatrics 94: 508–513.

Slifkin RT, Clark SJ, Strandhoy SE, Konrad TR. 1997. Public-sector immunization coverage in eleven states: the status of rural areas. Journal of Rural Health 13: 334–41.

Szilagyi PA, Rodewald LE, Humiston SG, Hager J, Roghmann KJ, Doane CB, et al. 1994. Immunization practices of pediatricians and family physicians in the United States. Pediatrics 94: 517–523.

University of Minnesota Rural Health Research Center. 1997. Rural Managed Care: Patterns & Prospects. Minneapolis, MN: University of Minnesota.

Zimmermann RK, Medsger AR, Ricci EM, Raymund M, Mieczkowski TA, Grufferman S. 1997. Impact of free vaccine and insurance status on physician referral of children to public vaccine clinics. JAMA 278: 996–1000.

14

Rural Mental Health and Substance Abuse

DAVID HARTLEY, DONNA C. BIRD, AND PATRICIA DEMPSEY

Current trends, including active consideration of parity for mental health benefits and the increasing role of managed care in the delivery of mental health services, may be breaking down some of the historic barriers between the mental and physical health care delivery systems. Unfortunately, the concerns of rural mental health and substance abuse service consumers and providers are often overlooked as these systems undergo financial and organizational changes. While system changes raise many concerns about quality, appropriateness, cost, and equity, this chapter will focus only on rural-specific issues with implications for policy, financing or organizational initiatives.

Clearly, the dramatically lower supply of specialty mental health professionals in rural areas, and corresponding reliance on primary care practitioners to deliver needed mental health care, are among the distinguishing features of the rural mental health system. According to the federal Bureau of Primary Health Care (BPHC), as of January 1997 more than three quarters of the country's designated Mental Health Professional Shortage Areas (MHPSAs) were nonmetropolitan, representing over 70% of the population residing in underserved areas (Plate 14.1). Thus, to a large extent, any discussion of the state of rural mental health services must include an assessment of the availability of mental health professionals.

Although primary care practitioners have demonstrated some success in treating a number of mental health problems, they are typically quick to recognize the need for a mental health specialist when faced with major psychoses. In many cases, this means referring patients to a psychiatrist located in an urban area. For rural people-experiencing serious and persistent mental illness, this lack of specialty services in their home communities may result in a permanent change of residence. For many such individuals, the downsizing of state hospitals that began in the late 1960s was the first step along this path. Those with less serious mental illness may not have found it necessary to relocate to receive services, but here too, the lack of specialty mental health services is associated with lower overall use of mental health services (Lambert and Agger, 1995).

This chapter presents information on the comparative mental health and substance abuse status of rural and urban residents, as well as what is known about the availability of mental health and substance abuse treatment services and personnel in rural areas. In addition, it includes a discussion of the role of community mental health centers and primary care practitioners in providing mental health services in rural areas. Finally, the chapter discusses two trends that are affecting the long-standing problems of personnel shortages in rural areas: innovative models for the integration of mental health and primary care, and the increasing role of large national managed behavioral health organizations in addressing availability, access, and quality issues in rural areas.

PREVALENCE OF MENTAL ILLNESS AND SUBSTANCE ABUSE IN RURAL POPULATIONS

Adults

Although the evidence is not entirely conclusive, the most recent national data available suggest that the over-

Table 14.1 Lifetime and 12-Month Prevalence of Psychiatric[a] Disorders by Urbanicity, 1991 (percent of respondents with problem)

		Any Affective Disorder	*Any Anxiety Disorder*	*Any Substance Use Disorder*	*Any Disorder*
National average	12-month	11.3	17.2	11.3	29.5
	Lifetime	19.3	24.9	26.6	48.0
Rural (n = 2000)	12-month	10.0	16.6	10.6	28.6
	Lifetime	16.7	25.2	25.3	46.2
Other urban (n = 607)	12-month	10.9	19.1	11.8	30.8
	Lifetime	19.4	25.2	27.2	48.6
Major metro (n = 5491)	12-month	11.8	17.2	11.5	29.7
	Lifetime	20.2	24.8	27.0	48.6

Source: Kessler et al. 1994.
[a]According to University of Michigan Composite International Diagnostic Interview and DSM-III-R. Rates shown are weighted percentage of those responding to National Comorbidity Survey, 1991, N = 8098.

all prevalence of clinically defined mental health problems among rural and urban adult populations is similar (Kessler et al., 1994). Analysis of data from the National Comorbidity Survey (Table 14.1) indicates that, if anything, the 12-month prevalence of any affective or anxiety disorder is slightly lower in rural than in urban areas. The lifetime prevalence of any affective disorder is likewise lower in rural than in urban areas, whereas the lifetime prevalence of any anxiety disorder appears to be roughly equivalent regardless of residence location. These findings are consistent with those from the National Household Survey on Drug Abuse (Table 14.2), which likewise notes no major differences in prevalence by urbanicity of residence for a variety of common psychiatric diagnoses.

As a check against survey data, which relies completely on the recollection and honesty of respondents, suicide deaths are often used as a proxy measure of the prevalence of mental illness. This is based on an understanding that suicides represent an extreme reaction to stressful situations of the sort that might be more effectively handled by other means, including visits to a mental health professional. Mortality data from the National Center for Health Statistics (Table 14.3) show variations in adult suicide rates between regions of the United States and within metro and nonmetro areas in the same regions.

As noted previously, rural residents whose mental health problems are so persistent that they require ongoing professional care must often move to urban areas where these services are readily available. This practice could be expected to lower the prevalence of serious and persistent mental illness in rural areas somewhat, but available data do not support this supposition (Kessler et al., 1997). In fact, studies completed to date indicate that approximately one quarter of individuals served by the public mental health system in both rural and urban areas have a serious and persistent mental illness (Greenley et al., 1992).

The overall prevalence of alcohol and other substance use among adults also does not appear to vary appreciably between rural and urban areas, although the types of preferred substances may differ somewhat. The National Comorbidity Survey found comparable lifetime and 12-month prevalence rates for any substance abuse disorder among its respondents regardless of residence. A survey conducted by the Monitoring the Future Study (Table 14.4) found that young adult residents of rural areas generally experienced lower rates of use of alcohol, marijuana, stimulants, and cocaine than their urban counterparts, although they did indicate higher use of cigarettes. Many of the rural-urban differences that are observed in these studies may be attributable to factors such as the socioeconomic status or ethnicity of residents, or to population density or adjacency to urban areas (Conger, 1997).

Again acknowledging the problem of respondent bias in surveys about alcohol and other substance use and abuse, other measures can and should be used as proxies. Arrests for driving under the influence (DUI) are an im-

Table 14.2 Adults 18 and Older Reporting Mental Health Problems by Urbanicity (percent with problem)

Urbanicity	*Major Depressive Episode*	*Generalized Anxiety Disorder*	*Agoraphobia*	*Panic Attack*
Large metro	6.6	1.6	1.5	2.2
Small metro	7.8	2.0	2.1	2.9
Nonmetro	7.2	1.8	1.6	2.1

Source: Substance Abuse and Mental Health Service Administration National Household Survey on Drug Abuse, 1995.

Table 14.3 Adult[a] Suicide Deaths by Region and Urbanicity, 1995

Region	Metro		Nonmetro	
	Number	Rate per 100,000	Number	Rate per 100,000
United States	22,351	14.91	6,694	17.94
New England	973	11.40	222	17.49
Mid-Atlantic	2,851	11.20	351	14.58
East North Central	3,176	12.97	973	15.32
West North Central	1,158	15.10	873	16.47
South Atlantic	4,437	16.36	1,268	17.96
East South Central	1,060	16.17	822	16.78
West South Central	2,463	16.22	857	18.20
Mountain	1,850	23.59	818	26.94
Pacific	4,383	16.19	510	22.34

[a]People 20 years of age and older.
Source: Unpublished data from The National Center for Health Statistics, Vital Statistics System, and The Bureau of the Census.

portant indicator of alcohol and other substance abuse problems. Table 14.5 shows a considerably elevated rate of DUI arrests for rural counties in the United States compared with urban and suburban areas. Alcohol use is a factor in a substantial number of motor vehicle crashes. In 1994 alone, over 8,000 fatal motor vehicle crashes in rural areas could be attributed to alcohol use (Table 14.6).

Children and Adolescents

The federal Center for Mental Health Services classifies children and adolescents who have serious emotional disturbance as those under age 19 who have a disorder that meets diagnostic criteria specified in the DSM-III-R (*The Diagnostic and Statistical Manual of Mental Disorders*, Revised Third Edition) and that results in functional impairments that interfere with the child's roles in family, school, or community activities. Largely because of persistent measurement problems, no national epidemiological studies of serious emotional disturbance among children and adolescents have been conducted in the United States (Costello, 1989; Friedman et al., 1996). As a consequence, researchers and policy makers are dependent on regional studies, surveys, and proxy measures for prevalence information. This lack of data makes it difficult to compare rural, suburban, and urban populations of children and adolescents accurately. Most researchers are of the opinion that factors other than place of residence are more likely to predict mental health or substance abuse problems among children and adolescents (Oetting et al., 1997).

The 1995 National Household Survey on Drug Abuse included a series of questions intended to elicit information on the mental health status of adolescents aged 12 to 17. Findings from this survey suggest that adolescent males living in nonmetropolitan areas experience higher rates of delinquent and aggressive behavior than their urban and suburban counterparts (Table 14.7).

As is the case with adults, child and adolescent suicide is used as a proxy measure for mental health problems among this population. The rate of suicides among nonmetropolitan children and adolescents is indeed higher than the metropolitan rate (Table 14.8). This appears to be particularly the case in the New England, East North Central, Mountain, and Pacific census regions. Multiple years of data, which were not available for this report,

Table 14.4 Thirty-day Prevalence of Use of Alcohol and Other Drugs, Adults Aged 19–32, 1994

Population Density[a]	Approximate Weighted N	Percent of Population Using Each Substance				
		Alcohol	Cigarettes	Marijuana	Stimulants	Cocaine
Total	8,700	67.6	27.3	13.3	1.5	1.5
Farm / country	1,100	58.5	31.1	10.6	1.3	0.6
Small town	2,600	65.7	28.4	12.5	1.3	1.2
Medium city	1,900	68.9	26.5	14.2	1.8	1.9
Large city	1,800	71.6	26.2	13.6	1.8	1.6
Very Large city	1,200	72.4	24.3	15.7	1.5	1.9

[a]A small town is defined as having less than 50,000 inhabitants; a medium city has 50,000 to 100,000 people; a large city 100,000 to 500,000; and a very large city as having over 500,000 residents. Within each level of population density, suburban and urban respondents are combined.
Source: The University of Michigan Institute for Social Research, Monitoring the Future Study 1975–1994, Volume II, Table 5, pp. 72–73.

Table 14.5 Arrests for Driving Under the Influence by Urbanicity and Sex, 1995

Population Density	*Number of Arrests*	*Rate per 100,000*	*Percent Male*	*Percent Female*
Cities	618,759	465.47	84.9	15.1
Suburban areas	472,159	568.97	85.0	15.0
Rural counties	163,002	824.07	86.6	13.4

Source: U.S. Department of Justice, Federal Bureau of Investigation, *Crime in the United States, 1995*. Washington, DC: U.S. Government Printing Office, 1996, pp. 234, 252, 261.

would give a clearer picture of the stability of this trend. The Youth Risk Behavior Survey, conducted by state agencies with guidance from the federal Centers for Disease Control and Prevention, includes a number of questions related to suicide risk among adolescents. Selected findings from this survey indicate that although females appear to be generally at higher risk than males for committing suicide, there is no consistent pattern of difference between rural and urban youth on these measures (Table 14.9).

Prevalence of the use of alcohol and other substances among youth is also typically estimated from survey data. Not all of these surveys include information enabling analysis of urban-rural differences to be conducted. The Monitoring the Future Study found that the annual prevalence of substance use by nonmetro high school seniors was lower than or equal to that of metro high school seniors for all substances except stimulants other than cocaine, barbiturates, and steroids (Table 14.10). Nonmetro respondents to this survey also reported a slightly higher incidence of getting drunk. Table 14.11, based on the same survey but examining patterns of use over the most recent month, confirms that excessive alcohol use is a significant problem for nonmetro high school seniors, and it also points to problems with use of smokeless tobacco among rural youth.

Ethnic Minority Populations

Some rural ethnic minority populations may experience a higher than average prevalence of certain mental health and substance abuse problems. This may be due, in part, to the social and environmental stresses of poverty or cultural isolation (Neighbors et al., 1992; Rogler et al., 1991). In most instances, the data are inadequate to document the extent of these differences. In part this is because the prevalence data are often obtained from service utilization records. Although the reasons are not well documented, it is widely understood that ethnic minorities in the United States underutilize mental health services (Takeuchi and Uehara, 1996). This section briefly reviews available information on this subject. More research is clearly needed.

African Americans

Over half of the African Americans residing in the United States live in the South; many of these live in rural communities (Takeuchi and Uehara, 1996). Analyses of data from the Epidemiologic Catchment Area Study found that African Americans experienced higher 6-month prevalence rates for cognitive impairment, panic attacks, phobia, and drug abuse than whites or Hispanics (Griffith and Baker, 1992). The National Comorbidity Survey, on the other hand, found that African Americans experience lower rates of affective disorders, substance use disorders, and lifetime comorbidity than whites, even when income and education are controlled for (Kessler et al., 1994).

Most studies of psychological disorders in black adolescents have been conducted using urban samples (Gibbs, 1990). These suggest, for example, that black female adolescents who experienced stressful life events in the previous 12 months are more likely to suffer from depression, conduct disorder, post-traumatic stress disor-

Table 14.6 Fatal Motor Vehicle Crashes in which Alcohol was a Factor, by Type and Urbanicity, 1994

	Total Crashes		*Percent in Which Alcohol Was a Factor*	
Type of Crash	*Urban*	*Rural*	*Urban*	*Rural*
Single vehicle	4,589	10,024	51.4	50.7
Multiple vehicles	6,432	8,703	31.7	28.4
Nonoccupant fatality	4,378	1,877	43.7	46.5

Source: U.S. Department of Transportation, National Highway Traffic Safety Administration, Alcohol Involvement in Fatal Traffic Crashes, 1994. Table 14, p. 7.

Table 14.7 Adolescents Aged 12–17 Falling in Clinical Range on Achenbach Mental Health Scales, By Sex and Urbanicity, 1995

	Percent of Adolescents										
Sex and Urbanicity	*Total Problem Score*	*Emotional Composite Score*[a]	*Behavioral Composite Score*[b]	*Withdrawn*	*Somatic Complaint*	*Anxious/ Depressed*	*Social Problem*	*Thought Problem*	*Attention Problem*	*Delinquent Behavior*	*Aggressive Behavior*
MALE											
Large metro	17.3	13.0	15.7	3.2	6.7	4.2	4.4	6.4	3.5	9.2	6.6
Small metro	16.9	13.8	14.7	4.5	9.0	5.2	5.2	7.4	5.8	9.5	6.2
Nonmetro	15.7	10.8	18.1	2.8	8.1	3.9	4.9	5.0	4.8	10.7	7.4
FEMALE											
Large metro	17.5	11.7	20.9	3.4	7.0	4.8	5.2	9.3	6.0	13.4	8.1
Small metro	21.1	14.2	22.4	1.9	7.1	5.3	6.7	9.2	7.4	10.4	7.5
Nonmetro	18.6	11.6	18.6	1.8	7.7	3.1	5.0	9.0	6.8	12.0	7.3

Source: Substance Abuse and Mental Health Services Administration, National Household Survey on Drug Abuse, Main Findings, 1995, Table 12.1, p.156; Table 12.2, p.157.
[a]Emotional Problems refers to Achenbach's Internalizing Score, which sums up the scores on three syndrome scales: Withdrawn, Somatic Complaints, and Anxious/Depressed.
[b]Behavioral Problems refers to Achenbach's Externalizing Score, which sums up the scores on two syndrome scales: Deliquent Behavior and Aggressive Behavior.

der, and somatic complaints; black male adolescents are more likely than whites to exhibit aggression and other forms of conduct disorder (Hoberman, 1992). Studies of racially mixed groups of adolescents typically find that these differences in symptoms are not significant when controls are placed on the age, socioeconomic status, and sex of the study participants (Gibbs, 1990).

Hispanics

Hispanic populations reside in rural areas throughout the American West and Southwest, with the greatest concentrations in California and Texas (Takeuchi and Uehara, 1996). Those who make their living as migrant farm workers travel to other parts of the country as crops are ready for harvesting. Hispanic Americans appear to use mental health services at rates lower than the general population (Schreiber and Homiak, 1981). Yet a study of predominantly Hispanic children of migrant and seasonal farm workers in North Carolina found that about 15% of them evidenced diagnosable symptoms of emotional or behavioral problems (Martin and Kupersmidt, 1992). Findings from the National Comorbidity Survey indicate that Hispanics experience higher prevalence of affective disorders and active comorbidity than non-Hispanic whites but show no difference in rates of anxiety disorders (Kessler et al., 1994). Other studies have found Hispanic youth to be more prone to depression and suicidal behavior than their black or Anglo counterparts (Hoberman, 1992). Qualitative research done among Mexican-American migrant workers in Florida found that instruments typically used to measure presence of mental illness in this population may yield inaccurate findings due to cultural differences in the way physical and mental disorders are perceived and described (Baer, 1996).

Table 14.8 Child and Adolescent[a] Suicide Deaths by Region and Urbanicity, 1995

	Metro		*Nonmetro*	
Region	*Number*	*Rate per 100,000*	*Number*	*Rate per 100,000*
United States	1621	5.60	599	7.45
New England	65	4.50	15	8.00
Mid-Atlantic	178	3.97	26	5.40
East North Central	234	4.76	111	8.23
West North Central	115	7.22	87	7.43
South Atlantic	265	5.50	91	6.41
East South Central	90	7.01	70	6.55
West South Central	241	7.05	75	7.10
Mountain	146	8.80	91	11.76
Pacific	287	5.38	33	6.89

[a]People 10 to 19 years of age.
Source: Unpublished data from The National Center for Health Statistics, Vital Statistics System, and The Bureau of the Census.

Heavy alcohol consumption is common among some rural adult Hispanic males, for whom it appears to be a cultural norm and a test of manhood (Castro and Gutierres, 1997). This practice appears to be particularly the case among migrant workers who travel without their families (Trotter, 1985—cited in Castro and Gutierres, 1997). Members of intact Hispanic families that observe Catholic traditions and practices may be at less risk for using alcohol and other drugs (Oetting, 1992). Conversely, Hispanics who are more highly acculturated into

Table 14.9 High School Students Who Reported Serious Suicidal Thoughts and/or Behaviors, 1995 (percent of respondents)

	Thought Seriously about Attempting Suicide			*Made a Suicide Plan*			*Attempted Suicide*			*Suicide Attempt Required Medical Attention*		
	Female	*Male*	*Total*	*Female*	*Male*	*Total*	*Female*	*Male*	*Total*	*Female*	*Male*	*Total*
MOST RURAL STATESa												
Alabama	25.2	16.0	20.8	19.3	13.7	16.6	10.0	6.0	8.1	2.6	2.9	2.8
Alaska	32.3	16.2	23.9	24.9	13.1	18.7	13.8	5.3	9.4	4.4	1.3	2.9
Arkansas	30.4	17.8	24.0	23.1	12.8	17.8	13.0	4.6	8.8	3.9	1.5	2.7
Maine	30.4	20.0	25.1	21.2	15.8	18.5	9.8	6.1	8.0	3.2	2.2	2.7
Mississippi	30.3	18.1	24.2	22.1	10.2	16.1	13.5	4.2	8.9	2.9	1.7	2.3
Montana	26.5	17.5	21.8	22.4	16.2	19.2	10.7	6.3	8.5	3.7	1.9	2.8
North Carolina	24.2	15.3	19.8	17.4	11.6	14.5	11.6	5.3	8.5	4.1	2.8	3.5
North Dakota	30.3	20.3	25.4	23.1	16.5	19.9	9.0	5.5	7.5	3.4	1.6	2.6
South Dakota	30.7	20.7	25.7	21.4	18.4	19.9	11.1	8.2	9.6	2.1	3.1	2.6
Vermont	33.4	23.0	28.2	25.6	18.5	22.0	12.3	8.2	10.3	3.9	3.8	4.0
West Virginia	30.4	20.9	25.6	22.6	18.3	20.5	12.2	7.6	9.9	3.2	3.4	3.4
Wyoming	30.0	17.5	23.6	21.6	13.4	17.4	10.7	6.0	8.3	3.0	2.1	2.6
SELECTED CITIES												
Boston	26.4	16.1	21.2	19.4	12.9	16.2	16.0	9.4	12.9	3.9	5.2	4.6
Chicago	23.7	12.3	18.2	19.6	9.7	14.8	15.1	11.0	13.2	4.8	5.2	5.0
Dallas	25.5	13.3	19.6	18.7	10.1	14.5	12.7	4.8	8.9	4.4	1.7	3.1
Denver	26.3	11.1	18.9	19.1	10.5	15.0	12.1	5.1	8.9	4.6	1.3	3.2
Miami	25.5	16.5	20.8	17.5	12.1	14.9	11.9	7.2	9.7	2.1	2.9	2.5
San Diego	32.1	20.7	26.7	24.5	16.4	20.7	13.7	6.1	10.0	3.9	1.6	2.8
Seattle	21.3	15.8	18.6	17.8	16.0	16.9	11.3	7.6	9.6	4.1	3.5	3.8

[a]Selected from among participating states.
Source: Centers for Disease Control and Prevention, Youth Risk Behavior Survey, 1995.

Table 14.10 Annual Prevalence of Substance Use by High School Seniors by Urbanicity, 1993 (percentage of respondants)

	Percent by Residential Status (Total n = 16,300)		
Type of Substance	*Large MSA (n = 3,700)*	*Other MSA*[a] *(n = 7,800)*	*Non-MSA (n = 4,800)*
Marijuana	29.1	26.2	23.1
Inhalants[b]	7.4	7.3	6.0
Hallucinogens	7.3	8.1	6.3
LSD	6.7	7.6	5.6
Cocaine	2.7	3.9	2.7
Crack	1.3	1.8	1.4
Other cocaine[c]	2.6	3.6	2.0
Heroin	0.6	0.5	0.5
Other opiates	3.1	3.7	3.7
Stimulants	6.5	8.5	9.8
Barbiturates	2.6	3.1	4.3
Tranquilizers	2.9	3.6	3.7
Alcohol[d]	77.9	75.2	76.0
Been drunk[e]	49.1	49.1	51.0
Steroids	0.7	0.9	2.2

[a]County or group of adjacent counties with at least one city or two adjoining cities with a population of 50,000 or more.
[b]Question included on five of six questionnaire forms; n is five sixths of total.
[c]Question included on four of six questionnaire forms; n is two thirds of total.
[d]Question included on three of six questionnaire forms; n is one half of total.
[e]Question included on two questionnaire forms; n is one third of total.
Source: Johnston et al. 1994. *Monitoring the Future Study*, Vol. I: Table 7, pp. 56–58.

Anglo society appear to experience higher rates of alcohol and drug dependence (Martinez, 1992).

Native Americans

Rural Native Americans typically live on or near reservations composed of individuals sharing a common tribal heritage. They may periodically move back and forth between these homelands and nearby cities where they go to seek employment and perhaps anonymity (Takeuchi and Uehara, 1996). Most of the data on prevalence of mental health and substance abuse problems among Native Americans is based on Indian Health Service utilization records, which show considerable intertribal variation in prevalence (Thompson et al., 1992). In general, most knowledgeable observers believe that American Indians suffer from the same mental health and substance abuse problems that afflict any population living in poverty. Alcoholism remains a chronic and widespread problem among most Native American populations, with beer being the preferred substance (Cole et al., 1992). The degree of illegal drug use seems to vary among tribal groups. In general, Native Americans adolescents appear to drink more heavily and use marijuana and readily obtainable inhalants such as gas, spray paint, and glue at higher rates than other American teens (Donnermeyer, 1992; Stubben, 1997). They also appear to be more likely to commit suicide (Hoberman, 1992).

Table 14.11 Thirty-day Prevalence of Daily Substance Use by High School Seniors by Urbanicity, 1993 (percent of respondents)

Type of Substance	*Large MSA (n = 3,700)*	*Other MSA*[a] *(n = 7,800)*	*Non-MSA (n = 4,800)*
Marijuana	2.5	2.4	2.3
Alcohol[b]	2.7	2.3	2.5
Five or more drinks in a row	27.6	26.5	29.2
Cigarettes (1 or more daily)	17.3	19.7	19.2
Cigarettes (10 or more daily)	9.1	11.2	11.7
Smokeless tobacco[c]	1.7	3.0	5.2

[a]County or group of adjacent counties with at least one city or two adjoining cities with a population of 50,000 or more.
[b]Question included on three of six questionnaires; n is one half of total.
[c]Question included on one of six questionnaires; n is one sixth of total.
Source: Johnston et al. 1994. *Monitoring the Future Study*, Vol. I: Table 9, p. 62.

Comorbidities

Comorbidity refers to three distinct sets of conditions that may occur in the same individual: the presence of more than one mental disorder; mental illness combined with alcohol or other substance abuse; and mental illness combined with physical illness. These are not specifically rural problems and at the present time only limited national data are available to document their extent in rural areas. However, their presence implies the need for integrated service delivery systems if rural communities are to support individuals with these conditions.

Early analyses of the National Comorbidity Survey data found that over three fourths of the lifetime psychiatric disorders identified in the study population were comorbid (Kessler et al., 1994). Fourteen percent (14%) of respondents to this survey had experienced three or more lifetime psychiatric disorders. Kessler and colleagues also showed that rural rates for comorbidity were lower than that for urban residents.

Abuse of alcohol and other drugs is another significant problem among persons with serious and persistent mental illness. People with this type of comorbidity are often called mentally ill substance abusers (MISAs) or dually diagnosed. A survey of clients using 10 rural community mental health centers in Wisconsin found that nearly one quarter had experienced problems with alcohol or other drugs in the past, and one fifth had current substance abuse problems (Barry et al., 1996). Another study of persons with mental illness conducted in two small Wisconsin cities and their surrounding rural areas found that 39.5% of those studied met diagnostic criteria for alcohol abuse (Greenley et al., 1992). An analysis of Massachusetts Medicaid claims for people with diagnosed mental illness found that those with comorbid substance abuse problems had psychiatric treatment costs nearly 60% higher than those without substance abuse problems (Dickey and Azeni, 1996). Most of this observed difference in cost was the result of the higher use of acute inpatient care by the mentally ill substance abusers.

People with psychiatric disorders also seem to experience higher rates of mortality from all causes and suffer disproportionately from a variety of serious illnesses (Goplerud, 1981). Frequently, they have physical symptoms related to their mental illnesses (a phenomenon known as *somatization*) and use medical care services at a higher rate than those without psychiatric disorders (Katon et al., 1990). Their physical symptoms often mask their underlying psychological distress and may make it more difficult for primary care physicians to diagnose and treat them correctly (Schulberg, 1991).

THE MENTAL HEALTH SERVICES INFRASTRUCTURE

As noted in the introduction to this chapter, most rural areas of the United States have fewer mental health services than the national average (Human and Wasem, 1991). As of 1990, only 79.5% of nonmetro counties in the United States had any mental health services, leaving the other 20.5% with no mental health services of any kind (Table 14.12). The average *number* of specialty mental health organizations in nonmetro counties is also substantially lower than the average number in metro counties. In general, we associate lower *availability* of services with lower *access* to services. For example, a study conducted in Maine found that *supply* of mental health professionals explained much of the observed difference in access to and use of mental health services (Lambert and Agger, 1995). Data in this section show consistently lower availability of hospital-based inpatient and outpatient services, both psychiatric and substance abuse, in rural areas.

Inpatient Services

Historically, most mental health inpatient care, whether acute or long term, was provided by state psychiatric hospitals. Since the 1960s, as these hospitals have been closed or downsized, responsibility for the care of those with serious and persistent mental illness has shifted to communities (Bachrach, 1977; Grob, 1992; Rochefort, 1984). On the outpatient side, this task has largely fallen to community mental health centers. However, both acute and longer term inpatient care is still needed. These services are typically provided by private psychiatric hospitals or by general community hospitals with inpatient psychiatric units (Redick et al., 1996). As a measure of the geographic availability of such care, Table 14.13 presents the 1995 rate of inpatient psychiatric beds per 100,000 population for metro and nonmetro areas by census region. The rate is consistently and—in the Mid-Atlantic, East South Central, and Pacific regions—dramatically lower for nonmetro than for metro areas. This suggests that people with acute mental illness residing in rural communities may travel to urban areas to receive inpatient care or may not receive such care in a timely manner.

Table 14.12 Mental Health Services and Organizations by County and Urbanicity, 1983 and 1990

	1983		*1990*	
	Metro (n = 735)	*Nonmetro (n = 2,402)*	*Metro (n = 735)*	*Nonmetro (n = 2,402)*
Percent of Counties with any mental health services	95.1%	78.4%	95.7%	79.5%
Average number of specialty mental health organizations	10.0	1.5	13.3	1.9

Source: *Mental Health, United States, 1996*. Table 9.1, p. 229; Table 9.2, p. 230.

Table 14.13 Inpatient Psychiatric Beds[a] by Region and Urbanicity, 1995

Region	Metro		Nonmetro	
	Number of beds	Rate per 100,000	Number of beds	Rate per 100,000
United States	104,630	49.2	19,040	36.2
New England	5,106	42.3	409	32.2
Mid-Atlantic	24,595	70.5	1,624	48.4
East North Central	16,639	48.1	3,236	35.9
West North Central	6,982	63.8	4,380	58.2
South Atlantic	18,364	48.7	3,655	36.8
East South Central	6,406	68.6	1,739	25.4
West South Central	11,170	49.5	2,600	38.7
Mountain	3,545	30.1	1,099	25.3
Pacific	11,823	30.5	298	8.2

Source: American Hospital Association Annual Survey of Hospitals.
[a]Including state and county mental hospitals, private psychiatric hospitals, VA medical centers, and nonfederal general hospitals with psychiatric services.
Note: Data are missing for 17% of hospitals.

Inpatient care is also used to provide detoxification and other intensive treatment to persons with alcohol and other chemical dependency problems. Table 14.14 shows the 1995 rate of alcohol and other drug abuse treatment beds per 100,000 population for metro and nonmetro areas by census region. In this case, the pattern is different, with approximate parity between metro and nonmetro areas nationally and in the Pacific region, coupled with regional variations that include higher rates in some nonmetro areas (specifically West North Central and Mountain) and lower rates in the rest.

Table 14.14 Alcohol and Other Drug Abuse Treatment Beds per 100,000 Population. Metro and Nonmetro, 1995

Region	Metro		Nonmetro	
	Number of beds	Rate per 100,000	Number of beds	Rate per 100,000
United States	16,050	7.5	3,909	7.4
New England	714	5.9	68	5.4
Mid-Atlantic	3,184	9.1	156	4.6
East North Central	2,863	8.3	671	7.5
West North Central	1,098	10.0	1,013	13.5
South Atlantic	2,935	7.8	699	7.0
East South Central	1,383	14.8	445	6.5
West South Central	1,959	8.7	392	5.8
Mountain	669	5.7	345	7.9
Pacific	1,245	3.2	120	3.3

Source: American Hospital Association Annual Survey of Hospitals.
Note: Data are missing for 17% of hospitals.

Outpatient Services

From 1969 to 1992, the number of patient visits to outpatient psychiatric facilities and programs more than doubled (Redick et al., 1996). A substantial part of this increase took place during the 1970s, when federally funded community mental health centers were in their initial growth phase and the deinstitutionalization movement was accelerating. Managed care is now starting to exercise an influence on the shift from inpatient to outpatient care as well (Meyer and Sotsky, 1995). Outpatient mental health services remain less accessible in most rural communities than they are in urban locations. For example, as of 1995, hospital-based outpatient psychiatric care was offered by 13.3% of nonmetro hospitals compared to 33.4% of metro hospitals (Table 14.15). This metro/nonmetro difference is most pronounced in the East North Central states, as well as the two South Central regions. Similarly, less than 11% of nonmetro hospitals offer outpatient alcohol and other drug abuse treatment services, compared with 26.5% of metro hospitals (Table 14.16).

Mental Health Professionals

The mental health professions encompass several disciplines, including psychiatry, psychology, social work, marriage and family therapy, counseling, and psychiatric nursing. Professionals in these disciplines typically have a formal advanced degree and are licensed by their respective state boards. In most states, psychiatrists are the only mental health professionals licensed to write prescriptions, although many states now extend prescribing privileges to psychiatric nurse practitioners. Many other mental health treatments—such as counseling or group therapy—can be provided by various other mental health professional (Edmunds et al., 1997). Substance abuse treatment services are typically provided by licensed substance abuse counselors. Some of the mental health professions also provide training and credentialing to enable their members to receive reimbursement for providing substance abuse treatment. In some settings, laypeople without professional training or paraprofessionals with associate's degrees may provide mental health or substance abuse treatment services under the supervision of a professional (Ivey et al., 1998). This becomes an especially important option in rural communities, which may lack specialty mental health professionals, or among cultural groups that may resist receiving care from a professional from outside the community (Bierman et al., 1997). Rural ethnic minorities, in particular, are more likely to seek needed mental health or substance abuse

Table 14.15 Hospital-Based[a] Outpatient Psychiatric Services by Region and Urbanicity, 1995

	Metro (n = 3997)		*Nonmetro (n = 2451)*	
Region	*Percent of Hospitals*	*Percent No Response*	*Percent of Hospitals*	*Percent No Response*
United States	33.4	19.0	13.3	12.7
New England	42.5	19.7	32.8	6.9
Mid-Atlantic	34.3	19.5	18.9	12.2
East North Central	43.2	13.1	16.0	8.6
West North Central	42.5	8.9	36.4	7.4
South Atlantic	31.9	21.6	15.4	15.4
East South Central	32.2	17.2	8.1	17.3
West South Central	25.3	14.3	6.4	11.2
Mountain	39.5	22.8	15.1	15.9
Pacific	22.3	29.4	7.1	26.9

Source: American Hospital Association Annual Survey of Hospitals.
[a]Including state and county mental hospitals, private psychiatric hospitals, VA medical centers, and nonfederal general hospitals with psychiatric services.

treatment for themselves or their children if the service providers are from the same ethnic group and speak the same language (Snowden and Hu, 1996).

Historical shortages of specialty mental health professionals in most rural areas of the United States persist even today (Keller et al., 1980; Knesper et al., 1984; Murray and Keller, 1991; Stuve, Beeson, and Hartig, 1989). As of December 31, 1997, 76% of the 518 designated Mental Health Professions Shortage Areas in the United States were located in nonmetropolitan areas with a total population of over 30 million. Table 14.17 summarizes the rate of mental health professionals per 100,000 population for each of the five core mental health professions. Because data were not available by county, urban-rural comparisons could not be provided. Instead, data are presented from the most rural states, with U.S. totals shown at the top for comparison. Here a relatively consistent pattern of lower supply of mental health professionals in states with large rural populations is visible. This table understates the urban-rural differences: the urban areas in these rural states typically have higher ratios of providers to population than the

Table 14.16 Hospital-based[a] Outpatient Alcohol and Other Drug Abuse Treatment Services by Region and Urbanicity, 1995

	Metro (n = 3997)		*Nonmetro (n = 2451)*	
Region	*Percent of Hospitals*	*Percent No Response*	*Percent of Hospitals*	*Percent No Response*
United States	26.5	19.0	10.7	12.7
New England	32.7	19.7	31.0	6.9
Mid-Atlantic	27.7	19.5	16.7	12.2
East N. Central	35.2	13.1	16.0	8.6
West N. Central	35.6	8.9	11.3	7.4
South Atlantic	24.9	21.6	10.2	15.4
East South Central	26.8	17.2	9.5	17.3
West South Central	19.0	14.3	4.3	11.2
Mountain	28.8	22.8	9.2	15.9
Pacific	17.6	29.4	7.7	26.9

[a]Including state and county mental hospitals, private psychiatric hospitals, VA medical centers, and nonfederal general hospitals with psychiatric services.
Source: American Hospital Association Annual Survey of Hospitals.

Table 14.17 Clinically Active[a] or Clinically Trained Mental Health Personnel per 100,000 Persons, Most Rural States, 1995–1996

	Psychiatry 1996	*Psychology 1995*	*Social Work 1996*	*Psychiatric Nursing 1995*	*Marriage and Family Therapy 1995*
Arkansas	6.6	13.6	18.2	0.5	2.8
Alabama	5.9	7.3	14.0	1.3	3.2
Alaska	10.0	15.3	98.8	5.5	11.8
Idaho	5.6	9.8	20.7	0.8	3.8
Iowa	5.2	19.2	26.1	1.3	5.5
Kansas	9.9	13.3	35.4	1.8	12.1
Kentucky	7.6	9.8	19.8	1.7	6.7
Maine	11.6	25.2	58.4	6.0	5.3
Mississippi	4.6	5.2	11.3	0.7	3.2
Montana	7.1	17.2	25.6	2.0	3.4
Nebraska	7.5	13.9	22.2	2.0	4.2
New Mexico	11.0	15.8	29.8	3.7	6.1
North Carolina	9.0	13.7	24.7	1.6	6.6
North Dakota	8.4	12.6	14.2	2.7	2.5
Oklahoma	6.1	10.1	20.2	0.8	22.4
South Dakota	7.3	15.1	17.4	1.0	4.5
Vermont	19.6	55.6	50.3	7.9	5.6
West Virginia	7.0	17.3	16.1	1.8	1.3
Wisconsin	8.7	14.8	30.8	0.9	8.4
Wyoming	5.6	16.3	20.4	1.9	7.1
United States	11.3	20.2	35.9	2.6	17.6

[a]For Psychiatry and Marriage and Family Therapy, we report clinically active professionals; for others we report clinically trained professionals because data are more accurate.

Source: Substance Abuse and Mental Health Services Administration, *Mental Health United States, 1996*, Table 10.3, pp. 195–198.

Table 14.18 Distribution of Psychiatrists Engaged in Patient Care by Region, Urbanicity, and Practice Location

	Metro			*Nonmetro*		
Region	*Number*	*Rate per 100,000*	*Percent Office-Based*	*Number*	*Rate per 100,000*	*Percent Office-Based*
United States	30,977	14.6	78.7	2,046	3.9	72.3
New England	2,950	24.4	78.7	183	14.4	77.6
Mid-Atlantic	7,352	21.1	72.4	202	6.0	64.9
East North Central	3,923	11.3	80.3	293	3.3	72.7
West North Central	1,374	12.6	79.6	250	3.3	64.4
South Atlantic	5,209	13.8	78.2	430	4.3	69.1
East South Central	1,043	11.2	77.9	163	2.4	79.8
West South Central	2,250	10.0	83.2	130	1.9	70.0
Mountain	1,349	11.5	82.7	189	4.4	78.3
Pacific	5,527	14.3	83.6	206	5.6	81.1

Source: American Medical Association Physician Masterfile, 1996.

state as a whole, as evidenced by Table 14.18, which presents these ratios for psychiatrists. This table also demonstrates that psychiatrists in rural areas are less likely to be office-based and thus more likely to be based in hospitals. Thus the availability of these specialty mental health professionals in rural areas is in part dependent on the presence of rural hospitals (Human and Wasem, 1991).

Rural mental health professionals may require special training above and beyond that appropriate to their disciplines if they are to be successful at their work (Beeson, 1991). Such training should emphasize the realities of the rural *environment,* such as physical distance, cultural factors, and resource limitations and of the rural practice—for example, the need to establish a relationship with the whole community, to assume the role of a generalist, to accept the lack of anonymity and the accompanying ethical dilemmas, and to cope with professional isolation and the potential for burnout (Beeson 1991; Sawyer and Beeson 1998). Training programs that place the student into rural settings appear to hold the most promise in this regard (Wagenfeld et al., 1993). Another strategy, most recently recommended by the Ad Hoc Rural Mental Health Provider Work Group sponsored by the federal Center for Mental Health Services, involves an increased use of interdisciplinary training (Pion, Keller, and McCombs 1997).

Child and Adolescent Mental Health Services

The Great Smoky Mountains Study of Youth (GSMS) funded by the National Institute of Mental Health found that children with diagnosed mental health problems receive related services in a variety of settings, including not only the mental health and general health care systems but also schools, child welfare agencies, and the juvenile justice system (Burns et al., 1995). Guidance counselors and psychologists working within school systems were most likely to serve children with mental health problems. A comparison of the rural and urban areas included in the study indicates that youths in urban areas were significantly more likely to use some type of service to address an emotional, behavioral, or substance use problem than youths in rural areas (Table 14.19). However, rural and urban youths participating in the study were also somewhat different demographically (Table 14.20). There were more African-American youths in the urban areas, and urban youths were more likely to be living in poverty. Urban youths also showed a somewhat higher prevalence of psychiatric diagnoses.

Comorbidity may affect overall service use among children and adolescents. A survey of high school students in one rural Arkansas county found that those experiencing symptoms of depression and/or problem drinking were also more likely to use hospital emergency departments and public health or school-based clinics for medical problems than their peers who did not report such problems (Rickert et al., 1996).

Table 14.19 Rural and Urban Youth Who Received Mental Health Services

Service Sector	*Percent Rural*	*Percent Urban*
Specialty mental health	13.0	16.8
General medicine	22.7	25.5
Education	8.6	11.3
Child welfare	2.7	5.0
Juvenile justice ($p < .01$)	2.3	6.1
Use of any sector ($p < .01$)	30.1	38.6

Source: Unpublished data from Great Smoky Mountains Study of Youth, 1995.

Rural communities present particular challenges to the implementation of prevention and treatment programs related to child and adolescent mental health and substance abuse (Bierman, 1997). They are often geographically large regions with widely dispersed populations, lacking in public transportation apart from that provided by the school systems. Such communities are typically tight-knit in terms of interpersonal relationships and are not always willing to trust the interventions of outside experts. Rural families are especially wary of services that might set their children apart from others or identify them as deficient in some way.

Mental Health Services in the Primary Care Sector

An estimated two thirds of U.S. patients with clinical symptoms of mental illness receive no care at all for such symptoms. Of those who do receive formal treatment, approximately 40% receive care from a mental health specialist and 45% from a general medical practitioner (Regier, 1993). Because of the documented lack of spe-

Table 14.20 Demographic and Clinical Characteristics of Rural and Urban Youth

	Percent Rural	*Percent Urban*
Sex (male)	52.4	49.0
Race (African American) ($p > .01$)	2.3	16.5
Poverty ($p < .05$)	24.8	31.5
DSM-III (R) Diagnosis	20.8	25.1

Source: Unpublished data from Great Smoky Mountains Study of Youth, 1995.

cialty mental health services, primary care practitioners (PCPs) probably provide an even more significant portion of mental health care in rural America. In fact, rural residents under continuing treatment for mental health conditions have been found significantly more likely to receive this care exclusively from a general medical practitioner (Rost et al., 1998).

The debate over the appropriateness and effectiveness of having primary care practitioners (PCP) provide basic mental health care has raged for years and covered a number of issues without fully resolving any of them. PCPs have long been criticized for underrecognition of mental health problems (Eisenberg, 1992; Gonzales et al., 1994). Rost and colleagues (1995), for example, found that rural family practice physicians were about half as likely as their urban counterparts to detect depression in patients. Others argue that PCPs may choose not to enter a psychiatric diagnosis into the medical record, because of the increased stigma rural residents associate with mental illness (Hoyt et al., 1997; Susman, 1995). PCPs with appropriate training and interest in mental health problems such as depression appear to be willing to assume responsibility for treating those problems in their patients (Hartley et al., 1998; Main et al., 1993). Rost and colleagues (1995) noted that rural PCPs were likely to prescribe medications at levels below those recommended by the AHCPR Guidelines (1993); on the other hand, research conducted by Olfson and colleagues (1995) suggests that PCPs in general engage in informal psychological interventions with patients considerably more often than is typically assumed.

Concerns about the quality and effectiveness of mental health care provided by PCPs have led some to conclude that mental health treatment should be provided by specialty mental health professionals, despite the fact that many areas have an undersupply of such professionals (Mechanic, 1990). In 1997, Montana's new Medicaid managed behavioral health plan required that all services be provided by licensed mental health and substance abuse treatment professionals. The plan's failure to accept PCPs as legitimate providers of mental health services meant that Medicaid patients in 24 rural counties had no local mental health services at all (Lambert et al., 1998).

Crisis Services

A lack of services or professionals in the immediate area does not always mean a complete lack of access. Rural residents are often willing to drive to urban areas for some services. On the other hand, when a psychiatric or substance abuse crisis occurs, local services are essential to prevent escalation of the problem to a level that requires more intensive care (Wilson et al., 1995). Unfortunately, the lack of professionals often means that rural hospitals cannot provide crisis services. Table 14.21 shows the percent of hospitals providing emergency psychiatric services in 1995. Among nonmetro hospitals nationwide, 18.6% offer such services, compared with 37.4% of metro hospitals. Some areas of the country are more severely underserved than others, with the South

Table 14.21 Hospital-Based[a] Emergency Psychiatric Services by Region and Urbanicity, 1995

	Metro (n = 3997)		*Nonmetro (n = 2451)*	
Region	*Percent of Hospitals Reporting Service*	*Percent No Response*	*Percent of Hospitals Reporting Service*	*Percent No Response*
United States	37.4	19.0	18.6	12.7
New England	44.5	19.7	41.4	6.9
Mid-Atlantic	40.8	19.5	35.6	12.2
East North Central	47.4	13.2	23.1	8.6
West North Central	49.0	8.9	18.1	7.4
South Atlantic	34.3	21.6	21.5	15.4
East South Central	39.3	17.2	11.3	17.3
West South Central	30.5	14.3	10.1	11.2
Mountain	38.1	22.8	17.1	15.9
Pacific	24.2	29.4	21.8	26.9

[a]Including state and county mental hospitals, private psychiatric hospitals, VA medical centers, and nonfederal general hospitals with psychiatric services.
Source: American Hospital Association Annual Survey of Hospitals.

Self-Help In Rural Areas: Reducing the Use of Crisis and Hospitalization Services

RUTH RALPH, Ph.D.

Evolution of Self-Help Groups

The movement toward consumer/survivor-run services began in the early 1970s, when groups of consumers began to share their experiences with the mental health system, particularly psychiatric hospitals. Some of these groups developed a patients' bill of rights that they then used to advocate for system change. Other groups developed consumer-run services as alternatives to those provided in the mental health system (Chamberlin, 1978). Over time, consumers were able to advocate with the mental health system for opportunities to participate as equals in the planning process and to provide alternative services. This success began to have an impact at the policy level. Recipient involvement in mental health services has been mandated by federal law since 1986 (Public Law 99-660) and actively promoted by projects at the state and federal levels (Parrish, 1989; NIMH, 1991). However, consumer involvement was often limited, and resistance to the belief that consumers could make decisions about their lives and service needs persisted (Ridgeway, 1988).

Who Participates in Self-Help Groups?

Studies in a variety of settings show the diversity of the people who use self-help. A study of participants in four self-help agencies in San Francisco found that nearly half (46%) of the respondents were currently homeless, another 13% were at risk for being homeless, and three out of four (78%) had been homeless at least once in the past 5 years (Segal, Silverman, and Tempkin 1995). The majority of respondents were male (72%), African American (64%), and had co-occurring conditions such as substance abuse or physical health problems. Their average age was 38. Another study of six self-help organizations across the United States yielded a somewhat different profile (Chamberlin, Rogers, and Ellison, 1995). The majority of participants were also male (60%) and the average age was 40. In contrast to the San Francisco study, over half the respondents (56%) were white and only 15% were homeless. Nearly 15% were married, and more than half (53%) reported they had children. Nearly half (48%) lived in private homes or apartments.

In a cross-sectional study in New York State, Carpinello and colleagues (1995) compared participants and nonparticipants of mental health self-help groups. Participants were slightly older and were more likely to be white, to be married, and to have higher levels of education than nonparticipants. Participants were also more likely than nonparticipants to be living in a private residence than in a community group setting or in public housing. Participants were less likely to have been hospitalized in the past 5 years for mental health problems and had higher confi-

Central states again showing the lowest rates in rural areas, and the greatest urban-rural differentials.

Changes in the Mental Health Delivery System

As mentioned elsewhere in this chapter, one of the major trends that has shaped the mental health services delivery system over the past 40 years is the *deinstitutionalization* of persons with severe and/or chronic mental illness who previously had been clients of state institutions. Many were hospitalized in urban areas and when deinstitutionalized remained there. Others migrated to urban areas where community-based services are logistically easier to provide. Another effect of this trend has been to focus the efforts of *community mental health centers* and state offices of mental health on the needs of the deinstitutionalized population. This population, usually referred to as the "seriously and persistently mentally ill," is the principal group for which categorical funding has been provided to these publicly funded agencies. Figure 14.1 shows sources of funding for state mental health authorities. Two-thirds of these funds come from state sources, but the ability of states to target these funds to community-based services is compromised by the high cost of inpatient care. Figure 14.2 shows the distribution of state mental health authority dollars by type of service, with a majority of this funding continuing to be spent on inpatient care, despite declining numbers of hospitalized patients.

dence in their ability to advocate for themselves and for others.

Effectiveness of Self-Help Groups

There is little empirical evidence on the effectiveness of self-help groups (Segal, Silverman, and Temkin, 1995; Blanch, 1994). A survey of mental health self-help group leaders in New York State suggests areas of outcome that should be studied further (Carpinello and Knight, 1993). Group leaders reported that participants had greater self-esteem, more hopefulness about the future, and a greater sense of well-being as a result of participating in the groups. The vast majority of group leaders reported that as a result of being in the group, participants got along better with others, assumed more responsibility, were more connected to peers, were more assertive, lived more independently, and were more empowered to make their own decisions. A number of other positive effects were reported as well, including improved listening skills, better speaking skills before a group, and better problem solving. Participants were also reported to be better able to hold a job and to be able to stay out of the hospital longer.

Special Concerns for Rural Self-Help Groups

In addition to the lack of services, rural residents often experience other barriers to the use of mental health services, including lack of adequate health insurance coverage; concerns about their reputation; lack of knowledge about service availability and effectiveness; and the belief that one must bear one's own problems. Of particular concern is confidentiality. In response to this, many rural people take their need for privacy and independence to the extreme point of isolating themselves even when their needs are great (Ziegler, 1995).

Interviews with rural mental health consumers reveal that some managed care organizations (MCOs) recognize the value of self-help and consumer involvement in reducing the use of crisis services and hospitalization, and thus reducing the costs of mental health services (Ralph, 1998). These MCOs have hired some consumers and appointed other consumers and family members to advisory and quality improvement committees. The consumers interviews also indicated that transportation is probably the greatest barrier to the development, implementation, and continuance of self-help groups. When transportation is provided, consumers in rural areas consistently attend self-help activities. In Tennessee, MCOs are trying a rotating self-help group, where consumers meet at different locations, with the people who live in that location acting as hosts. MCOs also are providing van transportation for groups from other areas.

In Kansas, the Self-Help Network at Wichita State University assists in developing self-help groups in rural areas for both physical and mental health problems (Ziegler, 1995). Little is currently known about the presence or activities of such groups in other states, what their successes and difficulties have been, and whether they have found that self-help does, indeed, reduce the use of crisis services, psychiatric hospitalization, or other mental health services. It is also not currently known how other managed care organizations or state offices of mental health view the value of self-help groups.

State Medicaid agencies have emerged as the other major state-level player in the changing structure of the mental health services system. While state mental health offices devote their limited resources to planning, operating, and/or regulating programs and services for seriously and persistently mentally ill adults and seriously emotionally disturbed children, the state Medicaid agency pays for most of these programs and services. As states have moved their Medicaid populations into managed care programs, they have often "carved out" the mental health benefits and transferred the management of those benefits to specialty firms known as *managed behavioral health organizations* (MBHOs). One effect of this trend on rural areas has already been noted: when MBHOs develop provider panels, they sometimes overlook the role of PCPs who provide mental health services in rural areas. This phenomenon caused serious access problems in Montana in 1997 (Lambert et al., 1998).

Some states that have expanded Medicaid mental health benefits while implementing Medicaid managed care have incorporated CMHCs into new *managed behavioral health* delivery models (e.g., Colorado, Utah, Oregon). As CMHCs have developed their managed care expertise to handle new financing arrangements and new populations, their role is once again changing (Christianson et al., 1995; Lambert et al., 1998).

Another effect of mental health carve-outs has resulted from the fact that as states demand that MBHOs reduce mental health costs for the Medicaid population, a common cost-saving strategy has been to reduce inpa-

Mental Health in the U.S. "Frontier"

JAMES CIARLO, Ph.D.

At the extreme of the "rural" dimension, however defined, lie areas in the western continental United States and Alaska that have few residents, encompass enormous amounts of land within their geopolitical (e.g., county) boundaries, and are distant from regional population and trade centers. The crux of most definitions of "frontier-ness" is low population density, usually considered to fall between 2 and 20 persons per square mile. Almost all frontier counties lie between the Pacific Coast mountains and the 98th meridian, a line running from about the middle of North Dakota through mid-Texas. Since late 1994, these western frontier areas have been monitored by the Frontier Mental Health Services Resource Network (FMHSRN), a "technical assistance center" supported by the U.S. Center for Mental Health Services, with the aim of increasing and improving the mental health services available to area residents. After examining available mental health literature on such areas, and also conducting focus-type "study groups" with frontier-area residents, caregivers, and public officials to generate additional information on frontier-related mental health issues, FMHSRN experts have generated a number of papers and brief communications for use in formulating mental health–relevant policies and in offering suggestions for future research. Some key points from these products are listed below; more details can be found in documents posted on the FMHSRN website (www.du.edu/frontier-mh/).

With respect to "need" for mental health services, data from the statewide epidemiologic Colorado Social Health Survey (Ciarlo et al., 1992) suggest that frontier populations have somewhat lower prevalence rates of diagnosable mental disorders and dysfunctions than higher-density rural towns or urban/suburban area populations. However, the availability of mental health services in the frontier is vastly inferior to other areas. For example, though need approximates 80% to 85% of the rate for more densely settled areas, availability of psychiatrists and child psychiatrists in 1994 was less than 10% of the per capita rate for other areas (Holzer et al., 1998). Further, most of what little mental health care is currently available in these areas is delivered by primary care medical doctors rather than mental health specialists, with at least those concurrent limitations in accurate problem elicitation and treatment options noted in the literature (Geller and Muus, 1997).

The FMHSRN is also urging western state mental health officials to help make more mental health services available to their states' frontier areas in two specific ways. First, given that many states are moving to serve their Medicaid populations through contracts with managed behavioral healthcare organizations (MBHOs), it is critical that these contracts require monitoring of services data for specific frontier counties, in order to show how adequately an MBHO is serving its sparsely populated areas (Keller, 1998). Second, FMHSRN is urging and assisting western states to move toward implementing "telemental health services" (TMHS) to supplement face-to-face services in their rural and frontier areas. TMHS seems to be especially useful in long-distance assessments of mental health problems and associated referrals or case dispositions in frontier settings, and in behavioral or medication-type follow-ups of persons released from psychiatric hospitals back to their remote home communities (LaMendola, 1996).

tient lengths of stay. Earlier discharge may not be a problem in urban areas, where community services such as partial hospitalization can support patients recovering from serious mental illness, but these services are rarely available in rural areas. Thus, rural residents hospitalized for mental illness may be at increased risk for relapse and readmission. Thus far, research has neither supported nor refuted this scenario.

A third effect of the growth of managed behavioral health is the organization of independent mental health practitioners into *behavioral health networks*. In several states, providers have formed these groups to make competitive bids on managed care contracts. In Oregon, for example, Greater Oregon Behavioral Health Incorporated (GOBHI), a private nonprofit consortium covering 19 rural counties, was selected as a provider orga-

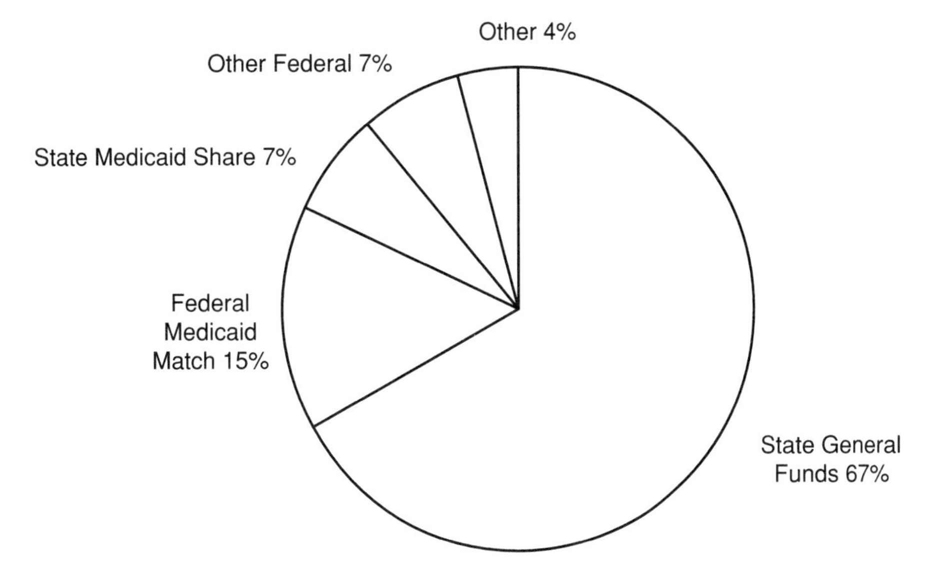

Figure 14.1. State mental health authority funding sources for mental health programs, fiscal year 1993. Source: National Association of State Mental Health Program Directors Research Institute. Revenue and expenditure study. Fiscal year 1993.

nization serving Oregon Health Plan beneficiaries in those counties (Lambert et al., 1998).

Seemingly running counter to the mental health carve-out trend, many rural communities have implemented innovative programs that *integrate mental health and substance abuse services with primary care.* By colocating these services, the stigma often associated with mental health services is overcome (Bird et al., 1998). Moreover, having mental health practioners on site can improve the diagnostic capabilities of PCPs, provide them with ready access to consultation, and help to assure that patients follow through with referrals. While one would expect carved-out managed care to place barriers between behavioral health and primary care services, early evidence from studies of managed behavioral health in rural areas indicates that where these integration models were already working well, behavioral health carve-outs have not been harmful (Lambert et al., 1998).

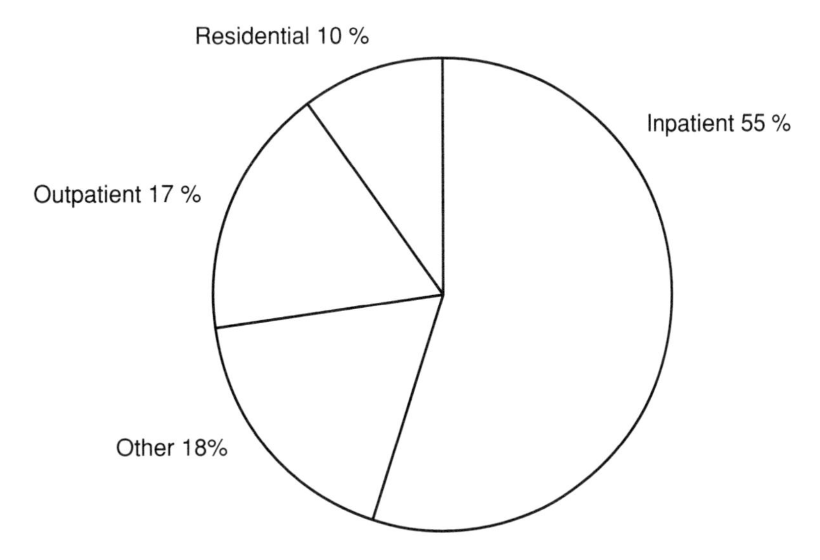

Figure 14.2. State mental health authority-controlled mental health expenditures by service, fiscal year 1993. Source: National Association of State Mental Health Program Directors Research Institute. Resource and expenditure survey. Fiscal year 1993.

SUMMARY AND CONCLUSIONS

Rural residents continue to have difficulty finding mental health providers, due to chronic shortages. The solution to this long-standing problem may lie in the increased role of managed behavioral health organization, behavioral health networks, and, to some extent, consumers. The willingness of MBHOs to use nonphysician mental health providers (as in Oregon), to add new services (as in Iowa), and to develop innovative strategies for bringing crisis and other services to rural areas (as in Colorado), combined with increased awareness of the role of self-help groups, may hold promise for improving the delivery of mental health services in rural areas.

REFERENCES

Bachrach LL. 1977. Deinstitutionalization of mental health services in rural areas. Hospital and Community Psychiatry 28(9): 669–672.

Baer RD. 1996. Health and mental health among Mexican American migrants: implications for survey research. Human Organization 55(1): 58–66.

Barry KL, Fleming MF, Greenley JR, Kropp S, Widlak P. 1996. Characteristics of persons with severe mental illness and substance abuse in rural areas. Psychiatric Services 47(1): 88–90.

Beeson PG. 1991. The successful rural mental health practitioner: dimensions of success/challenges and opportunities. Rural Community Mental Health 18(4): 4–7.

Bierman KL. 1997. Implementing a comprehensive program for the prevention of conduct problems in rural communities: the fast track experience. American Journal of Community Psychology 25(4): 493–514.

Bird DC, Hartley D, Lambert D, Coburn AF, Beeson P. 1998. Rural models for integrating primary care and mental health services. Administration and Policy in Mental Health 25(3): 287–308.

Blanch A. 1994. Importance of research on the involvement of consumers in services. Proceedings: The Fourth Annual National Conference on State Mental Health Agency Services Research and Evaluation, Alexandria, VA.

Burns BJ, Costello EJ, Angold A, Tweed D, Stangl D, Farmer EMZ, Erkanli A. 1995. Children's mental health service use across service sectors. Health Affairs 14(3): 147–159.

Carpinello SE, Knight E. 1991. A Qualitative Study of the Perceptions of the Meaning of Self-Help, Self-Help Group Processes and Outcomes. Albany, NY: New York State Office of Mental Health.

Carpinello SE, Knight EL. 1993. A Survey of Mental Health Self-Help Groups in New York State: Summary Results. Albany, NY: New York State Office of Mental Health.

Carpinello SE, Knight EL, Videka-Sherman L, Sofka C, Blanch A, Markowitz F. 1995. A Contrasting Profile: Participants and Nonparticipants of Mental Health Self-Help Groups. Proceedings, The Fifth Annual National Conference on State Mental Health Agency Services Research and Program Evaluation.

Castro FG, Gutierres S. 1997. Drug and alcohol use among rural Mexican-Americans. Robertson EB, Sloboda Z, Boyd GM, Beatty L, Kozel NJ, eds. Rural Substance Abuse: State of Knowledge and Issues. Rockville, MD: National Institute on Drug Abuse: 498–530.

Chamberlin J. 1978. *On Our Own: Patient-controlled Alternatives to the Mental Health System.* New York, NY: McGraw-Hill Co.

Chamberlin J. 1990. The ex-patient's movement: Where we've been and where we're going. Journal of Mind and Behavior 11: 323–336.

Chamberlin J, Rogers ES, Ellison ML. 1995. Self-help programs: a description of their characteristics and their members. Psychiatric Rehabilitation Journal 19: 3.

Christianson JB, Manning W, Lurie N, Stoner TJ, Gray DZ, Popkin M, Marriott S. 1995. Utah's Prepaid Mental Health Plan: The First Year. Health Affairs 14(3): 160–171.

Ciarlo JA, Shern DL, Tweed DL, Kirkpatrick LA, Sachs-Ericsson N. 1991. The Colorado social health survey of mental health service needs. Evaluation and Program Planning 15: 133–187.

Cole G, Timmreck TC, Page R, Woods S. 1992. Patterns and prevalence of substance use among Navajo youth. Health Values 16(3): 50–57.

Conger RD. 1997. The special nature of rural America. In: Robertson EB, Sloboda Z, Boyd GM, Beatty L, Kozel NJ, eds. Rural Substance Abuse: State of Knowledge and Issues. Rockville, MD, National Institute on Drug Abuse: 37–52.

Costello EJ. 1989. Developments in child psychiatric epidemiology. Journal of the American Academy of Child and Adolescent Psychiatry 28(6): 836–841.

Dickey B, Azeni H. 1996. Persons with dual diagnosis of substance abuse and major mental illness: their excess costs of psychiatric care. American Journal of Public Health 86(7): 973–977.

Donnermeyer JF. 1992. The use of alcohol, marijuana, and hard drugs by rural adolescents: a review of recent research. In: Edwards RW, ed. Drug Use in Rural American Communities. New York: The Haworth Press Inc: 31–75.

Edmunds M, Frank R, Hogan M, McCarty D, Robinson-Beale R, Weisner C, eds. 1997. Managing Managed Care: Quality Improvement in Behavioral Health. Washington, DC: National Academy Press.

Eisenberg L. 1992. Treating depression and anxiety in primary care. New England Journal of Medicine 326(16): 1080–1084.

Friedman RM, Katz-Leavy JW, Manderscheid RW, Sondheimer DL. 1996. Prevalence of serious emotional disturbance in children and adolescents. In: Manderscheid RW, Sondheimer DL, eds. Mental Health, United States, 1996. Washington, DC: Center for Mental Health Services; 71–89.

Frontier Mental Health Services Resource Network, Univ. of Denver, Colo. Brief electronic versions of each paper are available as "letters to the field," and can be found at the FMHSRN website (www.du.edu/frontier-mh/).

Geller JM, Muus K. 1997. Frontier mental health care and the integral role of the primary care physician. (Letter to the Field 5) Letter to the Field #5, Denver, CO, Frontier Mental Health Services Resource Network. Internet http://www.du.edu/frontier-mh/letter5.html

Gibbs JT. 1990. Mental health issues of black adolescents: implications for policy and practice. In: Stiffman AR, Davis LE, eds. Ethnic Issues in Adolescent Mental Health. Newbury Park, Sage Publications: 21–52.

Gonzales JJ, Magruder KM, et al. 1994. Mental disorders in primary care services: an update. *Public Health Reports* 109(2): 251–258.

Goplerud EN. 1981. The Tangled Web of Clinical and Epidemiological Evidence. Linking Health and Mental Health. Broskowski A, Marks E, Budman SH, eds. Beverly Hills, CA: Sage Publications: 59–76.

Greenley JR, Barry K, Fleming M, Greenberg J, Hollingsworth EJ, McKee D, Schulz R. 1992. Rural mental health services: research at the

Mental Health Research Center, University of Wisconsin. Outlook 2(3): 24–25.

Griffith EEH, Baker. FM 1992. Psychiatric care of African Americans. In: Gaw AC, ed. Culture, Ethnicity, and Mental Illness. Washington, DC: American Psychiatric Press Inc: 145–173.

Grob GN. 1992. Mental health policy in America: myths and realities. Health Affairs 11(3): 7–22.

Hartley D, Korsen N, Bird D, Agger M. 1998. Management of depression by rural primary care practitioners. Archives of Family Medicine 75(4): 563–588

Harvard Mental Health Letter. 1993. Self Help Groups. Vol. 9, No. 9.

Hoberman HM. 1992. Ethnic minority status and adolescent mental health services utilization. Journal of Mental Health Administration 19(3): 246–267.

Holtzer CE, Goldsmith HF, Ciarlo JA. 1988. The availability of health and mental health providers by population density. Letter to the Field #11. Denver, CO, Frontier Mental Health Services Resource Network. Internet http://www.du.edu/frontier-mh/letter11.html

Hoyt DR, Conger RD, et al. 1997. Psychological distress and help seeking in rural America. American Journal of Community Psychology 25(4): 449–470.

Human J, Wasem C. 1991. Rural mental health in America. American Psychologist 46(3): 232–239.

Ivey SL, Scheffler R, Zazzali JL. 1998. Supply dynamics of the mental health workforce: implications for health policy. The Milbank Quarterly 76(1): 25–58.

Jacobs MK, Goodman G. 1989. Psychology and self help groups: Predictions on a partnership. American Psychologist, 44: 536–545.

Katon W, Von Korff M, Lin E, Lipscomb P, Russo J, Wagner E, Polk E. 1990. Distressed high utilizers of medical care: DSM-III-R diagnoses and treatment needs. General Hospital Psychiatry 12: 355–362.

Kaufmann CL, Ward-Colasante C, Farmer J. 1993. Development and evaluation of drop-in centers operated by mental health consumers. Hospital and Community Psychiatry 44: 675–678.

Keller A. 1998. Managed behavioral healthcare in the frontier: Will the frontier manage and how? Letter to the Field #9. Denver, CO, Frontier Mental Health Services Network. Internet http://www.du.edu/frontier-mh/letter9.html

Keller PA, Zimbelman KK, Murray JD, Feil RN. 1980. Geographic distribution of psychologists in the Northeastern United States. Journal of Rural Community Psychology 1(1): 18–24.

Kessler RC, McGonagle KA, Zhao S, Nelson CB, Hughes M, Eshleman S, Wittchen H-U, Kendler KS. 1994. Lifetime and 12-month prevalence of DSM-III-R psychiatric disorders in the United States. Archives of General Psychiatry 51: 8–19.

Kessler RC, Zhao S, Blazer DG, Swartz M. 1997. Prevalence, correlates, and course of minor depression and major depression in the National Comorbidity Survey. Journal of Affective Disorders 45: 19–30.

Knesper DJ, Wheeler JR, Pagnucco DJ. 1984. Mental health services providers' distribution across counties in the United States. American Psychologist 39(12): 1424–1434.

Lambert D, Hartley D, Bird D, Ralph R, Saucier P. 1998. Medicaid mental health carve-outs: impact and issues in rural areas. Working Paper 9, Maine Rural Health Research Center, University of Southern Maine, Portland, Maine.

Lambert D, Agger MS. 1995. Access of rural AFDC Medicaid beneficiaries to mental health services. Health Care Financing Review 17(1): 133–145.

LaMendola WF. 1996. Telemental health services in U.S. frontier areas. Letter to the Field #3. Denver, CO, Frontier Mental Health Services Resource Network. Internet http://www.du.edu./frontier-mh/letter3.html

Main DS, Lutz LJ, Barrett JE, Matthew J, Miller RS. 1993. The role of primary care clinician attitudes, beliefs, and training in the diagnosis and treatment of depression. Archives of Family Medicine 2: 1061–1066.

Martin SL, Kupersmidt JB. 1992. Rural children at risk: mental health service utilization among children of migrant and seasonal farmworkers. Rural Mental Health Services: Research at the Mental Health Research Center, University of Wisconsin. Outlook 2(3): 26–28.

Martinez C. 1992. Psychiatric care of Mexican Americans. In: Gaw AC, ed. Culture, Ethnicity, and Mental Illness. Washington, DC: American Psychiatric Press Inc: 431–466.

Mechanic D. 1990. Treating mental illness: generalist versus specialist. Health Affairs 9(4): 61–75.

Meyer RE, Sotsky SM. 1995. Managed Care and the Role and Training of Psychiatrists. Health Affairs 14(3): 65–77.

Murray JD, Keller PA. 1991. Psychology and rural America: current status and future directions. American Psychologist 46(3): 220–231.

Narrows WE, Regier DA, Rae DS, Manderscheid RW, Lock BZ. 1993. Use of services by persons with mental and addictive disorders. Findings from the National Institute of Mental Health Epidemiological Catchment Area Program. Archives of General Psychiatry 50: 95–107.

Neighbors HW, Bashshur R, Price R, Selig S, Donabedian A, Shannon G. 1992. Ethnic minority mental health service delivery: a review of the literature. Research in Community and Mental Health 7: 55–71.

NIMH. 1991. Caring for People with Severe Mental Disorders: A National Plan of Research to Improve Services. DHHS Pub. No. (ADM)91–1762. Washington, DC: U.S. Government Printing Office.

Oetting ER. 1992. Planning programs for prevention of deviant behavior: a psychosocial model. Drugs and Society 6: 313–344.

Oetting ER, Edwards RW, Kelly K, Beauvais F. 1997. Risk and Protective Factors for Drug Use Among Rural American Youth. Rural Substance Abuse: State of Knowledge and Issues. Robertson EB, Sloboda Z, Boyd GM, Beatty L, Kozel NJ, eds. Rockville, MD: National Institute on Drug Abuse: 90–130.

Olfson M, Weissman MM, Lean AC, Higgins ES, Barrett JE, Blacklow RS. 1995. Psychological Management by Family Physicians. Journal of Family Practice 41(6): 543–550.

Parrish J. 1989. The long journey home: accomplishing the mission of the community support movement. Psychosocial Rehabilitation Journal 12: 107–124.

Pion GM, Keller P, McCombs H. 1997. Mental Health Providers in Rural and Isolated Areas: Final Report of the Ad Hoc Rural Mental Health Provider Work Group. Rockville, MD: Center for Mental Health Services.

Powell T. 1987. *Self-Help Organizations and Professional Practice.* Silver Spring, MD: National Association of Social Workers.

Public Law 99–660. 1986. Title V—State Comprehensive Mental Health Services Plans. Drug Export Amendments Act, PL 99–660, 100 stat. 3795.

Ralph, RO. 1998. Consumer issues. In Hartley, D (ed.) Best Practices in Rural Medicalid Managed Behavioral Health. Working Paper #15. Portland, ME: Maine Rural Health Research Center, University of Southern Maine.

Redick RW, Witkin MJ, Atay JE, Manderscheid RW. 1996. Highlights of organized mental health services in 1992 and major national and state trends. In: Manderscheid RW, Sonnenschein MA, eds. Mental Health, United States, 1996. Rockville, MD: Substance Abuse and Mental Health Services Administration; 90–111.

Regier DA, Narrow WE, et al. 1993. The de facto US mental and addictive disorders service system. Archives of General Psychiatry 50: 85–94.

Rickert VI, Pope SK, Tilford JM, Wayne J, Scholle SH, Kelleher KJ. 1996. The effects of mental health factors on ambulatory care visits by rural teens. Journal of Rural Health 12(3): 160–168.

Ridgeway P. 1988. The voice of consumers in mental health systems: a call for change. Center for Community Change Through Housing and Support, University of Vermont. Burlington, VT.

Rochefort DA. 1984. Origins of the "Third Psychiatric Revolution": the Community Mental Health Centers Act of 1963. Journal of Health Politics, Policy and Law 9(1): 1–30.

Rogler LH, Cortes DE, Malgady RG. 1991. Acculturation and mental health status among Hispanics: convergence and new directions for research. American Psychologist 46(6): 585–597.

Rost K, Williams C, et al. 1995. The process and outcomes of care for major depression in rural family practice settings. Journal of Rural Health 11(2): 114–121.

Rost K, Owen R, Smith J, Smith GR. 1998. Rural-urban differences in service use and course of illness in bipolar disorder. Journal of Rural Health 14(1): 36–43.

Share SC. 1995. National Directory of Mental Health Consumer and Ex-patient Organizations and Resources, South Carolina Share.

Sawyer D, Beeson P. 1998. Rural Mental Health: 2000 and Beyond. Saint Cloud, MN: National Association for Rural Mental Health.

Schreiber J, Homiak J. 1981. Mexican Americans. In: Harwood A, ed. Ethnicity and Health Care. Cambridge: Harvard University Press; 264–336.

Schulberg HC, Coulehan JL, Block MR, Scott CP, Imber SD, Perel JM. 1991. Strategies for evaluating treatments for major depression in primary care patients. General Hospital Psychiatry 13: 9–18.

Segal SP, Silverman C, Temkin T. 1995. Characteristics and service use of long-term members of self-help agencies for mental health clients. Psychiatric Services 46: 3.

Snowden LR, Hu T-W. 1996. Outpatient service use in minority-serving mental health programs. Administration and policy in mental health 24(2): 149–159.

Stubben J. 1997. Culturally competent substance abuse prevention research among rural native American communities. In: Robertson EB, Sloboda Z, Boyd GM, Beatty L, Kozel NJ, eds. Rural Substance Abuse: State of Knowledge and Issues. Rockville, MD: National Institute on Drug Abuse: 459–482.

Stuve P, Beeson PG, Hartig P. 1989. Trends in the rural community mental health work force: a case study. Hospital and Community Psychiatry 40(9): 932–936.

Susman JL. 1995. Mental health problems within primary care: shooting first and then asking questions? Journal of Family Practice 41(6): 540–542.

Susman JL, Crabtree BF, et al. 1995. Depression in rural family practice. Archives of Family Medicine 4: 427–431.

Takeuchi DT, Uehara ES. 1996. Ethnic minority mental health services: current research and future conceptual directions. In: Levin BL, Petrila J, eds. Mental Health Services: A Public Health Perspective. New York: Oxford University Press: 63–80.

Thompson JW, Walker RD, Silk-Walker P. 1992. Psychiatric care of American Indians and Alaska Natives. In: Gaw AC, ed. Culture, Ethnicity, and Mental Illness. Washington, DC: American Psychiatric Press Inc: 189–243.

Trotter RT. 1985. Mexican-American experience with alcohol: South Texas examples. In: Bennett LA, Ames GM, eds. The American Experience with Alcohol: Contrasting Cultural Perspectives. New York: Plenum Press: 279–296.

Wagenfeld MO, Muray JD, Mohatt DF, DeBruyn JC. 1993. Mental Health and Rural America: 1980–1993: An Overview and Annotated Bibliography. Washington, DC: Office of Rural Health Policy.

Wilson NZ, Wackwitz JH, Demmler J, Coleman SC. 1995. The Colorado Rural Crisis Study and a General Discussion of Issues Involved with Research in Rural Settings: A Rural Research Roundtable. Proceedings from the Fifth Annual National Conference on State Mental Health Agency Services Research and Program Evaluation. National Association of State Mental Health Program Directors, San Antonio, Texas.

Ziegler S. 1995. Self-help groups in rural Kansas: shelters from the storms of rural life. Helping Hands, A Newsletter Serving Self-Help Groups and Helping Professionals of Kansas. Wichita State University, Kansas.

15

The Rural Elderly and Long-Term Care

ANDREW F. COBURN AND ELISE J. BOLDA

The aging of America will have dramatic implications for the health care system. Approximately one fifth of the elderly—defined as persons over the age of 65—reside in rural places, accounting for 8.2 million people in 1995. Although in the past rural areas have had higher concentrations of older people, this trend appears to be changing.

The rural elderly differ in a number of important respects from the stereotypical image of the rural older person living in an idyllic home in a quaint country setting surrounded by a large multigenerational family. Compared with urban elders, the rural elderly have lower incomes, they are more likely to be poor, and they are less educated (Coward et al., 1994b). Although they are more likely to own their homes, those dwellings are more likely to substandard; that is, they are more likely to have inadequate heating and plumbing systems and to be in need of costly repairs (Coward et al., 1994b). The rural elderly are more likely to be in poorer health than their urban counterparts (Coward et al., 1994b). Yet they are less likely to have their health and long-term care needs met, because of problems in the availability of health and social services and the obstacles to delivering services in rural areas, including low population densities, limited transportation, and longer travel distances (Krout, 1994). Many rural-urban comparisons show significant rural differentials in health status and access to services, but it is always important to remember the diversity of rural places and people. There are, for example, significant differences among rural farm and nonfarm populations in many indicators. Likewise, the size of rural places and their proximity to more urbanized areas are often critical in understanding the nature of rural-urban differences in health status, access to care, and other important indicators. Unfortunately, national data do not always allow for comparisons at this level of geographic detail.

Patterns in the availability and use of health and long-term care services among the rural elderly suggest a number of important policy challenges. Federal and state efforts to shift the use of services away from costly, institutionally based care in hospitals and nursing homes will be particularly difficult to achieve in rural areas. The rural long-term care service system is characterized by a larger supply (per elder) of nursing home beds than in urban areas and fewer community-based, in-home service, and residential care options. These and other factors may undoubtedly contribute to the higher than usual rates of institutional service use among rural elders.

Changes in federal and state policies, consumer preferences, and other factors are transforming the landscape of our long-term care system. These changes are reflected in the increased reliance on private funding for services, the expansion of nonmedical residential care alternatives, the growth of in-home care options, and the greater integration and management of services across the primary, acute, and long-term-care systems. Whether and how these trends are affecting the rural elderly and the health and long-term care systems that serve them remain important questions.

This chapter compares the demographic and health characteristics of the rural and urban elderly (and trends in those characteristics), and assesses important differences in the availability, organization and use of health and long-term care services in rural areas. In the concluding section, we discuss the implications of these analyses in the context of the rapidly changing health and long-term-care policy environment and identify barriers to, and options for, improving the rural long-term-care system.

THE RURAL ELDERLY: POPULATION TRENDS AND CHARACTERISTICS

Population Trends

In general, rural areas have had a higher proportion of persons aged 65 and older than urban areas. In 1995, the elderly comprised 14.6% of the population in nonmetropolitan counties compared with 12.6% in metropolitan counties (Fig. 15.1). Nonmetropolitan areas generally have a higher proportion of older persons than metro areas (Table 15.1). Nonmetropolitan areas of fewer than 2,500 persons consistently have the highest proportion of older persons across all of the age categories.

Consistent with national trends, the elderly population has been growing in rural counties since the 1960s. Nationally, the elderly population rose from 9.2% of the total population in 1960 (16.6 million) to 12.6% (31.2 million) in 1990 (Fuguitt et al., 1997b). Growth rates for the elderly population were higher in nonmetropolitan counties during the 1980–1990 period than in metropolitan counties (Fig. 15.2). Recent estimates, however, show a reversal for the period 1990–1995, with a declining elderly growth rate in nonmetropolitan counties. As indicated, current estimates indicate that the population over age 65 actually declined by 0.12% between 1990 and 1995 in nonmetropolitan counties compared with metro counties, where the population of elderly grew by slightly less than one percent (0.68%). Estimates by Beale (1997) indicate that a third of all nonmetropolitan counties had declining older populations since 1990. Analyses by Fuguitt and colleagues (1998) suggest that this "deconcentration" of the elderly in rural areas is caused by two primary factors: an increase in the immigration of younger persons (under age 65) into nonmetropolitan counties and the simultaneous emigration of the elderly population away from rural areas.

Significant regional differences exist in the proportion of elderly residing in nonmetropolitan counties and in population growth rates in this age cohort. Specifically, the concentration of older persons in nonmetropolitan counties is greater in the Midwest and the South than in the West and the Northeast (Van Nostrand, 1993). There are also important differences across regions in the nature of the concentration of older persons in nonmetropolitan counties. In the Midwest, for example, growth in the population over age 65 is largely attributable to an increase in the elderly population "aging in place," combined with a net outmigration of younger people from these counties (especially farm counties in the Plains and western Corn Belt). In contrast, growth in the over 65 population in nonmetropolitan counties in southern and

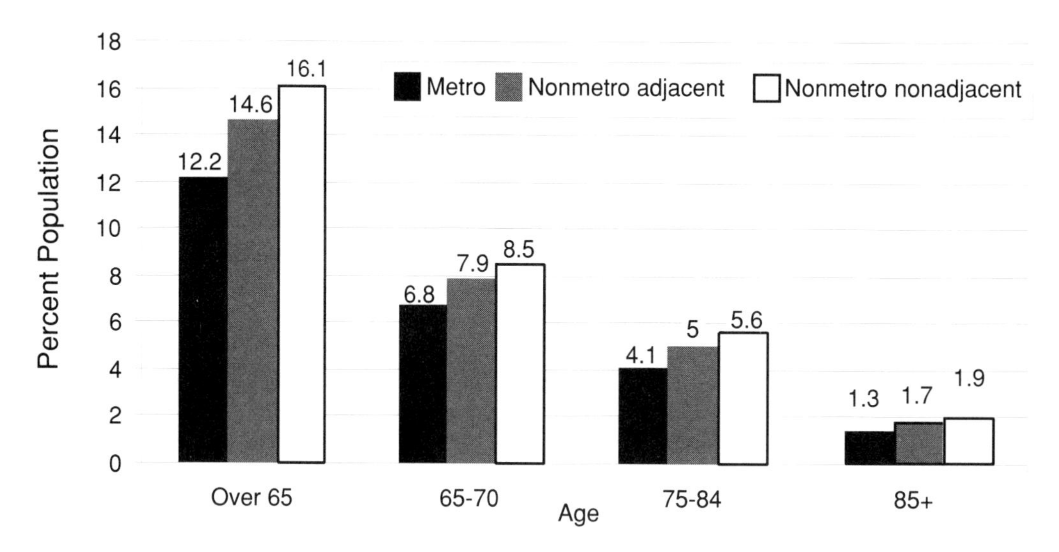

Figure 15.1. Age distribution of rural and urban residents older than 65 years of age, 1996. Author's calculations based on population estimates from Bureau of Census, Department of Commerce. Residence defined by urban influence codes. See, "A County-Level Measure of Urban Influence." Linda M. Ghelfi and Timothy S. Parker. Rural Economy Division, Economic Research Service, U.S. Department of Agriculture. ERS Staff Paper No. 9701. February 1997. Source: Bureau of the Census, 1996.

Table 15.1 Elderly Population by Urban and Rural Residence, 1996[a]

Urban Influence Code[b]	*Percent Population 65 and Older*	*Percent Population 65 to 74*	*Percent Population 75 to 84*	*Percent Population 85 and Older*
METRO				
Large city	11.81	6.55	3.95	1.30
Small city	12.86	7.16	4.31	1.39
NONMETRO, ADJACENT				
To large w/city	14.13	7.75	4.84	1.54
To large w/out city	15.46	8.41	5.33	1.73
To small w/city	14.21	7.68	4.90	1.63
To small w/out city	15.70	8.48	5.42	1.80
NONMETRO, NONADJACENT				
City, 10,000+	13.39	7.19	4.61	1.59
City, 2,500–9,999	15.75	8.34	5.53	1.89
Rural <2,500	17.27	9.07	6.08	2.12

[a]From U.S. Bureau of the Census. 1997 Estimates of the Population of Counties by Age, Sex, Race, and Hispanic Origin: 1990 to 1996. Washington, DC: Department of Commerce.
[b]From Ghelfi LM, Parker TS. 1997. A county-level measure of urban influence. Staff paper, AGES-9702, Economic Research Service, U.S. Department of Agriculture.

western states is largely attributed to the migration of older persons to retirement destinations from the northern states (Fuguitt et al., 1998).

Income and Poverty

Elderly residents of nonmetropolitan counties have lower incomes and are more likely to be classified as "poor" or "low income" than older persons residing in metropolitan areas. Lower incomes among the rural elderly are attributable to a variety of factors, including lower Social Security payments, lower lifetime earnings and savings, lower income from private retirement funds, and fewer opportunities for part-time work (Krout, 1994).

Data from 1995 indicate that 14.2% of elderly in nonmetropolitan counties were classified as "poor," with incomes below the federally designated poverty level ($7,309); 10.8% of the metropolitan elderly were so classified (Fig. 15.3). Nearly half (49.8%) of the elderly in nonmetropolitan counties were considered "low income"—defined as having incomes below 200% of the federal poverty level—compared with 37.9% of the metropolitan elderly.

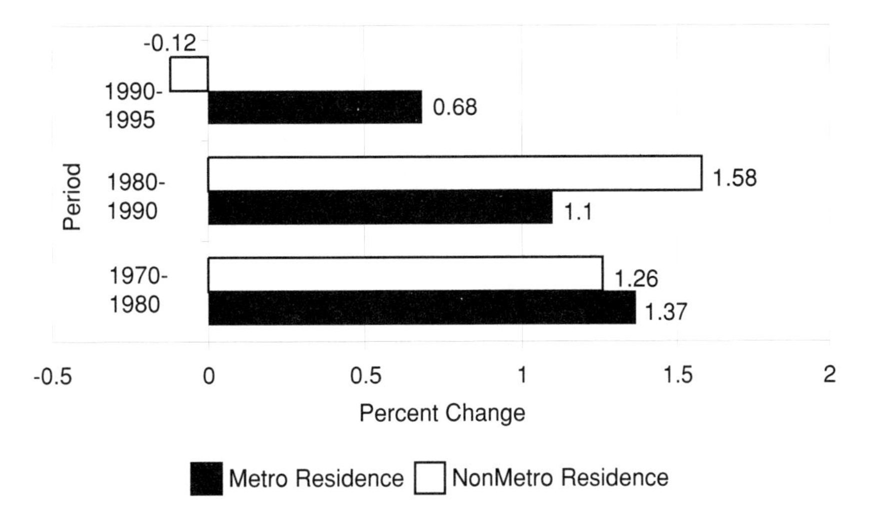

Figure 15.2. Percent change in population of those older than 65, 1970 to 1995, metropolitan and nonmetropolitan residence. Source: Fuguitt, Gibson, and Tordella, 1998.

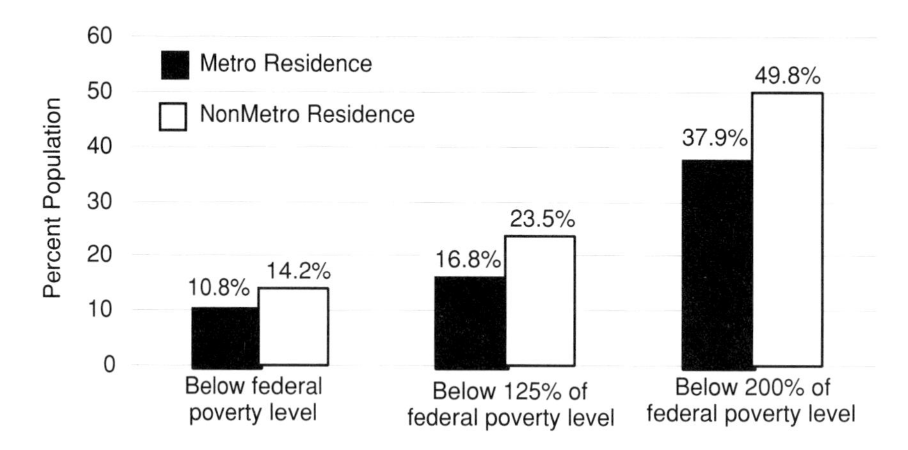

Figure 15.3. Income of rural and urban persons older than 65 years, 1995. Source: Bureau of the Census and Bureau of Labor Statistics. 1997. Current Population Survey, March 1997. Washington, DC: Department of Commerce.

Data from the Social Security Administration (SSA) indicate that the rural elderly receive lower average monthly Social Security benefits than those living in urban locations. This reflects the lower incomes and lifetime earnings of rural people prior to retirement (Krout, 1994). In 1990, benefits averaged $539 for persons living in nonmetropolitan areas compared with $599 for those living in metropolitan locations (Van Nostrand, 1993). A disproportionate share of rural residents receive income support under the Supplemental Security Income program (SSI): in 1990, rural residents made up 30% of all beneficiaries of this program, even though they make up only 20% of the nation's population (Van Nostrand, 1993). Moreover, rural elders—poor and non-poor—receive a higher proportion of their income from Social Security.

Minority Status

In general, minorities represent a smaller proportion of the older population in nonmetropolitan than metropolitan areas. In 1996, minorities represented 7% of the population over age 60 in nonmetropolitan areas compared with 12% in metro areas. In 1996, nearly 10% of those aged 60 to 74 in metro areas were African American, compared with 6% of nonmetro elders (Rogers, 1997). In contrast, more than half of older Native Americans live in rural places (Van Nostrand, 1993).

Living Arrangements and Housing

The living arrangements of the elderly in nonmetropolitan and metropolitan counties do not differ much (Fig. 15.4). The rural elderly, and especially those living on farms, are more likely than the urban elderly to be married and living with their spouses. In 1996, 71% of nonmetro and 66% of metro elders aged 60 to 74 were married (Rogers 1997). By age 75, however, the likelihood of living alone was somewhat higher in 1996 among nonmetro elders (51%) compared with their metro counterparts (48%) (Rogers, 1997).

The rural elderly are more likely to own their own homes, free of any mortgage, but those homes tend to be of lower value and are in poorer condition than those of urban elderly residents (Van Nostrand, 1993).

THE HEALTH AND FUNCTIONAL STATUS OF THE RURAL ELDERLY

Despite the stereotype of the hale and hardy older rural person, a higher proportion of rural elderly rate their health as fair or poor. This global measure of health status is usually considered critical because it is associated with mortality, quality of life, and other important measures of health status. Data from the National Health Interview Survey (1990–1994) indicate that rural elders, and especially those living in the most remote rural places, are more likely to rate their health as "fair" or "poor." As indicated in Table 15.2, 35% of rural elders between the ages of 65 and 69 who live in the smallest and most remote rural areas (<2,500 population) rate their health as fair or poor. This compares with 23.8% of elderly in the same age cohort who live in metropolitan areas and 28.3% of the elderly who live in nonmetropolitan areas adjacent to a metro area and 27.8% of the elderly living in nonmetro areas nonadjacent to a metro area. There are similar differences in self-assessed health ratings among the elderly living in

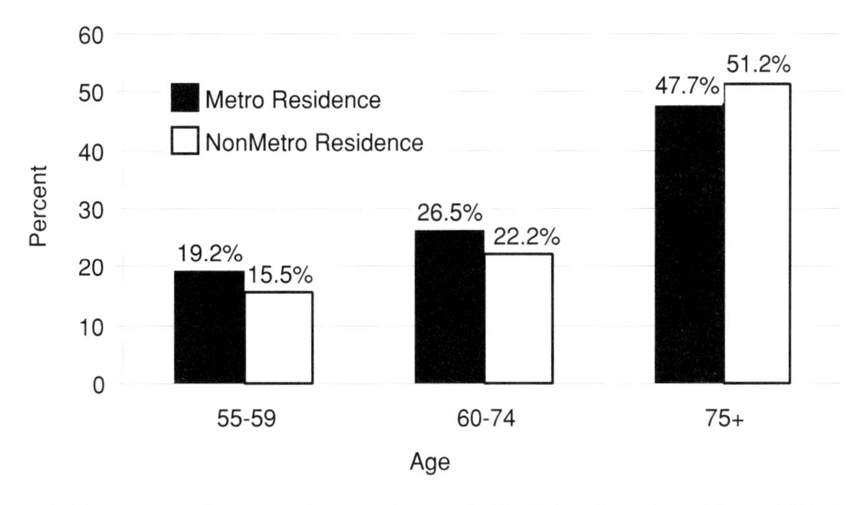

Figure 15.4. Percentage of persons 55 years of age and older living alone, by residence, 1996. Source: Rogers, 1997.

the most rural and most urban counties in the 70 to 74 and 75 and older age categories. These data suggest that older persons in nonmetropolitan areas are more likely to have a higher risk of mortality and lower level of life satisfaction than the elderly living in metropolitan areas.

As illustrated in Table 15.2, differences in health status vary by the size and adjacency characteristics of rural areas. Additionally, other studies have shown significant differences between farm and nonfarm elders in many health status measures. In general, farm-residing elders are more likely to be in better health than their nonfarm counterparts (Coward and Cutler, 1989).

Prior studies have shown few differences among elders living in metropolitan and nonmetropolitan areas in days of restricted activity (Van Nostrand, 1993). Analyses of data from the National Health Interview Survey from 1990 to 1994 show few differences among the elderly living in nonmetropolitan and metropolitan counties in their activity levels (not shown).

A higher proportion of elders in nonmetropolitan counties than in metropolitan counties reported a functional status problem—40.5% in adjacent nonmetropolitan areas and 37.6% in nonadjacent nonmetropolitan areas versus 34.3% in metro areas (Fig. 15.5). Elders living in nonmetropolitan areas adjacent to a metro area were somewhat more likely than those living in metropolitan areas to report having a limitation in at least one activity of daily living (ADL) or instrumental activity of daily living (IADL).

HEALTH INSURANCE COVERAGE

In general, elders living in nonmetropolitan counties rely more heavily on the Medicare and Medicaid pro-

Table 15.2 Self-assessed Health Status of the Elderly by Age and Urban Influence Codes, United States 1990–1994[a]

	Percent Reporting Health Status[b]					
	65–69 Years of Age		*70–74 Years of Age*		*75+ Years of Age*	
Urban Influence Code[c]	*Excellent/Very Good/Good*	*Fair/Poor*	*Excellent/Very Good/Good*	*Fair/Poor*	*Excellent/Very Good/Good*	*Fair/Poor*
Metro	76.1	23.8	74.1	25.9	68.8	31.2
Nonmetro adjacent	71.7	28.3	68.9	31.4	63.8	36.3
Nonmetro, nonadjacent	72.3	27.8	70.7	29.3	65.4	34.6
Rural <2,500	64.7	35.3	62.8	37.2	55.5	44.5

[a]From National Health Interview Survey, 1990–1994.
[b]The percentages are based on weighted frequencies and may not round to 100%.
[c]From Ghelfi LM, Parker TS. 1997. A county-level measure of urban influence. Staff paper, AGES-9702, Economic Research Service, U.S. Department of Agriculture.

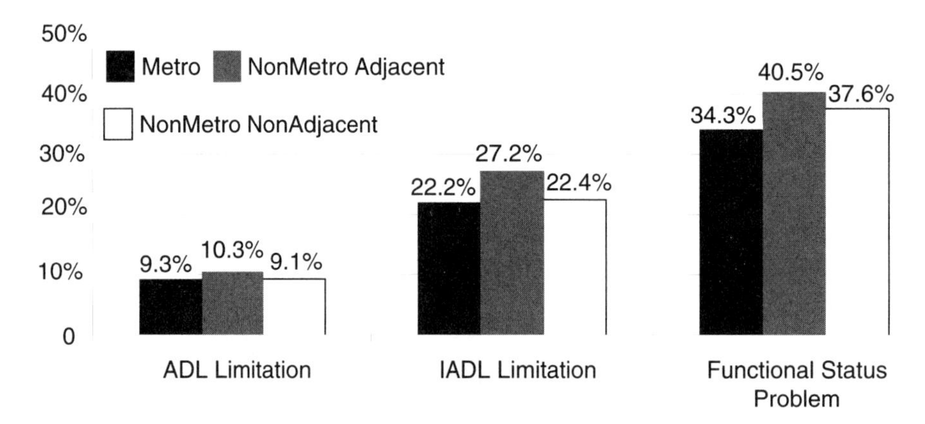

Figure 15.5. Percentage of persons aged 65 years and over with at least one activity of daily living (ADL), instrumental activity of daily living (IADL), or functional status problem, by residence, 1994. Source: National Health Interview Survey, 1990–1994.

grams and are less likely to have supplemental, private insurance coverage than those living in metropolitan counties (Fig. 15.6). The proportion of elders with supplemental private insurance coverage is lower in nonmetropolitan areas, and especially those not adjacent to a metro area. Only 67.8% of persons over the age of 65 living in nonmetropolitan areas, nonadjacent to a metro area, have access to private health insurance coverage; this compares with 70.7% of the rural elderly living in nonmetropolitan areas adjacent to a metro area, and 71.9% of elders living in a metropolitan area.

Not surprisingly, given their lower incomes and higher participation rates in the SSI Program, the rural elderly are more likely to receive Medicaid or public assistance than their urban counterparts. Nearly 10% of older persons living in nonmetropolitan areas, nonadjacent to a metro area, are receiving Medicaid or other public assistance. This compares with 5.8% of elders living in metropolitan areas.

HEALTH CARE ACCESS AND USE OF HEALTH SERVICES

As discussed in Chapter 3, Access to Care for Rural Patients, the more limited availability and accessibility of health professionals and services in rural areas are among the most recognized barriers to the appropriate use of health services among rural people. These and other access barriers, especially the lack of affordable and available transportation, limited income, and less health insurance coverage, are critical for the rural elderly who face additional problems with physical frailty and the lack of social support.

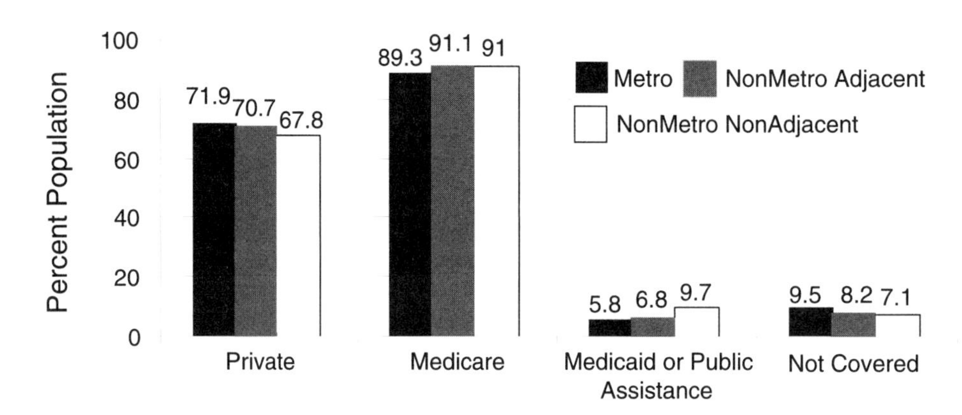

Figure 15.6. Source of insurance coverage for persons aged 65 years and older by residence, 1994. Source: NCHS, 1994.

Table 15.3 Mean Annual Doctor Visits and Hospital Stays Per Person by Age and Urban Influence Codes, United States 1990–1994[a]

	Mean Number per Person[b]					
	65–69 Years of Age		*70–74 Years of Age*		*75+ Years of Age*	
Urban Influence Code[c]	*Mean Number of Doctor Visits per Person for 12 Months*	*Mean Number of Short-stay Hospital Episodes per Person for 12 Months*	*Mean Number of Doctor Visits per Person for 12 Months*	*Mean Number of Short-stay Hospital Episodes per Person for 12 Months*	*Mean Number of Doctor Visits per Person for 12 Months*	*Mean Number of Short-stay Hospital Episodes per Person for 12 Months*
Metro	10.8	.19	10.8	.22	16.5	.27
Nonmetro, adjacent	9.8	.20	13.7	.25	23.3	.30
Nonmetro, nonadjacent	12.9	.25	9.12	.24	15.8	.31
Rural <2,500	11.2	.22	5.7	.17	21.9	.33

[a]From National Health Interview Survey, 1990–1994.
[b]The mean numbers are estimated using weighted NHIS data.
[c]From Ghelfi LM, Parker TS. 1997. A county-level measure of urban influence. Staff paper, AGES-9702, Economic Research Service, U.S. Department of Agriculture.

Physician Services

Data from the 1990–1994 National Health Interview Survey do not indicate a consistent pattern of differences across geographic areas in the average number of doctor visits per person in the past year (Table 15.3). Among elders aged 65 to 69, visit rates were lowest among rural elders living in nonmetropolitan areas adjacent to a metro area (9.8). In contrast, among elders aged 70 to 74, physician visit rates were lowest among elders living in nonmetropolitan areas of fewer than 2,500 population (5.7). Interestingly, rural elders over the age of 75 had similar or higher physician visit rates than urban elders in this same age cohort.

Not surprisingly, the rural elderly are more likely than those in urban areas to have to travel more than 30 minutes to obtain services; they are also more likely to have to wait more than 30 minutes at the site of care for their appointments (Van Nostrand, 1993).

Hospital Use

On average, the rural elderly have similar or higher rates of hospitalization compared with those living in urban areas. The average annual number of short-stay hospital episodes is the same or higher among the rural elderly in each of the three age cohorts (Table 15.3). Medicare discharges were approximately 14% higher in 1988 among the elderly living in nonmetropolitan areas compared with those in metropolitan areas. The number of days of care per 1,000 Medicare beneficiaries is lower, however, in nonmetropolitan than metropolitan counties (Van Nostrand, 1993).

THE RURAL LONG-TERM-CARE SYSTEM

Most elderly rely on their spouses, children, family members, and/or informal support networks to help them with their financial, household, and other needs. Only a small minority of older persons use formal, paid health and social support services (e.g., home health services). The family and social support characteristics of the rural and urban elderly are critical, therefore, to understanding differences that may exist in their long-term-care needs. As indicated earlier, there are few differences among the elderly living in nonmetropolitan and metropolitan areas in their likelihood of living alone (the most significant risk factor for use of formal long-term-care services); in fact, rural elders under the age of 75 years are somewhat more likely than their urban counterparts to be married and living with their spouses.

A body of literature suggests that the rural elderly are less likely than those living in urban places to use formal, in-home long-term-care services (Coward and Cutler, 1989; Kenney, 1993a,b). This phenomenon is usually attributed to the more limited availability and accessibility of formal services in rural communities. Moreover, among those using services, significant differences exist among the rural and urban elderly in the mix of services used. On the one hand, studies have shown a higher use of nursing home services (especially custodial level care) among the rural elderly and lower rates of home health and other community-based, in-home services (Shaughnessey, 1994; Coward et al., 1995; Coward, Horn, and Peek, 1996). The larger supply of nursing homes in rural areas, combined with the more limited availability of community-based, in-home services, are often suggested as reasons for these higher nursing home use rates (Greene, 1984).

The pattern of findings is not consistent, however. For example, one study has shown that the rural elderly are more likely to use the services of senior centers than the urban elderly (Krout, 1994). Moreover, a study focusing on those newly admitted to nursing homes found no difference among rural and urban nursing home residents in their use of formal support services prior to their admission to the nursing home (Coward, Duncan, and Freudenberger, 1994).

Federal and state policies continue to encourage shifts away from costly institutional-based care in hospitals and nursing homes to community-based, in-home services. The effects of these policies in rural areas, and especially those dominated by the availability and use of nursing homes as the primary source of long-term-care services, may be significant. The remainder of this section provides an overview of what is known about the availability and use of long-term-care services among the rural elderly.

Nursing Homes

According to the most recent data from the Nursing Home Component of the Medical Expenditure Panel Survey (MEPS) conducted in 1996, the supply of nursing homes and nursing home beds is nearly 43% greater in nonmetropolitan than metropolitan areas. In 1996, there were nearly 70 beds per 1,000 persons over the age of 65 in nonmetropolitan areas compared with 47.6 in metropolitan areas (Fig. 15.7).

The MEPS data also show that nursing homes located in nonmetropolitan areas are less likely than those in metro areas to have certified skilled nursing beds or special care units (Rhoades, Potter, and Krause, 1998). These findings are consistent with prior research suggesting that rural nursing homes are more likely to offer a custodial level of care than urban nursing facilities (Shaughnessey, 1994). Nursing homes in nonmetropolitan areas are also less likely to have non-nursing beds (i.e., personal care or independent living beds). Not unexpectedly, rural nursing homes tend to be smaller than those located in urban areas: nearly half (46%) of all nursing homes in nonmetropolitan areas have fewer than 75 beds compared with 29.1% in metro areas. Conversely, only 13.9% of homes in nonmetropolitan areas have more than 125 beds, compared with 31.5% of homes in metro areas (Rhoades, Potter, and Krause, 1998). Largely because of the Medicare swing-bed program, a high proportion of nursing homes in rural areas are hospital-based (16.4% compared with 8.3% in metro areas).

Rates of institutionalization are somewhat higher among the rural elderly. Six percent (6%) of the rural elderly in 1990 lived in institutions, compared with 5.1% of those living in metropolitan areas (Fig. 15.8). Rates of institutionalization were highest among those rural elderly living in communities larger than 10,000 people, and those with populations between 2,500 and 10,000 people (U.S. Bureau of the Census, 1992).

Using 1987 data, Dubay (1993) showed that Medicare beneficiaries living in nonmetropolitan counties have higher admission rates to skilled nursing facilities (SNF) than those living in metropolitan counties. In 1987, there were 9.8 Medicare skilled nursing facility benefit admissions per 1,000 urban Medicare enrollees versus 11.3 admissions per 1,000 rural Medicare enrollees (a 15.3% difference). In general, admission rates in rural counties were inversely related to population size, with those living in thinly populated nonmetro counties, not adjacent to a metropolitan area, more likely to have an admission to a SNF than other Medicare beneficiaries.

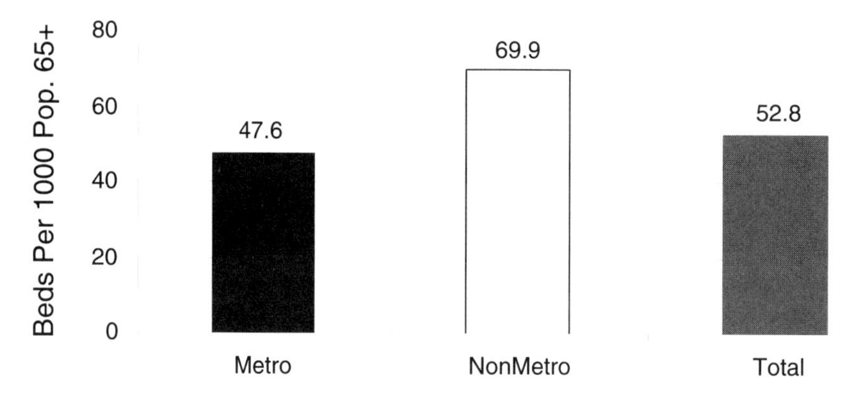

Figure 15.7. Nursing home bed supply in rural and urban areas, 1996. Source: Agency for Health Care Policy and Research, Medical Expenditure Panel Survey (MEPS)—Nursing Home Component, 1996

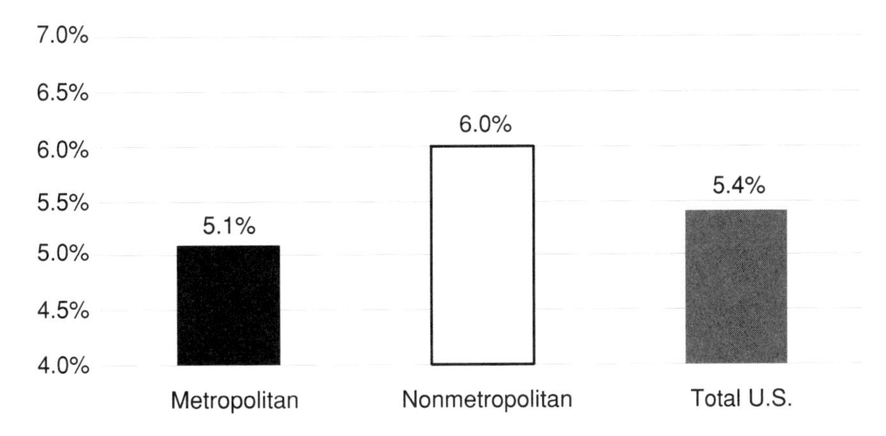

Figure 15.8. Percent of population aged 65 years and over living in institutions by location, 1990. Source: Bureau of the Census, 1990.

Using data from the Longitudinal Study on Aging (1984–1990), Coward and colleagues (1996) have shown that a higher percentage of residents of both urbanized and less urbanized, nonmetropolitan counties were admitted to nursing homes than those living in a metropolitan county. This study provides strong evidence that the rural elderly are at greater risk than urban elders of entering a nursing home in the course of their life; however, the authors were unable to account fully for the differences using the usual factors that predict nursing home use, such as sociodemographic and health characteristics of the population. They speculate that the supply of long-term-care services, the attitudes of the rural elderly toward nursing homes, and other factors may be potentially important determinants of higher nursing home use rates among the rural elderly.

Use of Home Health and Other Formal Services

Evidence shows that rural Medicare beneficiaries have lower home health use rates than urban beneficiaries. In a study using 1987 data, Kenney (1993a) showed that the rate of Medicare home health use is lower among rural than urban Medicare beneficiaries (44.5 users per 1,000 rural Medicare beneficiaries versus 50.6 for urban beneficiaries). The difference between the rural and urban rates has been narrowing over time. Interestingly, the number of visits per beneficiary is higher among rural Medicare enrollees than urban enrollees. The type of services used by rural and urban beneficiaries varies, however. Among those who use Medicare home health services, rural users are more likely to use skilled nursing and home health aide services; in contrast, urban users have higher rates of use for therapy and medical social service visits.

As discussed earlier, evidence conflicts regarding differences among the rural and urban elderly in their use of other formal long-term care services. Although there is little doubt that many rural areas have a more limited supply of community-based services and that access to these services may be compromised by distance and transportation, affordability and other problems, there is also evidence that among those most in need—the frail and infirm elderly—the use of services may be comparable among the rural and urban elderly (Coward et al., 1993). The reasons for this are not well understood. One explanation may be that the limited supply of community-based services in rural areas is better targeted to those most in need. We also know little about the rates of use of in-home services among the rural and urban elderly, and in particular, whether and to what degree the more limited supply of specialized therapists or other health personnel in rural areas may restrict the availability and use of in-home services. Nor is it known whether the higher cost of providing services in rural areas may affect the ability of agencies to provide care to rural elderly in their homes.

SUMMARY AND CONCLUSIONS

Although the proportion of older persons has generally been higher in rural than urban areas, trends in the 1990s suggest a potential reversal in this pattern: between 1990 and 1995, rural areas actually experienced a slight decline in the elderly population. The degree of concentration of older persons varies, however, by region, with greater concentrations in the Midwest and South compared with the Northeast and the West. The dynamics of the demographic shifts also differ, with older people more likely to "age in place" in the Midwest and Plains states. In contrast, the increasing population of the South and parts of the Southwest are largely attributable to in-migration of older retirees from the northern states. Naturally, the degree and nature of the concentration of older persons in rural communities and regions has important implications for rural health and long-term-care systems. The well-documented deficiencies in the availability and accessibility of health and long-term-care services in rural areas will make it hard to meet the needs of older people in rural communities.

It is not clear that important differences between the rural and urban elderly in income, health status, or other characteristics have changed significantly over the past decade: the rural elderly continue to be poorer and less healthy than their urban counterparts. Although the rural elderly also face barriers to health and long-term-care services because of more limited service availability, distance, and transportation problems, their rates of use of health and long-term-care services are not as different from the urban elderly as one might expect. There are, for example, few differences in their use of physician and hospital services. However, the rural and urban elderly differ in the mix of long-term care services they use. The rural elderly are significantly more likely to use institutional nursing home care and less likely to use home health and other in-home services. We know very little about the effects of service supply, financial barriers, cultural attitudes, or other factors on these patterns of long-term care service use. Nor do we know what implications differences in service access and use might have on the health and well-being of older rural residents.

There are numerous barriers and challenges to reducing the differences in health and long-term care access and use for older persons living in rural places. Two are especially important. First, the current financing of long-term care generally, and in rural areas in particular, limits the availability of services (and therefore their use) in rural areas. With a more limited capacity to pay for long-term care services out of their own pockets, rural elders are more dependent on Medicare, Medicaid and other public programs for funding to meet their long-term care needs. Yet, as evidenced in recent provisions in the Balanced Budget Act of 1997 reducing Medicare post-acute care expenditures, continuing pressures on public programs may limit access to critical services for older people living in rural communities. Moreover, the smaller economies of scale, higher costs of developing and providing services, and lower supply of therapists and other critical health personnel represent significant barriers to the development of adequate long-term-care services in rural areas.

A second challenge will be to develop better models for delivering health and long-term care services in rural communities. This problem is especially important in the light of the limited financing for long-term care and the competition for health personnel. Incentives are needed in new and existing programs to encourage rural providers and communities to expand available services and develop better-integrated service models. The development of partnerships and service networks among rural and urban health and long-term-care providers may be needed to achieve these objectives, for it is unlikely that smaller rural communities can support the full service network that may be needed. The expansion of managed care financing and delivery models in rural areas may provide the necessary incentives for service expansion and integration among acute and long-term-care providers. Achieving this objective is critical for developing a more adequate long-term-care service system to meet the needs of older people in rural communities.

REFERENCES

Beale C. 1997. Nonmetro population growth rebound of the 1990's continues, but at a slower recent rate. Rural Conditions and Trends 8(2): 46–50.

Coward RT, Duncan RP, Freudenberger KM. 1994a. Residential differences in the use of formal services prior to entering a nursing home. The Gerontologist 34: 44–49.

Coward R, McLaughlin D, and Duncan RP. 1994b. An overview of health and aging in rural America. In: Coward R, Brill G. Kukulka, Galliher Health Service for Rural Elders, New York: Springer Publishing; Chapter 1.

Coward R, Lee G, Dwyer J, Seccombe K. 1993. *Old & Alone in Rural America*. Washington, DC: American Association of Retired Persons.

Coward R, Netzer J, Mullens R. 1996. Residential differences in the incidence of nursing home admissions across a six-year period. Journal of Gerontology: Social Sciences 51B(5): S258–S267.

Coward R, Horne C, Peek C. 1995. Predicting Nursing Home admissions among incontinent older adults: a comparison of residential differences across six years. Gerontologist 35(6): 732–743.

Coward R, Cutler S. 1989. Informal and formal health care systems for the rural elderly. HSR: Health Services Research 23(6): 785–806.

Dubay L. 1993. Comparison of rural and urban skilled nursing facility benefit use. Health Care Financing Review, 14(4): 25–37.

Fuguitt G, Gibson R, Beale C, Tordella S. 1998. Elderly population change in nonmetropolitan areas: from the turnaround to the rebound. Washington, DC: U.S. Department of Agriculture.

Greene VL. 1984. Premature institutionalization among the rural elderly in Arizona. Public Health Reports 99: 58–63.

Kenney G. 1993a. Rural and urban differentials in Medicare home health use. Health Care Financing Review 14(4): 39–57.

Kenney G. 1993b. Is access to home health care a problem in rural areas? American Journal of Public Health 83(3): 412–414.

Krout J. 1994. An overview of older rural populations and community-based services. In: Krout J, ed. Providing Community-Based Services to the Rural Elderly, Thousand Oaks, CA, Sage Publications.

Rhoades J., Potter D., Krause N. 1998. Nursing Homes—Structure and Selected Characterisitics, 1996. Rockville, MD: Agency for Health Care Policy and Research. MEPS Research Findings No. 4, AHCPR Pub. No. 98–0006.

Rogers C. 1997. Nonmetro elders better off than metro elders on some measures, not on others. Rural Conditions and Trends 8(2): 55.

Shaughnessy PW. 1994. Changing institutional long term care to improve rural health care. In: Coward RT, et al., eds. Health Services for Rural Elders. New York: Springer Publishing.

U.S. Bureau of Census. 1992. 1990 Census of Population: General Population Characteristics, U.S. 1990: CP-1–1) Washington, DC: U.S. Government Printing Office.

Van Nostrand JF, ed. 1993. Common Beliefs About the Rural Elderly: What Do National Dat188a Tell Us? National Center for Health Statistics, Vital Health Statistics 3(28), April.

Epilogue: Rural Health Policy and Data

THOMAS C. RICKETTS III

Rural health policy is clearly nested within the larger domain of national health policy. The core issues of access, costs and quality frame the primary concerns of policy makers and citizens alike in rural communities as well as urban and transitional places. As a nation we are concerned with our performance in these three important dimensions of health care. To this end, we have created data systems, information structures, and indicators that we can track and use to inform policy making. It is at this point that one of the most important differences between rural and other health policy making becomes apparent: the data to assess changes in the rural portion of America's population are often not available whereas there is a relative wealth of data describing the nation as a whole and especially its urban portion.

THE HEALTH CARE DELIVERY PROBLEMS OF RURAL AMERICA

The picture that emerges from an overview of the chapters is of a nation with a clearly uneven distribution of health care resources but a less clear picture of the health effects of that skew. Rural people have lower potential access to physicians, with the availability of primary care physicians half that of urban places and approximately one third for specialists. For groups for which data are readily available, such as Medicare beneficiaries, the data show that rural residents use less care—40% less in the case of cardiology visits. Rural residents have fewer resources to enable them to make use of health care services, they are slightly more often uninsured, and they have lower total incomes. National surveys show that rural people report being unable to see a doctor when they need to slightly more often than urban residents, but the differences were not statistically significant. Finally, a small but significant difference exists in the proportion of rural people who were in poor or fair health who had not seen a doctor in the previous 12 months.

The programs developed to address the problems of access to care for rural populations have been generally successful in keeping the differences between urban and rural areas from widening but often their consequences are unintended and unwelcomed. The Rural Health Clinics program, for example, attracted negative attention from the media when entrepreneurs used its benefits for economic advantage rather than to alleviate access disparities. The immense promise of telemedicine systems to distribute services and skills to rural communities is finding slower than anticipated diffusion, partly due to infrastructure costs and conflicting policies over payments for services and licensure of professionals. Managed care is feasible in rural places but the degree to which rural places fit into or can have their own plans survive alongside very large integrated networks is an open question.

The problems associated with rural medical care often capture more attention than other important parts of the health care system. Mental health care access for rural people, for example, has been shown in these pages to be a severe problem. Supportive services for children with disabilities and developmental problems are largely missing from rural areas. When a small rural community faces the need to support a family in which a rare but costly chronic disease occurs, there is often the very difficult choice of whether or not the local government, the county or township, can manage the expense of that case and still provide other necessary services. The fragility of social services systems in rural places is not often considered in state or federal programs.

THE DATA THAT SUPPORT RURAL HEALTH POLICY

The preceding chapters present data intended to support the contention that health care delivery and health status in rural America are different from the rest of the country. There are health care delivery problems specific to rural areas that may not be considered in national policies. And certain health problems become more intense in rural communities due to problems of access. The data used to support these arguments have been drawn from a very wide range of sources, but where possible, the authors have depended on major national health, economic, and census surveys.

The United States uses several national surveys and data sets to understand the health status of its citizens—the National Health Interview Survey (NHIS), the National Long Term Care Survey (NLTCS), and the Medicare Current Beneficiary Survey (MCBS)—and the performance of its health care delivery system, a prime example being the Medical Expenditure Panel Survey (MEPS). These surveys are not as useful for rural areas as they are for urban places or the nation as a whole for three reasons: confidentiality, sample size, and the lack of access to data in the surveys (Schur, Good et al. 1998).

The issue of confidentiality is real and rural health research access to data that might identify individuals in small towns or rural areas is considered too risky to permit. National survey data could, potentially, be used to do analyses of general types of rural communities. An example would be persons living in the most rural nonmetropolitan counties as classified by the Urban Influence Codes described in Chapter 1. However, these analyses are not a high priority for the federal agencies that control the data and their limited resources mean that studies looking specifically at rural populations are seldom done.

The use of national survey data to represent populations at levels smaller than major regions is complicated by the sample design of the national surveys. Rural populations are, by definition, spread thinly across all regions and the characteristics that make for differences in health, such as isolation and occupation, are those that create the greatest difficulty in identifying people for surveys in an efficient and effective manner. For most national surveys, the nonmetropolitan sample is scattered across the nation in a limited number of clusters, and in any given region there would not be enough people to allow for stable estimates of the characteristics of the rural population of that region.

This problem has no easy solution. The funds to support national surveys are severely limited and more so in a time when the trend is to smaller government and fewer intrusions on privacy. On the other hand, we are hearing that information is vital to allow market mechanisms to reduce costs and improve quality. When managed care firms enter rural markets they seek information concerning the burden of illness in the community, the costs that will be incurred to deliver care in these sparsely populated areas, and they seek to understand how well their delivery units have done their job. Data systems that feed these types of needs are emerging in the form of registries, report cards, community health information networks (CHINs), and real or virtual warehouses for data sharing and use (Shortell, Gillies et al. 1996). At one time it was argued that the reason benefits of cost efficiencies and quality control brought on by managed care could not enter rural places was due to small populations (Kronick, Goodman et al. 1993), an assertion rebutted by observation of competitive behaviors (Ricketts 1994; Slifkin, Ricketts et al. 1996) and the actual spread of managed care systems into rural communities (Christianson, 1998). The staying power of these data-dependent systems is yet to be confirmed, but one element that can make it more difficult to achieve system efficiencies in rural communities is the lack of usable information on populations and the lower level of information technology found in rural community health care delivery systems (Alexander and Ricketts, 1996).

Policy making for rural America, both public and private, is hindered by the availability and quality of basic information describing the rural population. This volume has tried to fill the gap in a summary sense but the many special situations and regional issues that occur would require a book many times the size. It is this need for more useful information to help us make the decisions necessary to meet the growing health care problems of rural places that motivates this book, but the result cannot be that this becomes a static reference or an end in itself. The real value of this book will be whether it stimulates more questions that demand the development of new information—that the information presented here leads to the development of more and better data, that is superceded by a much superior, future report: *Rural Health in the United States in the Twenty-First Century*.

REFERENCES

Alexander J, Ricketts TC. 1996. Assessing Managed Care Preparedness in Rural Community-Based Practices in North Carolina. Chapel Hill, NC: Rural Health Research and Policy Analysis Center, University of North Carolina.

Christianson J. 1998. The growing presence of managed care in rural areas. Journal of Rural Health **14**(3): 166–168.

Kronick R, Goodman DC, Wennberg J, Wagner E. 1993. The marketplace for health reform: the demographic limitations of managed competition. New England Journal of Medicine **328**(2): 148–152.

Ricketts TC. 1994. Geographic methods for health services research: a focus on the rural-urban continuum. Lanham, Md.: University Press of America.

Schur CL, Good CD, Berk ML. 1998. Barriers to Using National Surveys for Understanding Rural Health Policy Issues. Bethesda, MD: Project HOPE Walsh Center for Rural Health Analysis: 7, 4 appendices.

Shortell SM, Gillies RR, Anderson DA, Erickson KM, Mitchell JB. 1996. Remaking Health Care in America: Building Organized Delivery Systems. San Francisco: Jossey-Bass Publishers.

Slifkin RT, Ricketts TC, Howard HA. 1996. Potential effects of managed competition in rural areas. Health Care Financing Review **17**(4): 143–56.

Index